Advance praise for *Beyond the Medical Gaze*

Informed by our personal and family experiences, many of us enter the medical field with the goal of helping people through compassionate care. However, training is focused primarily on the scientific underpinnings of disease and the biological, mechanical, and surgical therapies to treat conditions. Practicing in the current highly demanding healthcare environment risks burnout and compassion fatigue that may result in emotional distance between providers and those they care for. In this groundbreaking book, Dr. Morton reminds us, "Behind every step forward in medical progress lie countless human stories of people who must find the courage to live on the edge of medicine and often survival." As we discover new routes to survival for patients with complex congenital heart disease and other previously lethal conditions, this book provides a map of how to walk with those affected and their loved ones to maintain recognition of their whole person, not just their condition. There is an acknowledgment that while appropriate boundaries are necessary, the small things we can do, such as asking which music should be playing in the procedure room, make a difference. In addition to treating illness, providing information to increase understanding of why a medical condition has developed is essential for life outlook and planning. This book and the many quotes from those who have undergone extensive medical care detailing dehumanizing moments will give healthcare professionals the courage to counter historical norms in medical education and practice.
—Elena Amin, MBChB, Associate Professor of Pediatrics, Division of Pediatric Cardiology, University of California, San Francisco

As a psychologist working with complex PTSD as the result of chronic and repeated trauma, the suffering associated with long-term health conditions is one of the most common difficulties faced by my clients. Most often, the pain is the result of having their feelings and needs be invalidated or dismissed. Dr. Liza Morton offers a deeply compassionate discussion that includes the complex needs of patients and medical professionals by focusing on the cultivation of relational safety within healthcare delivery. Through her own lived experience, professional expertise, knowledge of polyvagal theory, and countless case examples, Dr. Morton brings essential and transformational guidance that has the power to create lasting and meaningful change. This should be required reading for all medical professionals. Moreover, this is a gift to patients with long term conditions looking for ways to advocate for healthcare rooted in the psychobiological wisdom inherent in us all.

—**Dr. Arielle Schwartz, clinical psychologist and author of** *The Complex PTSD Workbook* **and** *The Post-Traumatic Growth Guidebook*

This book takes the reader on a fascinating journey through the research evidence and multidisciplinary knowledge relating to psychologically informed health care. We travel through psychology, medicine, nursing, and, most importantly, we get to hear human stories from patients who have traveled through healthcare services. Liza Morton's work is important as it highlights the need for a shift in the culture of healthcare to address psychological well-being and safety alongside physical treatment.

—**Dr. Lucy Bray, Professor of Child Health Literacy, Edge Hill University**

In this innovative and heroic work, Dr. Liza Morton mentors us on a journey of discovery and empathy into the world of living with long-term health conditions (LTCs), revealing intimate truths that will transform how we think about chronic illnesses and the people who endure them. Her compelling storytelling weaves powerful patient narratives with a rigorous review of her own and others' research, offering clear-eyed yet tender insights into the hearts and minds of both children and adults living with congenital cardiac and other LTCs. Morton makes visible the often-unappreciated experiences of LTC patients at home and in clinic, testing, and treatment while providing a comprehensive blueprint for change through psychologically informed healthcare. For healthcare practitioners, educators, and policymakers, this book is nothing short of a revolutionary challenge to embrace a new ideal: starting now, we must consider, comprehend, respect, and care for all the ways that an LTC affects a person. For patients and families living with LTCs, Morton's work offers something even more valuable: the needed relief of simply being understood, perhaps for the first time. What sets Beyond the Medical Gaze apart is its remarkable scope and depth. Morton leaves no stone unturned—from evidence-based research to deeply moving personal accounts, from the polyvagal neuroscience of trust-building to the best in music and art therapy, from practical case studies to transformative reflections that readers can apply immediately. This tour de force doesn't just describe a better healthcare system; it starts us building one, providing the resources needed to support the emotional and relational well-being of patients, families, and providers alike. This isn't just another book about healthcare—it's a vital catalyst for change that will reshape how we think about, treat, and live with chronic illness. No matter how chronic illness may touch you, Beyond the Medical Gaze isn't just recommended reading—it's essential.

—George S. Thompson, MD, Chairman of the Board of Directors of the Polyvagal Institute, coauthor of *Polyvagal Theory and the Developing Child*, award-winning researcher on the climate of professionalism in medical education, and medical director for crisis services at ReDiscover in Lees Summit, Missouri, USA

Dr Morton shares her patient and psychologist lens, as she provides a walk-through account of her healthcare experience as an individual with a long-term condition (LTC)—guiding us across some of her key milestones seen within the lifespan framework. Her almost tangible patient account is candid and elicits thought-provoking feedback. True to the biopsychosocial framework, the impact of having an LTC is explored and unveils the impact of the LTC on the individual within their familial, societal, and historical context, heightening awareness of discrimination and disempowerment. Explicit in her intent, Dr. Morton calls for improvement in the provision of psychological and emotional support within healthcare. The book offers clarity to the practical implications of the bidirectional relationship held between mind and body and extends this further through promoting holistic practice. Appealing to different ways of learning, the book provides an array of models, case studies, reflective practice exercises, and specific ideas for intervention. A timely and fundamental read, that encourages compassion within self and toward others, on the shared endeavor to deliver psychologically informed and trauma informed healthcare.

—Pauline Aiston, Chartered Health Psychologist and Clinical Lead for the ACHD Psychology Service, Bristol Heart Institute (BHI), University Hospitals Bristol and Weston

Liza Morton's perspective and her professional knowledge as a gifted psychologist and researcher shine through as she provides a comprehensive, essential guide for those working in the medical field. The importance of psychologically informed healthcare is demonstrated throughout; however, this book also lays out significant, yet often overlooked steps to making a real difference in the lives of vulnerable individuals dealing with illness. The experiences of both the patient and provider are respectfully acknowledged, and the book is peppered with quotes to further demonstrate the importance of empathy, compassion and human connection. Liza clearly describes how this increased awareness and shift in practice, policy, and culture can lead to improved patient outcomes, both mentally and physically, and how it can often provide increased meaning and satisfaction to those in the field of medicine.

—Tracy Livecchi, Licensed Clinical Social Worker, Connecticut, New York, coauthor of *Healing Hearts and Minds: A Holistic Approach to Coping Well with Congenital Heart Disease*

In Beyond the Medical Gaze, Liza Morton examines medical care for chronic conditions, masterfully depicting the critical elements that influence both treatment and healing. From the essential relationship dynamics between healthcare personnel and patients, to the often-overlooked environmental factors of hospitalization, and complex biopsychosocial models for recovery, she offers a thorough reflection on holistic care. Drawing on her own and other patients' experiences, Morton presents a comprehensive framework for transforming hospital care. Her coined term "psychologically informed healthcare" heralds a new era of medicine—one focused on person, not illness. This book is an essential read for any healthcare institution committed to not only treating but also genuinely caring for its patients.

—Lene Osmundsen, CPsychol, Clinical Psychologist working in somatic hospital/field of health psychology, Norway, President of European Congenital Heart Disease Organisation (ECHDO)

I extend my heartfelt gratitude to Dr. Liza Morton for authoring this book, which advocates for a movement toward compassionate and psychologically informed healthcare, wherein patients, families, and clinicians feel safe, respected, and empowered. Alongside poignant vignettes, reflective exercises, and practical strategies, Dr. Morton adeptly interweaves her personal narrative into each section. Descriptions of her experiences as a patient, clinician, educator, researcher, and advocate will undoubtedly captivate readers from the outset. While advancements in modern medicine typically celebrate researchers and clinicians, this book equally honors patients and their families, whose contributions are indispensable to such progress. As artificial intelligence garners increasing attention within the healthcare sector, voices like Dr. Morton's are crucial in reminding us of the enduring importance of humanity in medicine. She underscores that compassion and empathy are skills that can be cultivated and enhanced, inspiring readers to challenge the status quo in ways that are both aspirational and attainable.

—Adrienne Kovacs, Clinical and Health Psychologist, Equilibria Psychological Health

While it is not especially uncommon for career choices to be shaped by childhood experiences, it's pretty rare for those to start at just 11 days old, as happened to Dr. Liza Morton when she became the then world's youngest recipient of a cardiac pacemaker—only for it to fail within 24 hours. Dr. Morton's is not only a remarkable life but one which gives her unique insights as both a lifelong patient and as a counseling psychologist and researcher. Beyond the Medical Gaze: Practicing Psychologically Informed Healthcare is beautifully written in an accessible style that is full of "aha" moments. It's also an incredibly important book for clinicians and other health professionals to gain a richer understanding of their patients' lived experiences of long term conditions; for policymakers to work past the cliches of favored but ineffective remedies to complex problems; and for academics to learn from someone who traverses the high hard ground of theory to the swampy lowlands of practical solutions with enviable ease. I sincerely hope it becomes the global bestseller in its field it deserves to be.

—**Professor Brian Dolan OBE, Director Health Service 360; Originator, Last 1000 Days and EndPJparalysis patient safety campaigns, Oxford**

Liza Morton is a true leader in this space. She captures what so many in our community are working to raise: you can physically save a life, but without fully addressing mental health, the journey remains incomplete. Liza brings forward the often invisible realities of living with congenital heart disease, from how hospital smells and gowns can trigger difficult memories, to the quiet weight of stigma and the effort not to seem different. Her work shows how deeply experiences shape patient outcomes in ways that are too often overlooked. As she writes, "The odds are that someone you know is living with CHD." Yet for so many, these stories remain unseen. Like many patients and families, Liza has turned her own experience into work that is making an extraordinary difference in Scotland and around the world. *Take a Chance on Me* was the song playing the year she was born, and we are so grateful that so many took a chance on her. An incredible song for a beautiful soul. I hope this book and these stories stay with you long after you read them, just like that song is probably playing in your head.

—**Kate Doherty-Schmeck, Executive Director, Global Alliance for Rheumatic and Congenital Hearts (Global-ARCH), United States**

"Beyond the Medical Gaze" is a powerful and timely contribution to the field of healthcare. Dr. Liza Morton's unique dual perspective as both a lifelong patient and a Counseling Psychologist allows her to illuminate the vital need for psychologically informed care with remarkable clarity and compassion. The book is accessible, full of insight, and rich with moments that make the reader pause and reflect.

While its relevance is global, its message resonates even more deeply in developing countries, where healthcare systems often face resource limitations and where many individuals lack awareness of their rights as patients. In such settings, the integration of psychological understanding into medical care is not just important—it is essential. This book is a must-read for clinicians, policy makers, and anyone committed to truly patient-centered care. I hope it receives the wide recognition it deserves.

—Sandra Mattos, MD PhD, Paediatric and Fetal Cardiologist, UCMF-Caduceus-CirCorReal Hospital Português de Beneficência, Pernambuco, Federal University of Pernambuco, Brazil

This book will be highly valued in the contemporary era marked by the rise of artificial intelligence and the increasing prevalence of insurance-based healthcare systems—contexts that may, at times, constrain clinicians' ability to deliver care aligned with best practices. It offers a compelling exploration of the evolving science of patient-centered care, a field that remains underdeveloped and inconsistently applied across much of the world. By incorporating the perspectives of patients, families, clinicians, and researchers, Dr. Liza Morton in this book integrates the latest evidence and lived experiences, rendering it both intellectually engaging and academically robust.

The importance of actively involving patients and families in care delivery—and the positive impact such engagement has on clinical outcomes—is clearly substantiated, particularly in the context of managing chronic and long-term conditions. The book underscores the necessity of educational approaches that extend beyond traditional medical curricula, advocating for experiential learning and emphasizing the value of understanding each patient as a unique narrative. This enriches the comprehension of both medicine and the management of disease.

Furthermore, the discussion of moral, ethical, financial, and quality-of-care dimensions—within the framework of Psychologically Informed Healthcare and the latest advancements in patient-centered care—illuminates the shared benefits for both healthcare providers and recipients. As such, this book stands as an essential reference for the implementation of rights-based patient care, will be useful in the context of low- and middle-income countries (LMICs), where significant epidemiological and demographic transitions are reshaping healthcare delivery.

—Dr. Sreehari Madhavankutty Nair, Department of Health Services, Government of Kerala

Beyond the Medical Gaze

Beyond the Medical Gaze

Practicing Psychologically Informed Healthcare

Liza Morton

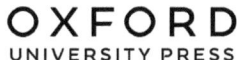

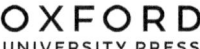

Oxford University Press is a department of the University of Oxford.
It furthers the University's objective of excellence in research, scholarship,
and education by publishing worldwide. Oxford is a registered trade mark of
Oxford University Press in the UK and in certain other countries.

Published in the United States of America by Oxford University Press
198 Madison Avenue, New York, NY 10016, United States of America.

© Liza Morton 2025

All rights reserved. No part of this publication may be reproduced, stored in a retrieval system, transmitted, used for text and data mining, or used for training artificial intelligence, in any form or by any means, without the prior permission in writing of Oxford University Press, or as expressly permitted by law, by license or under terms agreed with the appropriate reprographics rights organization. Inquiries concerning reproduction outside the scope of the above should be sent to the Rights Department, Oxford University Press, at the address above.

You must not circulate this work in any other form
and you must impose this same condition on any acquirer.

Library of Congress Cataloging-in-Publication Data
Names: Morton, Liza, 1978- author
Title: Beyond the medical gaze : practicing psychologically informed
healthcare / Liza Morton.
Description: New York, NY : Oxford University Press, [2025] |
Includes bibliographical references and index. |
Identifiers: LCCN 2025019558 (print) | LCCN 2025019559 (ebook) |
ISBN 9780197804964 hardback | ISBN 9780197804988 epub | ISBN 9780197804995
Subjects: LCSH: Chronic diseases—Psychological aspects | Chronically ill
Classification: LCC RC108 .M67 2025 (print) | LCC RC108 (ebook)
LC record available at https://lccn.loc.gov/2025019558
LC ebook record available at https://lccn.loc.gov/2025019559

DOI: 10.1093/9780197804995.001.0001

The manufacturer's authorized representative in the EU for product safety is
Oxford University Press España S.A. of Parque Empresarial San Fernando de Henares,
Avenida de Castilla, 2 – 28830 Madrid (www.oup.es/en or product.safety@oup.com).
OUP España S.A. also acts as importer into Spain of products made by the manufacturer.

Dedicated to my mum, husband Craig, son Dylan, and nieces Emma and Alice

And my dogs, over the years, Carbonyl, Rigby, Luke, Louis, and wee Lass

For their unconditional love and support

For anyone affected by a long term health condition, especially those gone to soon.

No society can legitimately call itself civilised if a sick person is denied medical aid because of lack of means.
—**Aneurin (Nye) Bevan**[1]

Without mental health there can be no true physical health.
—**Dr. Brock Chisholm**[2]

Contents

Foreword: Seeing Life from Both Sides Now	xvii
Preface: Take a Chance on Me	xxi
Positionality Statement	xxxi
Acknowledgments	xxxiii
Quick Reference: Core Principles of Psychologically Informed Healthcare	xxxv

PART 1. THE MEDICAL GAZE

1. The Mind–Body Connection — 3
 On Feeling Ill and the "Patient Role" — 7
 Survival Mode: How the Body Responds to Traumatic Medical Experiences — 13
 The Impact of LTCs on Parenting and Birth Trauma — 18
 Childhood Illness: Medical Interruptions to Secure Attachment and Loss of a Normal Childhood — 25
 Finding Connection in an Ableist World — 31
 The Person Beyond the Condition: Self-Esteem and Body Image — 37
 The Psychological Impact of Working in Healthcare Settings — 39
 Perfect Storm: Understanding the Impact of Living with an LTC on Mental Health, Recovery and Well-being — 40

2. The Cartesian Problem in Healthcare — 43
 Survival-Focused Healthcare — 44
 The Doctor Is Ready for You Now: Disempowering Aspects of Medical Care — 46
 Patiently Waiting Across the Healthcare Journey — 47
 Hospital Attire — 49
 Disease Prestige — 52
 Epistemic Injustice — 54
 The Compassion Crisis in Healthcare — 57
 An Inhospitable Environment — 61
 Poor Sleep — 62
 Psychologically Informed Healthcare: A Culture Shift — 63

PART 2. PSYCHOLOGICALLY INFORMED HEALTHCARE

3. Good Bedside Manner: Relational Safety In Healthcare — 69
- Relational Safety: Our Innate Need for Social Connection — 71
- Compassion as a Cornerstone of Psychologically Informed Healthcare — 73
- Psychological Safety and Co-Regulation — 82
- Beyond Bravery Stickers: Providing a Safe Space for Feelings — 87
- Active Listening: Sitting with Distress — 89
- Delivering Difficult News — 94
- Establishing Trust with Children — 95
- Caring for Teenagers — 96
- Seasons of Life: Transition to Adult Care — 98
- Caring for Older Adults — 100
- Hidden Patients: Supporting Carers — 100
- Trauma-Informed Healthcare — 101
- Recognizing Mental Health Difficulties — 103
- Recognizing Health Anxiety — 104
- Recognizing PTSD — 105
- Recognizing Medically Related Trauma — 106
- Recognizing Phobias — 107
- Recognizing Obsessive Compulsive Disorder — 108
- Recognizing Panic Disorder — 109
- Recognizing Generalized Anxiety — 109
- Recognizing Depression — 110
- Empowerment: A Seat at the Table: Working in Partnership — 111
- Shared Decision-Making — 112

4. Conditions for Healing — 117
- Environment: Healing Healthcare Spaces — 117
- Addressing Poor Sleep — 119
- Soothing Presence — 120
- Green Spaces in Healthcare Settings — 122
- Empowerment: Challenge Disempowering Aspects of Healthcare — 123
- Enabling Access to Clinical Information — 125
- Ward Rounds — 126
- Holistic Care and Embedding Psychological Support — 127
- Autistic SPACE — 129
- Emotional Preparation for Surgery — 133
- Pain and Pain Management Programs — 134
- iSupport International Rights Based Standards to Support Children During Medical Procedures — 134
- Managing Pediatric Pain — 137
- Holistic Support — 138
- Child Life Specialists and Play Therapists — 138

Virtual Reality	140
Healing Power of Music	141
Listening Therapy	144
Therapy Animals	144
Art Therapy in Hospitals	145
Cinemas	146
Giving Back: Volunteers	147

5. Healing the Healer: You Cannot Pour from an Empty Cup — 149

Overview	149
Establishing Healthy Boundaries	150
Organizational Responsibilities	151
Burnout, Compassion Fatigue, and Vicarious Trauma	151
The Cost of COVID-19	153
Building Self-Care and Resilience at Work	154
Psychologically Safe Working Environments	155
Compassionate Leadership	156

6. Culturally Sensitive Healthcare — 161

Overview	161
Social Inequalities and Intersectionality	162
A Long Time Coming: History of Discrimination and Stigma	165
Abuse in Hospitals	169
Change Is Gonna Come: Strategic Action	171
Safeguarding in Healthcare	172
Patient Rights	172
Children's Rights	175
Narrative Humility, Unconscious Bias and Bridging the Empathy Gap	177

PART 3. EMOTIONAL HEALING

7. Working with Clients Therapeutically — 183

Overview	183
Evidence-Based Treatment Modalities	185
Respecting Diversity, Recognize and Validate the Wider Impact	188
Mental Health Disparities	189
Promote Self-Care	191
Processing Medically Related Trauma	192
When the Mind Feels Safer than the Body	193
A Polyvagal Approach to Dealing with Medical Trauma	194
Neuroception of Psychological Safety Scale (NPSS)	197
Gendlin's Focusing and Felt Sense	198
Gabor Mate's Seven A's of Healing	199
Emotional Regulation	201
Cognitive Defusion	203

Enhancing Self-Compassion ... 204
Recognizing Grief, Loss, and Anger ... 207
Story Writing ... 208
Therapeutic Letter Writing ... 208
Reintegration and Connection ... 209
Empowering Self-Management ... 215
Helping Your Client Prepare for Medical Experiences ... 215
An Invincible Summer: Spirituality, Finding Meaning and
   Post-Traumatic Growth ... 216
Finding Meaning, Purpose, and Hope ... 219
Savoring ... 220

APPENDICES: FURTHER RESOURCES AND HANDOUTS

Appendix 1: Grounding and Mindfulness Exercises ... 227
Appendix 2: Sleep Hygiene Tips ... 229
Appendix 3: Dealing with Emotions ... 231
Appendix 4: Somatic Exercises ... 233
Appendix 5: Loving Kindness Meditation ... 235
Appendix 6: Nurturing Self-Compassion ... 237
Appendix 7: Self-Compassionate Letter Writing ... 239
Appendix 8: Self-Soothing Touch ... 241
Appendix 9: Shaking It Off ... 243
Appendix 10: SOBER: Stress Interruption Technique ... 245
Appendix 11: Patient Prompt Sheet ... 247
Appendix 12: Managing Anxiety About Seeing the Doctor ... 249
Appendix 13: Pacing, Planning, and Prioritizing ... 251
Appendix 14: Building Resilience ... 253
Appendix 15: European Association for Children in Hospital (EACH) Charter ... 255
*Appendix 16: ISupport Rights Based Standards for Children Having
   a Health Care Procedure (Test, Treatment, Examination, or Intervention)* ... 257
*Appendix 17: Neuroception of Psychological Safety Scale—Generic
   Version (NPSS-G)* ... 263
*Appendix 18: Neuroception of Psychological Safety Scale (NPSS):
   Manual and Scoring Guide* ... 265

Afterword ... 269
Notes ... 271
Index ... 303

Foreword

Seeing Life from Both Sides Now

Rows and floes of angel hair
And ice cream castles in the air
And feather canyons everywhere
I've looked at clouds that way
But now they only block the sun
They rain and snow on everyone
So many things I would have done
But clouds got in my way
I've looked at clouds from both sides now
From up and down, and still somehow
It's cloud illusions I recall
I really don't know clouds at all

From "Both Sides Now"
by Joni Mitchell
© June 19, 1967; Gandalf Publishing Co.

Joni Mitchell's song, "Both Sides Now," offers a poignant reflection on the complexity of human experience—the tension between ideals and realities, between what we assume and what we come to understand through lived experience. This theme echoes throughout the work of Dr. Liza Morton, who uniquely bridges the perspectives of both patient and professional. With insight and compassion, she critiques the medical gaze, which often prioritizes physical treatment while overlooking the psychological and emotional dimensions of care. Like the shifting perspectives in Mitchell's lyrics, Dr. Morton's book reveals how the same medical experience can be understood in profoundly different ways depending on one's vantage point. Her remarkable journey—from a child reliant on pioneering cardiac interventions to a polyvagal-informed psychologist—offers a vital and transformative lens through which to rethink modern healthcare.

Born in 1978, as ABBA's "Take a Chance on Me" topped the charts—a fitting anthem for the medical pioneers who would soon perform groundbreaking surgery on her tiny heart—Morton's life has been shaped by the intricate dance between medical innovation and human experience. At just 4 days old, she was rushed to Scotland's national children's hospital in congestive heart failure. The medical team, taking a chance on a groundbreaking intervention, attached her to an external cardiac pacemaker via leads threaded through an artery in her groin. When this restored her life, she became the first 11-day-old baby to receive an implantable pacemaker—a procedure that would define not only her survival but also her understanding of the complex relationship between medical advancement and human experience.

Those early years were marked by constant medical interventions. By age 7, Morton had undergone five cardiac surgeries involving thoracotomy—procedures that required breaking open her ribs to attach pacemaker devices directly to her heart. Each surgery, while necessary for survival, left not only physical scars but also deep impressions on her developing nervous system. Today, through the lens of polyvagal theory, we understand how such early experiences shape our neural platforms for safety and threat detection, influencing how we engage with the world, and particularly with medical environments.

Through Morton's eyes, we see healthcare from both sides now: the lifesaving interventions that enabled her survival, and the often-overlooked emotional landscape of the patient journey. Like Mitchell's clouds that "only block the sun" and "rain and snow on everyone," Morton reveals how medical care, despite its vital importance, can cast shadows over the psychological well-being of those it aims to heal. Her experience with early pacemakers, set to a fixed rate regardless of her body's needs, became a powerful metaphor for healthcare's tendency to prioritize survival over the subtle rhythms of human experience.

The technological limitations of those early devices meant her heart beat at the same predetermined pace whether she was sleeping or playing, afraid or excited—a stark contrast to the natural variability that our nervous systems require for optimal functioning. This lived experience would later illuminate her understanding of polyvagal theory's emphasis on how our autonomic state influences our capacity for social engagement, emotional regulation, and healing. As she describes, feeling perpetually out of sync with her body's natural rhythms created a profound disconnection that modern healthcare often overlooks.

Her journey took a transformative turn when she discovered polyvagal theory, which provided a scientific framework for understanding her lifelong experiences. The theory explained why she often felt tired, dizzy, and agitated, why physical exertion made her sick, and why her temperature regulation and sleep patterns were disrupted. These weren't just isolated symptoms but manifestations of an autonomic nervous system struggling to maintain balance without the natural variability of heart rate that supports flexible adaptation to environmental demands.

Morton's insights are particularly powerful because they bridge what philosophers call "hermeneutical injustice"—the gap in our collective understanding that often leaves patients unable to articulate their experiences. Through her work, she gives voice to the embodied experience of chronic illness, translating personal knowledge into professional insight. Her understanding of how the autonomic nervous system responds to medical environments has transformed our appreciation of what it means to provide truly comprehensive care.

What makes Morton's perspective so compelling is not just her ability to translate these experiences into psychological insight but also the profound compassion she extends to both patients and healthcare providers. She recognizes the dedication and skill of medical professionals while also illuminating the unintended emotional costs of a system that prioritizes survival over holistic well-being. Her courage in revisiting her own medical history, her self-compassion in acknowledging its impact, and her commitment to ensuring that others receive the psychological support she lacked as a child make this book not just a scholarly contribution, but a deeply humane one.

This understanding led to her groundbreaking development of the Neuroception of Psychological Safety Scale, a tool that quantifies what patients had long felt but struggled to express—how the range of environments and interactions influences their sense of safety and capacity for healing. The desire to create the scale emerged from her unique position straddling both worlds: the visceral knowledge of a patient who has navigated countless medical procedures and the professional insight of a psychologist trained in the nuances of human response to threat and safety.

The journey from patient to practitioner has allowed Morton to illuminate the critical role of psychological safety in healthcare settings. Her work demonstrates how the medical gaze, as a perspective, focuses primarily on physical symptoms and survival, often missing the profound impact of the patient's personal neuroception—the unconscious assessment of safety and threat—on healing and recovery. Through her research and clinical practice, she provides examples and suggestions informing the reader how healthcare environments and interactions can either support or hinder our natural capacity for healing through their impact on our nervous system's state.

Her experiences growing up without psychological support, returning to school just weeks after major surgeries, and navigating the complex emotional terrain of chronic illness alone, have shaped her vision of what healthcare could be. She shows us how understanding polyvagal theory can transform medical care from a series of interventions into a deeply human interaction that supports healing at all levels—from the cellular to the social.

In *Beyond the Medical Gaze*, Morton takes us on a journey through the clouds of modern healthcare, showing us what lies both above and below. Like Mitchell's reflection that "it's cloud illusions I recall," she helps us see through the illusion that medical care can be purely technical. Her work demonstrates that when we attend to psychological safety, we aren't just making healthcare more comfortable—we're making it more effective.

This book represents more than just a critique of current healthcare practices or a blueprint for improvement. It is a testament to the possibility of transformation when we view healthcare through both the medical and psychological "gaze." Morton's unique perspective—having looked at healthcare from both sides now—offers us invaluable insights into how we can create a healthcare system that honors both the technical excellence of modern medicine and the fundamental human need for safety, connection, and understanding.

—Stephen W. Porges, Distinguished University Scientist, Indiana University and Founding Director, Traumatic Stress Research Consortium, Kinsey Institute, United States, Founder of the Polyvagal Institute.

Preface

Take a Chance on Me

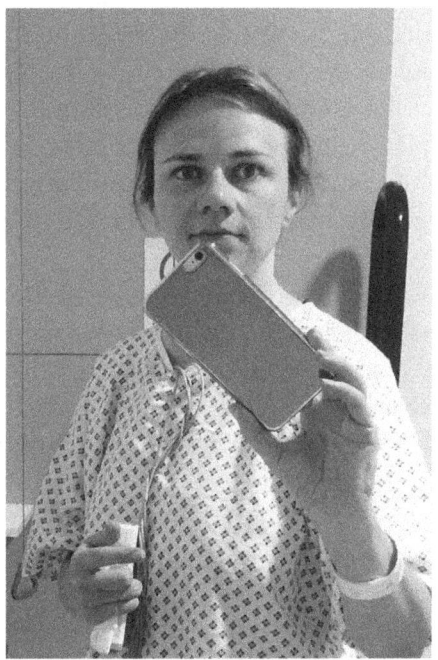

A selfie taken in the summer of 2018, during a month-long stay in hospital, wearing a hospital gown and on telemetry awaiting surgery for complex lead extraction and my 11th pacemaker. The photograph won Strathclyde University's Images of Research Impact Award for our work exploring the impact of backless hospital gowns on well-being. It was displayed for a year as part of an exhibition at the River Clyde outside Glasgow's Science Centre, across the water from Yorkhill Hospital, where I had all my childhood surgeries.

My motivation for writing this book is simply my life story; it is a response to my experiences in the hope of improving emotional and psychological support throughout the healthcare journey. I was born in March 1978, as ABBA's "Take a Chance on Me" fittingly topped the UK charts. My health started to decline as soon as I arrived in the world. I was separated from my mother who was also very unwell and when I was 4 days old, a medical team transferred me, by ambulance, from the maternity ward where I was born to the national children's hospital in Scotland. When I arrived, I was already in congestive heart failure. After assessing the situation, a pioneering pediatric cardiology team attached me to an external cardiac pacemaker, threading leads via an artery in my groin to my heart. When this restored life, I was diagnosed with complete heart block. In a world first for an 11-day-old baby at that time, they took a chance on me by fitting an implantable pacemaker.[1,2] I am tremendously grateful to the NHS, advances in medicine, and those innovators for my life.

Yet, my journey, dependent on pioneering medical care, has been tenuous. The first pacemaker failed and had to be replaced just 24 hours later, meanwhile I suffered a stroke, which temporarily paralyzed the left side of my body. Since, I have faced countless cardiac surgeries, treatments, complications, and hospitalizations. When I was 4 years old, my pacing device broke when I fell downstairs. By the age of just 7, I had been fitted with five cardiac pacemakers by thoracotomy—heart surgery that involves breaking open the ribs and fitting the device to the outside of the heart. I was relatively lucky. Not long before I was born, children that depended on a pacemaker had to carry around an external battery pack. Before that, an external pacing device had to be plugged into the mains electricity, leaving the child unable to move around.

Growing up with a heart condition was not easy. These early pacemakers were unreliable and often needed reprogramming. For a sense of how far technology has come, consider the substantial development of computers since the late 1970s to date. For comparison, the first computer, an HP3000, was installed in the White House by the Carter administration the same year that I was born. Back then, the programming ability of early pacemakers, to suit the individual's physiological needs, was limited. For me, these early pacing devices propelled my heart to beat at a preset, fixed rate all the time, rather than being physiologically responsive to my body. Further, battery life was a problem and pacing leads were prone to failure with little means to safely extract them (all the epicardial leads from my childhood pacemakers are still on my heart, as it was too risky to remove them, presenting risk of infection). Pacemakers were much larger and were challenging to fit on a tiny heart inside a small baby's body.

During countless hospital appointments, I remember lying still on a hospital bed, surrounded by a team of men in white coats armed with a large magnet, leads, gel, stethoscopes, and electrodes. A professor of physics came from Glasgow University to teach the cardiology team how to use the new innovative technology. They would place cold gel then a small metal plate on both of my wrists and ankles, wrap a rubber strip around them and then attach an electrode (until sticky electrode patches came into common use). Then they placed the magnet over the site of my pacemaker and made my heartbeat faster, then slower, as they learned how to interrogate the pacemaker. I felt very dizzy, almost fainting and gasping for breath when they turned it right down. I focused on counting the holes in the ceiling tiles and holding my mum's hand. I can still smell the distinctive hospital smell when I think back to those days.

Further to frequent pacemaker interrogations, living with a heart condition requiring experimental treatment involved lots of other regular medical procedures too. Some were less invasive scans such as X-rays, electrocardiograms (EKGs), and echocardiograms (ECHOS). Some were painful, including venograms, cardiac catheterizations, having a cannula or arterial line fitted, bloods taken, medical injections, or stitches, chest drains, and various drips extracted postsurgery. Many involved having to strip out of my clothing and keep quiet and still.

I was a medical curiosity. I was also a little girl who just wanted to do things other little girls took for granted. Because these early pacemakers propelled my heart to beat at a fixed rate whatever I did, I was physically limited. My heart was set at 70 beats per minute for most of my childhood, a compromise my team eventually found that best allowed me to both function during the day and sleep at night. My lips and fingertips turned blue when I was cold, I vomited on overexertion and often felt nauseous and dizzy. My talking and walking were delayed (I did not learn to walk until I was two and a half).

"Am I allowed to?" was a recurrent question throughout my childhood, as my mum, cardiologist, and I tried to balance the risks of damage to my device or health with trying to live as normal a life as possible. Skating, skateboarding, skipping games, skiing, elastics (a playground trend at the time), electric blankets, fairground rides, climbing, jumping, trampolining, horse riding, gymnastics, metal detectors, magnets, and active play were not recommended (besides, active play left me feeling unwell); however, I did learn to ride a bike and swim, occasionally tried skipping, and took the risk of getting my ears pierced! I could only dream about taking dance classes like the other girls in my class, who came to school with glitter on their faces from performing in a dance show the night before. I had to avoid being bumped by other children as they ran around the playground and jostled in the school corridor for fear of dislodging a lead. I sat and watched my classmates take part in gym class and sports day. I never complained and just got on with it, aware of the concern I already caused. I am Scottish; being stoic and pragmatic, viewing my life in the grand scheme of things, came naturally and kept things in perspective. I attended mainstream school and somehow got by. Although my mum frequently told me she wished she could "wrap me up in cotton wool," my parents raised me to focus on what I could do, and I was content. Life still had plenty to offer; I adapted and embraced it. I loved learning, reading, writing, music, arts, crafts, animals, nature, and imaginative play. It is only in writing this that I realize these activities liberated me from any physical limitations, leveling the playing field. My Barbie did not have a heart condition or scars, while reading, writing, and drawing allowed me to enact what I couldn't in real life. I had friends who were, for the most part, understanding, and my condition is "hidden," mostly protecting me from stigma from strangers. I was also grateful for the more inclusive 1980s playground fads such as yo-yos, collecting and swapping stickers, and Rubix cubes.

For me, issues arose when everyone else decided they were going to do something active that I knew I would find a struggle, such as going on a bike ride in the summer, swimming, or going out in the cold, during the winter, to play in the snow. Then I had to decide whether to push myself and feel unwell or to draw attention to my condition and risk being left out.

From an early age, I had a deep sense of how fragile life is, and appreciation for each moment of health. I also understood that life is not always fair, and it was up to me to make the best of the hand I had been dealt. I saw other children in hospital who sadly had it far worse, at least I got to come home and enjoy periods of reasonable health, and for this I was grateful. Feeling sorry for myself was a waste of precious time. Seeing what was happening to other children and their families, some of whom never got to experience life beyond the hospital, was difficult and has stayed with me. I also learned how strong, kind, and warm people can be when faced with life's hardest challenges. Aside from my hospital ward, I did not know any other children like me, there were none at my school or in books or magazines, on TV, or in films. I felt different and at times alone in the world.

Recommendations changed as technology improved. We learned together. I was known as a guinea pig, miracle baby, and bionic girl (labels that still make me cringe). Fortunately, the older I got the more I could do as technology advanced; I was far more limited as a young child than during adulthood, although I face increasingly complex pacing issues with lead extraction and implant. Recently, I sent my lovely pediatric cardiologist a copy of my coauthored book *Healing Hearts and Minds: A Holistic Approach to Coping Well with Congenital Heart Disease.* He thoughtfully replied, noting how I'd grown up with pediatric cardiology,

> You are indeed a pioneer and survivor. When I qualified in 1962, pediatric cardiology was still a toddler, but it was growing up and interest in the whys and wherefores and how to improve things was, I think, in good hands, and progress was steady with interchange of ideas from country to country . . . an astonishing intervention was Echocardiology pioneered at Glasgow . . . . *Healing Hearts and Minds* [our book] reminds me that while as doctors we did our best medically, surgically, anesthetically, intensive nursing care wise, and so on, we were less good at seeing our patients outwith their clinical visits as their very unique selves. This book is needed to broaden our minds.

In the mid-1980s, we were due to go on a family trip to stay with my aunt in the United States. The trip had been booked for months. My pacemaker broke about 6 weeks before we were due to leave. Faint and sick, I recall being bundled up by my mum in a large brown towel and rushed to hospital where I was taken straight to theater for a thoracotomy. Unfortunately, the new leads also failed. When I came around from surgery, I overheard distressed discussions between my team and parents as the heart monitor kept alarming. I remember feeling deeply unwell and sad that I was causing so much distress to the adults responsible for my care. When they came to tell me the bad news, I preempted them and told them that I knew that I needed to go back to the theater and that it was fine, I did not mind. I was 7 years old.

During this episode, my parents considered canceling our family trip, but that would mean disappointing my long-suffering brother (whose younger sister was always ruining everything by getting ill). Thankfully, the second surgery was a success, and my cardiologist recommended that we should go ahead with our holiday, noting that congenital cardiology care in America, if needed, was cutting-edge. I am grateful my parents were brave enough to take me, teaching me not to let my heart condition hold me back. Even though I spent it clutching my scars and healing ribs, we had a wonderful holiday in the sunshine with my American cousins. However, I remember being sent to the bottom of the garden each time my aunt used her new microwave oven, because in those days they interfered with pacemakers.

When I was 13 years old, I needed open heart surgery to repair a hole in my heart (atrial septal defect, ASD). The ASD had somehow escaped notice, and my heart had become enlarged. Leading up to this procedure I had to undergo two cardiac catheterizations. Local anesthetic was used, so I was awake throughout these procedures. I lay frozen to the spot as a team struggled to insert a thin tube through a vein into my groin to the heart, before they finally gave up and moved to my other side. I could feel everything they did, including using a scalpel to make the incisions. Lying on a cold, hard surgical bed in a hospital gown, I felt exposed, cold, in pain, and very distressed. The open-heart surgery itself took many hours, and afterward I woke up to find myself in intensive care, panicking because I could not breathe since I was still attached to the ventilator.

Around this time, I was fitted with my first variable-rate, endocardial pacemaker, meaning that my heart rate could now go up and down in response to my body. This enabled me to be more active. I required a further thoracotomy to remove the childhood pacing device. There followed issues with the leads and the requirement for a second system. Then for three consecutive years, just before Christmas, the pacing box, now placed under my collar bone, made its way through my skin. Each time I had to go back to the theater to have it reburied, until the decision was made to bury it under the pectoral muscle. I temporarily developed an occlusion in my vein that led to issues with my left arm becoming paralyzed. Throughout this time, the need for surgeries seemed relentless. I was also sitting exams (at times concealing a heart monitor) and juggling the normal challenges of teenage life, my growing collection of scars unwelcome.

Fixing the ASD and fitting me with a variable rate pacemaker should have given me more energy. Yet, paradoxically, by my mid-teens, I had developed chronic fatigue, a "medically unexplained" symptom I have battled daily ever since. The fatigue became so debilitating that I ended up missing almost a year of senior school. While I've always experienced nightmares about being in hospital, they also became more regular. During waking hours, cues such as the smell of toast (the first meal I was allowed after surgery) or disinfectant triggered flashbacks about my hospital experiences. I often felt tense, prepared for the next medical emergency, or exhausted from navigating my condition. At times, I felt low and anxious, despairing about how I would manage to complete my education, work, and function independently as an adult. My school did not offer any additional support for missed schooling, and my parents could not afford personal tutors. I wanted to go to university and study to become a psychologist, with the hope of improving understanding of the impact of living with a serious medical condition, but at times this seemed like an impossible dream. I knew learning was my best route to independent life. In desperation, when I was 17 years old, I asked my cardiologist to refer me to psychology or psychiatry, highly stigmatized during the 1990s. I was assessed by a very kind child psychiatrist who took a keen interest in my case and tried his very best, given understanding at the time. While he recognized my trauma history he surmised I was functioning well given my unique circumstances and was mystified by my chronic fatigue. While I was living on the edge of advances in cardiology care, the psychological insight I needed to support this trailed far behind. Eventually he prescribed a low dose of what was a relatively new medication, a selective serotonin reuptake inhibitor (SSRI), for its stimulating properties which improved my functioning enough to attend school part time. I studied hard, somehow gaining a place at a university close to home so I could drive back and forth to classes and accommodate my need for daytime naps. It was not until my early 30s that I found the therapeutic support I needed, which I sought privately.

I was fitted with my 11th pacemaker a few years ago when my pacing leads developed yet another intermittent fault. The surgery itself only required a 2-night hospital stay. Unfortunately, for a surgical slot with a complex pacing team, I had to wait for 2 months, a month of which I spent in hospital worrying what would happen if the leads broke completely. I remember a trainee doctor telling me that I would be an interesting case if I was not so terrifying! Although I have done my best to minimize it, the reality is that my condition affects the entire family; at the time, my son was 12 years old and on summer holiday from school. My husband had to take leave from work to take care of him. This was my third pacemaker surgery since my son's birth.

Despite everything, I have lived as full a life as possible. I am happily married with a wonderful son, and supportive friends and family. But my health condition has affected every facet of it, for better and worse. I have always been deeply appreciative of the good times, of the people who have stood by and supported me. I make the most of every opportunity. Witnessing my son grow up and being able to take part in the normalities of life that I was unable to, from childhood, has brought me tremendous pleasure. Watching him take part in his school sports days, jumping with his friends on a trampoline and enjoying fairground rides has brought me untold joy. Likewise, watching my nieces perform in their dance shows with glitter covered faces.

However, while I am grateful for the healthcare I have received, it has at times been brutal, frightening, and depersonalizing. I have benefited from compassionate care from world-class healthcare professionals. However, accessing the specialist care I need became more challenging when I reached adulthood adding to the burden of living with my condition. At times, I have been left traumatized because no one would listen to me—my symptoms were dismissed, my valid concerns ignored, leading to confusion, distress, and life-threatening situations.

Looking back, I can see I went through too much with little time for recovery between each medical crisis. There was a lack of support post-surgery in terms of rehabilitation, and when I returned to school just weeks after cardiac surgeries, my peers and teachers had no idea what I had been through. Adults with acquired coronary heart problems are offered more recovery time and support than I got as a child. Perhaps, this was partly my own doing. I did not want "special treatment," or to consider myself disabled at a time when this was highly stigmatized. I was fiercely independent (some might say stubborn), and I hated being pitied. I wanted to fit in and to live as normal a life as possible, but the scars were there. I was medically burned out without the reassurance that there would ever be an end to the need for further interventions. At any moment there may be another medical crisis, and sure enough at least every few years there has been.

As I was growing up, my family and I were not offered psychological support, this simply was not available during the 1980s–1990s. Over the last 47 years, I have never been offered emotional or psychological support during countless medical tests, surgeries, or on receiving difficult news. There has simply been an expectation to get on with it because, to quote a doctor during my last health crisis, "it's the nature of your condition." I remember looking in vain for books on the psychological impact of growing up with a heart condition to make sense of my unusual life experiences. This gap motivated my career as a psychologist, researcher, advocate, and eventually coauthor of *Healing Hearts and Minds: A Holistic Approach to Living Well with Congenital Heart Disease*, written with my dear friend Tracy Livecchi.

Even when I began training in my own field, I found little account of the experience of living with a serious health condition. Around 10 years ago, I came across Professor Stephen Porges's polyvagal theory. When I was a child, we were told that the heart was a simple pump and, even though my childhood pacemakers were set at a fixed rate, if the pacemaker was working, I should be able to function relatively normally. This was far from my lived experience. I often felt tired, dizzy, and agitated. I was physically sick on exertion and when I got excited or nervous. I got dehydrated easily, had poor temperature control and appetite, and restless legs when I tried to sleep. I did not keep well, catching every cold or virus on offer with a persistent cough. I watched other children in awe at their boundless energy, wondering why I could not keep up. When I tried, I failed, always trailing behind. I was "absentminded" often caught up in my own thoughts and losing or forgetting things, much to my poor mum's frustration. Looking back at photographs of me as a young child my cheeks betray the characteristic ruddy appearance of a heart condition, and I am small for my age. Even modern pacemakers are not truly physiologically responsive, and I have wondered if this contributes to the chronic fatigue I still experience daily.

For context, it is important to note that I suffer from the most serious type of heart block (third degree). This means the electrical signal from the top chamber of my heart to the bottom chamber does not get through, and I depend on my pacemaker for every heartbeat. This is quite rare, especially from birth; most people with a pacemaker only need it as a "back up" when their device senses the occasional missed heartbeat.

Polyvagal theory offered a framework to understand my embodied experience. If my heart, central to my autonomic nervous system (ANS), could not adaptively respond to my body's needs, then homeostatic control of my ANS in response to my environment would be compromised. Polyvagal theory proposes that homeostatic variability is shaped during our early years. Respiratory sinus arrythmia (RSA), a noninvasive measure of parasympathetic tone and the body's stress response, has been linked to emotional regulation and well-being lifelong (I still have not been able to establish exactly how RSA and heart rate variability are affected by congenital heart block and fixed rate pacing). Polyvagal theory seemed to have important implications for those of us who are pacemaker-dependent from infancy. On a whim, I emailed Professor Stephen Porges asking him if he thought this made sense. To my surprise, he replied right away saying, Yes! This validation of my embodied experience, growing up, was incredibly healing. We have kept in touch since, and I was privileged to contribute the chapter "Born with a Heart Condition: The Clinical Implications of Polyvagal Theory" to his and Deb Dana's edited book, *Clinical Applications of the Polyvagal Theory: The Emergence of Polyvagal Informed Therapies*.[3] I went on to colead a collaboration with him and a team of international colleagues to develop the Neuroception of Psychological Safety Scale (included in the Appendix) and became involved in the Polyvagal Institute (PVI), most recently presenting my work in at the PVI institute annual gathering in Berlin, 2024.

Over the last decade or so, there has been a welcome shift in recognizing the psychological impact of living with a chronic health condition. While the tide is turning, we are far from adequately addressing the psychological and emotional impact of living with long-term health conditions. The book's title is inspired by Michel Foucault's term "le regard médical" (the medical gaze) from his work *The Birth of the Clinic: An Archaeology of Medical Perception*.[4] Foucault argued that Western medicine has objectified the human body, which has become viewed as separate from personhood. This has led to the "patient" story becoming morphed to fit the biomedical paradigm with a focus on symptoms and test results at the cost of acknowledging emotions, idiopathic symptoms, and lived experience. While our understanding of pain, distress, and trauma has also revolutionized over the last half century we have still not successfully married this with healthcare provision. More and more of us are living with a long-term health condition dependent on medical care, yet even modern medical care can be painful, invasive, and frightening. The psychosocial impact of living with a long-term condition is extensive. This need not be inevitable, and contemporary understanding in psychology has much to offer the healthcare profession to improve care. Feeling as safe as possible, respected, and validated is fundamental to building resilience, recovery, and well-being and to prevent medical trauma. Compassionate care and effective communication skills are key to this. While this comes naturally to many health professionals, we can no longer risk leaving it to their individual "bedside manner." We need to move "beyond the medical gaze" to "practicing psychologically informed healthcare."

I know from hard-won personal experience that psychologically informed healthcare must be embedded in everything from hospital design, ward routines, and patient clothing to training all healthcare staff and providing psychological support for patients and healthcare professionals alike. Many of the challenges cannot be changed. There may be necessary surgeries, investigations, and procedures. Daily life can include managing chronic symptoms, and there can be personal costs in terms of the impact on relationships, life choices, and finances. But there are many factors that can mitigate these challenges, alleviate distress, and protect mental health and well-being. Further, given the multiple occupational challenges that healthcare professionals face, they also need to be supported to ensure their well-being.

I am indebted to and grateful for all the healthcare I have received, lifelong. I hope this book is a testament and contribution to modern healthcare. It is important to remember how far we have come in our collective understanding of pain, trauma, and psychology and of each era's cultural and social contexts and limitations. There is always an opportunity to learn from what has gone before and as "friendly critics" openly and honestly appraise what works and what needs to be improved. We need to work together in our common humanity to keep improving care for everyone and for those coming up. After all, any one of us may experience a serious health condition or bear witness to a loved one's suffering.

Positionality Statement

The importance of positionality statements from researchers in science production and writing is increasingly being recognized, in terms of ethics and validity. This allows the writer transparency about their sociocultural background and motivations and better enables the reader to understand how the writer's identity may have influenced their work.[1]

As described in the preface, and detailed throughout the book, I have lived with a serious heart condition from birth. I have drawn from my extensive personal experience—personal therapy; research training, activity, and publications; clinical training, practice, and supervision; and healthcare activism—to write this book. As a counseling psychologist and researcher, I am trained in reflective practice and critical evaluation. My shared identity with the subject of the book affords a unique insider perspective, facilitating a deeper understanding of the issues faced by people living with a long-term health condition. However, it also requires careful reflection to balance the potential for empathic understanding with the need to remain critical and objective. As both an "insider" and "outsider" in authoring this book, I aimed to be mindful of how my personal experiences of living with a chronic condition may influence this work. Further, I am a white, heterosexual, cisgender female from a working-class background in central Scotland and a married mother of one son.

Professionally, I am a chartered (British Psychological Society) and registered (Health and Care Professions Council [HCPC]) counseling psychologist with approximately 20 years of experience providing psychological therapy for adults presenting with a wide range of mental health difficulties in both NHS Scotland and independent practice. My career in psychology has been motivated, at least in part, by a passion to better understand the psychological impact of living with a serious medical condition from childhood and to improve healthcare to this end. I trained as a counseling psychologist through the British Psychological Society's independent route. Currently, I work part time as a senior lecturer in applied psychology, contributing to teaching on a counseling psychology doctoral program at Glasgow Caledonian University in Scotland. As a practice academic, I also hold a PhD in psychology from Glasgow University and I have been involved in applied psychology research for over 20 years, publishing and presenting widely on what

I have termed "psychologically informed healthcare" and on medical trauma and psychological safety.

Further, I have been involved in healthcare activism for over 10 years, successfully petitioning the Scottish Government for National Healthcare Standards for people living with congenital heart disease, across the lifespan. To this end, I sat on several health committees voluntarily for over a decade working with key stakeholders including policymakers, healthcare professionals, people with lived experience, and the media. For many years, I have promoted better understanding about the emotional and psychological impact of living with a congenital heart condition internationally through presentation, publication, and working with key stakeholders.

I have used the term "patient" in this book to refer to an individual with a health condition when they are in the "patient" role within the healthcare setting. Any one of us can find ourselves in this role, and I have used this term in recognition of this quite specific social position that I have spent much of my life in.

Acknowledgments

I would like to acknowledge the many individuals who have helped us to make this book possible. They include as follows:

Oxford University Press and my editors, Dana Bliss, and Sarah Ebel.

Professor Stephen Porges, for kindly providing the Foreword.

Maggie, Sarah, Hollie, Katerina, Richard, Lene, David, Roy, Sally, Connie, Yvonne, Lou, Becky, Alex, Sebastian, Karla, and Katie, for generously sharing their healthcare experiences through the moving quotes included throughout the book.

Karen Neaton, perioperative nurse, Gold Coast University Hospital, Australia; Meredith Kalbacker, LCSW, Mount Sinai Fuster Heart Hospital's Adult Congenital Heart Disease Center, New York; Ruth Stakeman, Dipl., music therapist, German Music Therapy Society, Soltau, Germany; Lucy Bray, professor in child health literacy, nursing and midwifery, Edgehill University, England; and my mum, Liz Paul, for providing the "Learning from" sections and sharing their experiences from life, clinical practice, and research.

Lucy Bray, professor in child health literacy, nursing and midwifery, Edgehill University, England; Pauline Aiston, chartered health psychologist and clinical lead for the ACHD Psychology Service, Bristol Heart Institute (BHI), University Hospitals Bristol and Weston; Elena Amin, assistant professor of pediatrics, University of California, San Francisco, and George S. Thompson, MD, chairman of the Board of Directors of the Polyvagal Institute and medical director for crisis services at ReDiscover in Lees Summit, Missouri, USA, for reviewing the manuscript and providing invaluable feedback.

I am deeply appreciative to everyone for sharing their insights and experiences that help to bring life to the book and offer examples of lived experience and innovative practice.

I am also thankful to the family, friends, teachers, mentors, and colleagues who have supported me and taken the time to understand, accommodate, and accept my health condition, while always seeing me.

Finally, I am deeply grateful for the National Health Service in the United Kingdom, which has provided me with free healthcare since birth, a testament to our shared humanity, and the countless dedicated healthcare professionals who have contributed to my care.

Quick Reference: Core Principles of Psychologically Informed Healthcare

Psychologically informed healthcare aims to embed contemporary understanding in psychological and emotional health into healthcare practice grounded in the core principles of R.E.S.P.E.C.T:

- **Relational safety**, providing mandatory training in and delivery of compassion-focused healthcare for all healthcare professionals (Chapter 3).
- **Empowerment**, supporting self-management and healthcare literacy and challenging disempowering aspects of healthcare (Chapter 4).
- **Soothing presence** of caregivers supported across the healthcare journey, as wanted by each individual patient (Chapter 4).
- **Psychological safety** (polyvagal informed) for patients and healthcare professionals, including emotional and psychological support that is preventative, embedded (not just reactive), and that acknowledges and validates a normal response to adverse circumstances, implementing coping strategies and support throughout healthcare delivery (Chapters 3 and 4 for supporting patients, Chapter 5 for healthcare staff, Chapter 7 for therapists).
- **Environment**, healthcare settings and policies that support healing and psychological safety (Chapter 4).
- **Culturally sensitive**, tackling ableism and discrimination and recognizing health inequalities and intersectionality (Chapter 6).
- **Trauma-informed healthcare** (Chapter 4).

PART 1
THE MEDICAL GAZE

1
The Mind–Body Connection

Considering how common illness is, how tremendous the spiritual change that it brings, how astonishing, when the lights of health go down, the undiscovered countries that are then disclosed, what wasted and deserts of the soul a slight attack of influenza brings to light, what precipices and lawns sprinkled with bright flowers a little rise of temperature reveals, what ancient and obdurate oaks are uprooted in us in the act of sickness, how we go down into the pit of death and feel the waters of annihilation close above our heads and wake thinking to find ourselves in the presence of the angels and the harpers when we have a tooth out and come to the surface in the dentist's arm chair and confuse his "Rinse the mouth—rinse the mouth" with the greeting of the Deity stooping from the floor of Heaven to welcome us—when we think of this and infinitely more, as we are so frequently forced to think of it, it becomes strange indeed that illness has not taken its place with love, battle and jealousy among the prime themes of literature.

—Virginia Woolf[1]

A decade ago, at an international medical conference, I attended a keynote lecture celebrating the 50th anniversary of Christiaan Barnard, the South African cardiac surgeon, performing the world's first heart transplant. The speaker took us on a fascinating journey through the history of cardiology from the first open-heart surgery, via the heart-bypass machine and pacemakers, to sophisticated contemporary surgical interventions including keyhole techniques. At the end of the presentation, the audience gave a standing ovation for the pioneers in their field, the broad shoulders on which they proudly stood, and rightly so. I stayed seated, paralyzed with emotion trying to hide the tears streaming down my face.

While I felt gratitude, I was overwhelmed thinking about the human stories briefly touched on in the talk. This included Louis Washkansky, recipient of the first heart transplant. He went on to regain full consciousness, before dying just 18 days later of pneumonia. In "an adventure in medical ethics," Baby Fae, born with hypoplastic left heart syndrome, became the recipient of a baboon heart transplanted by Dr. Leonard Bailey in 1984. She was just 12 days old and survived for only 3 weeks post-surgery.[2] A young mum was left brain damaged after being a human "heart-lung machine" to provide cross-circulation for her young child undergoing early heart surgery in the 1950s. The mother spent the rest of her life in an asylum while her child died.[3]

I thought of clients who have come to me for therapy over the years and of the friends that I have met through patient groups—survivors on paper faced with a lifetime of navigating the many added challenges of living with a complex medical condition. I also reflected on my own story—dependent on pioneering healthcare since birth, a "Guinea Pig" for pacing technology—and of the children from my childhood hospital. Behind every step forward in medical progress lie countless human stories of people who must find the courage to live on the edge of medicine and often survival.

The rapid development of surgical, anesthetic, pharmacological, interventional, and diagnostic techniques over the last century have led to people living longer and surviving with conditions they would previously have succumbed to in infancy. Of course, this should be celebrated. There is no doubt that medical science has alleviated untold suffering, gifting enlightenment and life to many of us. For many, life before modern medicine was undeniably short, harsh, and brutal. However, the psychological and emotional burden of feeling unwell, enduring invasive medical treatments, and living with long-term medical symptoms has been poorly addressed in healthcare practice.

Most of us will require healthcare at some point in our lives—when we are born, when we require treatment for common illnesses, following an accident, during pregnancy and childbirth, or for assistance as our health declines during older age. A growing proportion of us will also require added healthcare throughout our lives. Thanks to advances in medical care people are living longer, while birth rates have decreased, leading to an increasingly aging population.

As individuals live longer, the prevalence and cost of chronic disease is growing, presenting a growing socioeconomic burden globally. Chronic diseases, or long-term conditions (LTC), are health conditions that cannot, at present, be cured and that are controlled with medication, medical treatments, and symptom management. LTCs are estimated to affect one-third of the global population and are the leading cause of disability worldwide.

The estimated cost of LTCs is expected to reach $47 trillion worldwide by 2030.[4] Managing chronic health difficulties is a common experience affecting around a quarter of your neighbors, coworkers, friends, and family members.[5]

LTCs are associated with a heightened risk of depression, anxiety, medically related post-traumatic stress, and diminished life satisfaction and self-esteem. Further, healthcare professionals face occupational challenges to their emotional health and well-being, which can result in burnout, compassion fatigue, and vicarious trauma, negatively impacting on patient care. Yet, current healthcare policy and practice poorly address psychological and emotional well-being, for patients or practitioners. A cultural change in healthcare toward more holistic practice is long overdue to better support this growing population, who often face the "patient burden" of daily symptoms, medical monitoring, and invasive treatments.

This book aims to provide an innovative and comprehensive framework for anyone working in healthcare practice, policy, or education, grounded in the latest evidence base and the author's unique lifelong experiences, health advocacy, research, and psychology practice. *Psychologically Informed Healthcare* embeds contemporary understanding in psychological and emotional health into healthcare practice. While the book primarily aims to support healthcare professionals and policymakers it is also of relevance to psychologists, clinical social workers, counselors, and other mental health professionals working with people living with LTCs and includes a dedicated concluding chapter for these professionals. Finally, it may also help people living with LTCs, their families, and their friends to empower them throughout the healthcare journey.

Part 1 of the book outlines the need for *psychologically informed healthcare* by considering what it means to live with an LTC, how the body responds to traumatic medical experiences, childhood illness and developmental trauma, stigma, discrimination, and the possible impact of LTCs on social support, self-esteem, body image, and mental health. Chapter 2 considers how a predominately "survival focused" approach to healthcare policy and practice can, at times, create circumstances that exacerbate mental health risk factors including disempowering aspects of healthcare, waiting across the patient journey, hospital attire, disease prestige, epistemic injustice, the compassion crisis in healthcare, healthcare environments, and poor conditions for rest, sleep, and recovery in hospital settings.

In Part 2, a framework for *psychologically informed healthcare* is outlined which aims to embed contemporary understanding in psychological and emotional health into healthcare practice. Chapter 3 considers the core tenets of this framework and the importance of relational safety in building trust, psychological well-being, and recovery in healthcare practice. The chapter considers compassion as a cornerstone of psychologically informed healthcare including the science of compassion, and offers strategies to build trust, to provide a safe space for feelings, and to develop empathic listening, and offers recommendations for delivering difficult news. Considerations in establishing trust with children, teenagers, and older adults and the importance of neurodivergent-affirmative and trauma-informed healthcare are also outlined, while common mental health presentations are explored. Finally, empowering patients through self-management, healthcare literacy, and shared-decision making are considered. Chapter 4 explores conditions for healing by considering how the healthcare environment can better support emotional and psychological well-being, recovery, and feelings of psychological safety. Chapter 5 outlines the "cost of caring" by exploring the psychological and emotional challenges healthcare professionals can face, including burnout, compassion fatigue, and vicarious trauma, and offers strategies for supporting psychological well-being for healthcare professionals. In Chapter 6, cultural sensitivity is considered by exploring the interplay between social inequalities, intersectionality, and LTCs. Abuse in the hospital setting, safeguarding, and patient rights are explored, including reflective exercises to promote antidiscriminatory practice and cultural humility. A concluding chapter is included for mental health professionals who work with people living with LTCs individually or within a healthcare setting, for example as part of a healthcare team. This chapter provides a comprehensive overview for working therapeutically with this client group including consideration of evidence-based therapeutic modalities, cultural competencies, working with medically related trauma, emotional regulation, enhancing self-compassion, reintegration and connection, empowering self-management, preparing for medical procedures, and post-traumatic growth.

Reflective exercises, real-life testimonials, case studies, examples of innovative practice and research, and handouts are incorporated throughout the book to deepen understanding and learning, and can be used for discussion. A wide range of further resources and handouts are included in the Appendix to support this therapeutic work, including the Neuroception of Psychological Safety Scale (NPSS).[6]

> **Reflective Exercise for Healthcare Professionals: Psychologically Informed Healthcare**
>
> Before we begin, please take some time to reflect on your current practice, the organizational context you work in, and your training experience. It may be helpful to keep these reflections to look back on once you have read this book.
>
> - What is your current understanding about the psychological and emotional impact of living with a serious health condition?
> - How is this affected by your personal experience, or that of your loved ones?
> - What is your current understanding about the potential psychological and emotional impact of working in a healthcare profession?
> - Were these issues adequately covered in your training program?
> - Do you think they are adequately addressed in healthcare policy and practice?
> - What organizational and structural facilitators and barriers are there to acknowledging and meeting the emotional and psychological needs of people who are experiencing health difficulties and of healthcare staff, in healthcare settings?
> - How can we work to improve this individually, organizationally, and systemically?
> - What does practicing psychologically informed healthcare mean to you?

On Feeling Ill and the "Patient Role"

Volumes are now written and spoken upon the effect of the mind upon the body. Much of it is true. But I wish a little more was thought of the effect of the body on the mind.
—Florence Nightingale[7]

Most of us have experienced the discomfort of being unwell at some point, having dealt with the irritation of childhood chickenpox, a fitful fever and tender body while suffering from the flu, or struggling to breathe through a blocked nose from the common cold. During these periods of illness, uncomfortable symptoms and discomfort often reduce our ability to focus on the rest of life. Our sleep, work, and relationships may temporarily suffer. We tend to look to others for comfort, care, and rest; chicken soup from our grandma, hugs and treats from loved ones, respite or help with work and chores. Often our mood is affected too. We may feel anxious, low, easily irritated, and just a bit sorry for ourselves.

We can notice this in our children and pets too. When they are unwell, they are just not themselves, in fact this might be the first thing we notice even before any symptoms appear. If a child falls and grazes their knee, they will cry and want a soothing cuddle from their caregiver. A kiss to the injured knee will surely help its recovery. During a period of illness children often regress; a usually independent child might want more cuddles, be more emotional and cranky, be unable to sleep alone, and request comforting foods or a previously outgrown special toy. Pets feel sorry for themselves when they are not well too. They become clingy, avoid their food, and may become withdrawn.

We all know that feeling unwell impacts our mind and bodies, our ability to relate to others and carry out our usual daily tasks. Thankfully, for most people these episodes are not serious, and they are usually short and infrequent. However, many people must learn to manage symptoms related to chronic health problems daily, over months, years, and for some a lifetime. Having to muddle your way through life with symptoms such as persistent pain, fatigue, or limited mobility can feel overwhelming and relentless.

Thankfully, there are many things that can improve quality of life and emotional and psychological health for this growing population throughout the healthcare journey (explored further in Part 2). Further, many people living with an LTC demonstrate resilience, positive adaptation, and tremendous courage, finding ways to live full and meaningful lives. However, the path to well-being could be easier with improved understanding and support. To develop this, it is important to be mindful of the challenges such individuals can face, as outlined below. It is important to remember that not everyone with an LTC will face all these difficulties, which are highly variable depending on current health status, social circumstances, and available support.

Health is a state of complete physical, mental and social well-being and not merely the absence of disease or infirmity.

—World Health Organization[8]

Chronic health issues are commonly associated with the patient burden of debilitating daily symptoms such as fatigue, pain, and changes in mobility. For example, it is estimated that globally, 20%–25% of people will experience chronic pain in their lifetime. Chronic pain is an interplay between biological, psychological, and social factors and is associated with heightened stress responses, feelings of anxiety, and isolation.[9]

People with chronic health conditions can face other debilitating symptoms too. For example, multiple sclerosis can cause ambulation issues, imbalance, falls, urinary incontinence, fatigue, pain, and cognitive and memory problems.[10] Epilepsy, which affects between 40 and 70 people per 100,000, is associated with increased morbidity and mortality, other neurological problems, cognitive problems, and fatigue. Quality of life for people living with epilepsy is related to available social support, yet epilepsy is still highly stigmatized, which in turn can lead to increased anxiety, depression, low self-esteem, and poor medical adherence.[11]

The COVID-19 pandemic has, to date, left an estimated 65 million people worldwide living with long COVID. This debilitating chronic illness can affect multiple bodily systems with a wide range of symptoms including fatigue, nausea, loss of appetite, constipation, shortness of breath, chest pain, palpitations, brain fog, memory loss, cognitive impairment, sensorimotor symptoms, dizziness, autonomic dysfunction, and postexertional malaise, significantly impacting on psychosocial functioning.[12,13]

For people living with an LTC, symptoms can be highly unpredictable—there may be good days and bad, making it tricky to make plans and commitments. This can negatively affect understanding from others, because when someone sees you at your "best" it can be hard for them to understand the hidden cost.

> *I was diagnosed with Rheumatoid Arthritis in 2015, my joints were so swollen by then that I was diagnosed by my GP who took one look at me and diagnosed me. . . . I was urgently referred to a rheumatologist. Suddenly I was propelled into a world of heavy duty medications, steroid injections and hospital appointments. All the time I was thinking, this is not me, I am not a sick person, I am a professional person with a family, life, and career. I remember feeling scared, lost and very very angry that this happened to me.*
> —Connie, 48, living with rheumatoid arthritis, nurse, United Kingdom

Living with an LTC can also involve routine exposure to invasive medical tests and procedures, which can be painful, often occurring in the absence of loved ones. Routine care may involve injections to control diabetes, INR (international normalized ratio) checks for people on blood-thinning medication, remembering to take medication to manage chronic pain, and regular check-ups with healthcare providers. Specifically, diabetes, a chronic metabolic disorder, can affect physical, social, and psychological functioning. Effective self-management of diabetes is critical to supporting health. However, this requires commitment to strict daily medical routines often via checking blood glucose levels and self-injection of insulin with a pen. Yet, psychological support of this population is underresourced, contributing to reduced quality of life and well-being, which can affect self-management and medical adherence.[14]

Sometimes the cure can seem worse than the disease. There may be side effects of medications, which, depending on the required treatment, may include a dry mouth, weight gain, impotency, digestive discomfort, brain fog, fatigue, or even suppression of immunity, in the case of immunosuppressant therapy for autoimmune conditions such as lupus or rheumatoid arthritis.[15]

At times, living with an LTC can also involve invasive medical tests, hospital stays, surgery, living with implantable devices (such as an implantable cardioverter-defibrillator [ICD]), and facing medical uncertainty. For example, living with a colostomy negatively impacts on overall quality of life, affecting psychological and sexual health, body image, social life, routine, and travel. One recent qualitative research study, using semistructured interviews, found that people who had undergone a permanent colostomy reported experiencing it as a significant and traumatic life change.[16] Further, living with an ICD was associated with more threatening illness perception and lower quality of life, compared with controls, in an international cross-sectional study of over 3,000 adults with congenital heart disease from 15 countries.[17]

The administrative load of living with an LTC can also be extensive, requiring organizing and attending healthcare appointments; arranging time off work; obtaining and collecting prescriptions for medications; liaising with multiple healthcare professionals about appointments, tests, and results; seeking answers and referrals; and making sense of treatment regimens and recommendations. For people with private healthcare systems this can also include dealing with medical bills, insurance companies, and concerns over the impact on personal finances. These time-consuming tasks may contribute to patient burnout.[18]

Multidisciplinary communication is often significantly lacking, with clinicians wanting to just focus on their area and not considering the body as a whole. This really delayed understanding of my condition.
—Becky, 36, Ehlers-Danlos syndrome, postural orthostatic tachycardia syndrome (POTS), chronic fatigue, United Kingdom

Further, a growing number of people are living with multiple long-term conditions (MLTCs), or multimorbidity, with earlier age of onset in people living in deprived communities. MLTCs are also more common in women. Holland et al. report findings from a qualitative evidence synthesis study that aimed to develop a greater understanding of the effect of MLTCs on people's lives.[19] The study included coproduction involving patient and public involvement (PPI) with colleagues living with MLTCs in line with NIHR guidance.[20] The authors report that living with MLTCs was experienced as a complex workload comprising eight types of work, many of which are reciprocally linked: symptom work (e.g., managing symptoms), emotional work (e.g., dealing with associated feelings), investigating and monitoring (e.g., tests and procedures), health service and administration (e.g., attending appointments, dealing with services that focus on single conditions), medication work (e.g., polypharmacy and complex regimes), financial work (e.g., impact on finances), learning and adapting (e.g., loss of independence and roles), and accumulation and complexity (e.g., having to self-advocate) The authors note that much of this work, and the associated impact on people, may not be apparent to healthcare staff, and current health systems and policies are poorly equipped to meet the needs of this growing population. Further, a lack of integration and poor communication between different medical specialties adds to the burden of living with MLCTs.[21]

Initially Robert felt elated that he was in remission from bowel cancer and looked forward to getting back to his old self. However, he found it difficult to adjust to life with the colostomy fitted during bowel surgery and avoided socializing or traveling too far from home in case there were any issues. Over time, this led to him feeling low. Gradually, with the support of a district nurse and his partner, he became more confident about going out. However, he wished someone had better prepared him for the long-term psychological impact of his treatment.

Acute episodes of poor health can lead to abrupt and unexpected symptoms and involve medical emergencies, uncertainty, and a sense of vulnerability and life threat. To illustrate, sudden cardiac arrest is associated with depression, anxiety, post-traumatic stress, and the development of heart-focused health anxiety, which can undermine quality of life.[22]

A doctor ordered additional pain medication. The evening after the operation, I asked to be given these. The nurse told me that she had consulted with the other nurses and decided not to give me this medication. I was stunned and too weak to do anything about it. The next morning I was given the pills by another nurse. I will never forget that night and the feeling of helplessness and being at the mercy of others.
—**Lou, 48, bowel endometriosis, Germany**

During medical care, there is little choice but to entrust your life to your healthcare team. In this "patient role," many people report feeling vulnerable, dependent, frightened, and disempowered. It can be hard for others to understand what chronic illness and suffering feel like unless they have experienced it. Simple acts of empathy, humanity, and compassion matter as much as any medicine. Within this relationship dynamic, which has traditionally been paternalistic, there is an imbalance of power with regard to health status, medical knowledge, and access to, often lifesaving, medical care.[23] This can be worsened by socioeconomic disparities in terms of education, social status, and finances. It is important for healthcare providers to recognize this power imbalance, because it can result in a loss of agency, which can prevent patients from articulating concerns, asking key questions, or remembering what has been said after clinical encounters. Further, feeling disempowered is a risk factor for psychological distress and the development of medically related post-traumatic stress.

Reflective Exercise: The Impact of LTCs

While it is simply impossible to understand what serious illness and pain feel like unless you have experienced them firsthand, and this experience is highly variable depending on the condition and a multitude of other factors, it is useful to have some sense of what living with an LTC can feel like. Please only carry out this reflective exercise if you feel able to, bearing in mind it may be triggering if you have experienced serious ill health.

If you feel comfortable doing so, please consider the last time you felt unwell or in pain. How did this impact on:

- Your mood?
- Your sense of self?
- Feelings of autonomy?
- How you felt about your body?
- Your ability to carry out your normal daily activities?
- Your relationships?
- Your finances?

If these symptoms had persisted for days, weeks, months, and even years, consider what the impact would be on each of the above. What if you had experienced these symptoms persistently from childhood? How would you feel about regularly having to seek healthcare advice or hospitalization?

Survival Mode: How the Body Responds to Traumatic Medical Experiences

I have had to hold still for countless, invasive, often painful medical procedures. I learned as an infant not to "cause a fuss" and that if I protested when having a catheter inserted, cannula placed, or stitches removed it would hurt more and take longer. Besides, my life depends on these interventions. But my "bravery" does not mean that they do not hurt me, or that I am not anxious. It upsets me when staff say, "you must be used to this." During each medical procedure, each moment when I fear for my life, I freeze, a common response to trauma.

Research has consistently shown that people who are living with chronic health difficulties are more likely to feel anxious.[24] In many ways this is understandable, considering the added life stressors they can endure, both medically and beyond. Anxiety is a normal response to uncertainty and to situations that we find threatening or challenging. Further, traumatic experiences can result in a sense of threat and trigger symptoms of post-traumatic stress, particularly when exposure is repeated and cumulative.[25]

Stressful situations can trigger our body's alarm system, this is a normative response for self-protection. Three parts of the brain are involved in the stress response during traumatic experiences.[26,27] The prefrontal cortex, sometimes called the "primate brain," becomes less active. This part of the brain handles higher mental functions including executive function, regulating attention, feelings and desires, language, working memory, rational thinking, and impulse control. This is why people often report being unable to think clearly or articulate themselves during traumatic experiences. The hippocampus, responsible for processing memories, also becomes less active. As such, trauma memories are often fragmented and unprocessed. People often struggle to recall what happened to them, or experience this as piecemeal flashbacks and nightmares. Finally, the amygdala or "alarm center" becomes more active, setting an alarm off in the body by signaling the hypothalamic-pituitary-adrenal (HPA) axis to release the stress hormones cortisol and norepinephrine. This results in feelings of fear or anger and mobilizes the body to flee or fight the danger, or in the case of extreme threat to become immobilized. Our bodies act first and think later in response to traumatic events. While this is a normal defensive strategy that protects us from harm, severe traumatic stress can be associated with lasting changes in these brain areas resulting in our bodies becoming tuned to become more reactive to stress (Figure 1.1).[28]

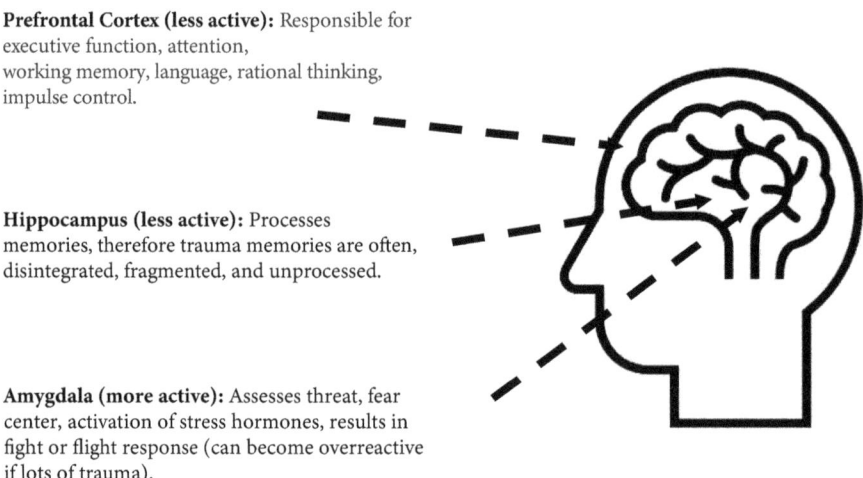

Prefrontal Cortex (less active): Responsible for executive function, attention, working memory, language, rational thinking, impulse control.

Hippocampus (less active): Processes memories, therefore trauma memories are often, disintegrated, fragmented, and unprocessed.

Amygdala (more active): Assesses threat, fear center, activation of stress hormones, results in fight or flight response (can become overreactive if lots of trauma).

Figure 1.1 Infographic depicting how the human brain responds to stressful and traumatic experiences

Professor Stephen Porges's *polyvagal theory* (PVT) offers a useful framework for understanding how our bodies respond to stress grounded in neurophysiology, psychology, and evolutionary theory.[29] PVT proposes that the autonomic nervous system (ANS) has three distinct physiological and behavioral states. These states are initiated by the two parts of the ANS: the sympathetic nervous system and the parasympathetic nervous system, the latter of which includes both the ventral vagal and dorsal vagal branches of the vagus nerve. Each state is associated with distinct functions and responses to the environment. To feel healthy, we need to be able to assess and flexibly respond to our environment when we are both safe and unsafe. PVT describes how the ANS continually and subconsciously assesses situations for safety or threat. This surveillance is termed "*neuroception*" (see Figure 1.2). Neuroception is a reflexive process, beneath our conscious awareness.

PVT proposes that in situations detected via neuroception as psychologically safe our bodies operate in the ventral vagal system of the parasympathetic nervous system. This activates physiological, affective, and cognitive processes that optimize social engagement and prosocial behaviors, including compassion for others. Porges refers to this mode of being as our "*social engagement system*," sometimes referred to as the "*rest and digest system*." In this mode, we feel calm, relaxed, and psychologically safe and our bodies are optimized for healing, learning, and social connection. For general health and well-being, we want to be in this mode most of the time.[30]

However, situations detected as unsafe shift our bodies into defense mode. Most commonly this happens via the sympathetic system, which leads to fight

The Mind–Body Connection   15

Neuroception of threat: Fight or Flight Mode (hyperarousal)

Sympathetic Nervous System (SNS)

Increases: Blood pressure, heart rate, fuel availability, adrenaline, oxygen to vital organs, blood clotting, pupil size, dilation of bronchi, defensive responses

Decreases: Fuel storage, insulin activity, digestion, salivation, relational ability, immune response

---

Neuroception of Psychological Safety: Social Engagement System

Parasympathetic Nervous System - Ventral Vagal Complex (VVC)

Increases: Digestion, immune response, rest & recuperation, health & vitality, circulation to nonvital organs, ability to relate & connect with others, eye movement & head turning, prosody in voice, steady breathing

Decreases: Defensive Responses

Neuroception of threat: Immobilization Response (hypoarousal)

Dorsal Vagal Complex (DVC)

Increases: Immobilization behavior(with fear), endorphins that help numb & raise the pain threshold, conservation of metabolic resources

Decreases: Blood pressure, heart rate, temperature, muscle tone, facial expressions & eye contact, depth of breath, social behavior, attunement to human voice, sexual responses, immunity

Figure 1.2 How the nervous system responds to safety and threat
Source: Adapted from Porges, S. W. (2022). Polyvagal theory: A science of safety. Front Integr Neurosci, 16, 871227.

or flight behaviors that are supported by increases in heart rate, shortened breathing, and increased muscle tension. During this *hyperarousal*, our bodies prepare to act to fight or flee the perceived danger. For example, when we approach a healthcare setting for a medical procedure, we may need to overcome an innate urge to flee the situation, leaving us feeling breathless and nauseous, with a pounding heart and sweaty palms.

If we perceive a threat to life, our most primitive threat response is activated via the dorsal vagal pathway. In this third "death feigning" mode, we go into *hypoarousal*, which is felt as dissociation. During this *immobilization* response our body *shuts down* rather than being activated, as the body plays dead for survival. Afterward, we may struggle to recall what happened to us because the parts of our brain that make sense of events and store memories are compromised. To illustrate, this may happen during invasive hospital procedures when the individual feels like they have no control, are unable to move, and feel very scared and vulnerable. *Hypoarousal* during a traumatic experience is linked to the development of post-traumatic stress disorder.[31]

A fourth response, the *"fawn response"* has recently been described in situations where we neurocept danger and both the fight/flight and immobilization responses are activated simultaneously. During this response, known as "appeasement," the sympathetic system provides the fuel for movements to meet the needs of others while the dorsal vagal circuit enables dissociation and disconnection to protect ourselves. This enables us to pacify interpersonal threats and is associated with "people pleasing," whereby we aim to regulate the other's nervous system to protect ourselves. For example, in a hospital setting a child may appear to happily comply with painful medical treatments and go along with narratives to be brave, strong, and a good patient, while feeling deeply distressed, because they want to keep the adults around them happy and do not feel safe enough to share their feelings or vulnerability. Over time this may lead to neglecting our own needs, and turning negative feelings toward the self in the form of self-criticism, self-loathing, or self-harming behaviors. In adulthood, an unresolved fawn response may lead to codependence, depression, or somatic symptoms of pain and illness.[32,33]

PVT states that our ANS is both expressive and receptive. In other words, not only do we constantly assess threats and safety in our environment but also we communicate this with each other. As mammals we have evolved a toolkit to broadcast the state of our ANS to others, and to respond to theirs. To this end, we are adept at reading social cues and the vagus nerve is involved in the control of facial expression, eye movement, vocalizations, and hearing. We literally "wear" the state of our nervous system on our face, in our voice and through our body language. Healthcare professionals may notice when a patient is particularly scared or anxious because they may be holding themselves tensely, sweating, breathing fast, fidgeting, speaking tersely, struggling with eye contact, and even displaying the characteristic high blood pressure associated with *"white coat syndrome."*[34]

Over time, when our nervous system is stuck in a heightened response mode, it elevates chronic levels of stress hormones such as cortisol and adrenaline in our body. This is linked to increases in weight gain, decreased immune function, and a detrimental effect on overall health, both physically and psychologically.[35]

As a species we are good at dealing with stressful situations. We have evolved to deal with threats from predators and competitors to protect our young and find resources for survival. However, in the modern world we seldom need to follow through on fight or flight when faced with everyday stressors, often leaving us sitting with bodies charged for action. Likewise, we no longer need to "play dead" for survival. Yet, we still live with the legacy of our ancestral history.

Nevertheless, even when we experience significant trauma, we usually recover from this in the days and weeks after the event, as our bodies adaptively return to a sense of safety. However, for some, exposure to trauma can lead to the development of post-traumatic stress, particularly when the stressors are prolonged and cumulative. There are several factors that can increase the risk for the development of post-traumatic stress, following exposure to adverse situations. These include feelings of powerlessness, a lack of personal agency and feelings of entrapment, preexisting physical and mental health difficulties, and poor social support during and after the event. Over time, exposure to trauma can lead to disconnection and alienation.[36]

It is important to note that neurodivergent individuals may be at increased vulnerability to trauma due to sensory sensitivities, social difficulties, and communication challenges. Further, trauma symptoms can overlap with or exacerbate existing neurodivergent traits, posing diagnostic and therapeutic challenges. Gajwani and Minnis describe the cumulative impact of childhood adversity and neurodiversity. They describe this intersectionality a *"double jeopardy"* because the increased health risks associated with both adverse childhood experiences and neurodevelopmental conditions combine to increase the risk of a maladaptive stress response and negative health outcomes.[37]

It is unusual to face a traumatic situation that you have already experienced, knowing that you will face it again. Yet, this is often the case for people living with LTCs,[38] particularly if they have faced exposure to potentially traumatic life events, such as surgery, poor health, and being separated from loved ones during extended periods of hospitalization. If we experience a lot of traumatic experiences, our nervous system can become attuned to interpreting situations as threatening. This is particularly true for childhood trauma. When you are raised in a more "hostile" environment it is important for your survival to have a more responsive threat system for protection. Over time this may narrow the window of feeling psychologically safe, biasing us toward expecting threats, compromising the nervous system, and contributing to "unexplained medical symptoms" such as fatigue, pain, and stomach complaints.

Medical conditions may also affect autonomic regulation more directly. For example, changes in autonomic functioning are present in fibromyalgia, characterized by chronic, widespread pain and symptoms of fatigue and dizziness.

Postural orthostatic tachycardia syndrome (POTS), a common abnormality of the autonomic nervous system often diagnosed with fibromyalgia, consists of autonomic failures such as dysregulated blood flow and orthostatic tachycardia.[39]

Jenna developed juvenile arthritis during childhood and needed to attend a clinic regularly for steroid injections. One day, her family got stuck in traffic and arrived late to the appointment. Jenna and her mother already felt stressed about being late on arrival. Her usual nurse was off sick, and the substitute nurse was in a hurry. She did not introduce herself to Jenna or prepare with her like her usual nurse. Jenna found the injection much more painful. She started to cry and felt unsupported by the nurse, who wrote something in her records about her being emotional and anxious. Afterward she found herself dreading having to go back for another treatment. Leading up to her next appointment she felt increasingly anxious. This started to impact on her schoolwork. She also felt isolated from her friends who did not understand because none of them had any health issues, so she started withdrawing socially.

The interaction between the immune system and the autonomic nervous system is increasingly being recognized. For individuals with type 1 diabetes mellitus, the effects of stress are influenced by aberrant regulation of stress hormones and relative presence of insulin at the time of stress. Researchers suggest that this can be attributed to the presence of autonomic nervous system abnormalities associated with diabetic neuropathy, as well as individual psychological differences.[40] Further, in multiple sclerosis (MS), an autoimmune disease involving dysregulation of both sympathetic and parasympathetic systems, when communication between the ANS and immune system is dysregulated, inflammatory responses may induce or worsen a flair of symptoms.[41]

The Impact of LTCs on Parenting and Birth Trauma

Growing up I did not really think about whether I wanted to be a mum. There was never an explicit conversation about it, but I got the impression that I should focus on other ambitions. It was not until my mid-20s that a doctor approached me about the topic. During a period of stress my chronic fatigue had become all-consuming, and I developed new symptoms including trigeminal neuropathy, painfully dry eyes, hypnotic jerks, a rash on my wrists, loss of appetite, and joint pain, while my voice reduced to a whisper. Frustrated and desperate for answers, I sought a private consultation, with

Dr. S, a highly recommended general consultant. At our first meeting, he told me it was likely that I was suffering from an autoimmune disorder, noting that my mum probably had Lupus or Primary Sjogren's syndrome because both are linked to the development of fetal heart block.[42] Dr. S explained that I was likely born anti-Ro-positive, suffering from neonatal lupus, and he conducted some blood tests which showed anomalies of my immune system. My mum also undertook medical testing and was diagnosed with both Primary Sjogren's and Lupus.

In light of this, Dr. S informed me, in his compassionate yet matter of fact style, that if I wanted children, I should have them soon, to mitigate any risk to the baby and myself. I am hugely grateful to him for not only giving us answers about why I was born with a heart condition but also by empowering me with information that enabled me to seek genetic counseling and make an informed choice about having a baby. My healthy son was born a few years later. Becoming a mother is a gift I never expected, and I have cherished every moment.

I received excellent care throughout my pregnancy, from a specialist obstetrician and an anesthetist who checked me regularly and worked with me to develop a birth plan. However, despite all these efforts, the birth itself was traumatic. Even with all the preparation and traveling to a specialist center for a planned birth, none of my team were present during the delivery. When I asked my midwife to follow my birth plan, 10 hours into labor, by requesting a planned epidural the head midwife told me "You young girls just can't deal with pain." At this point, to our horror, my husband and I realized she had not looked at my medical birth plan and had no knowledge of my heart condition. Not long after I ended up being rushed to the theater for an emergency caesarean section. Two days later, I was discharged from care but gradually felt unwell. The following day I was sent to emergency care by my family doctor and admitted to hospital. After undergoing tests, the on-call cardiologist diagnosed me with heart failure and my husband, and I were told I needed a heart transplant. I spent the night away from my new baby, inconsolably crying in the cardiology ward with a very compassionate nurse who just sat with me. The following day, a cardiology team with specialist knowledge of congenital heart disease conducted some other tests informing us there had been a misdiagnosis. My heart just looked different on an X-ray due to the surgical procedures I have had. I was not in heart failure. Much to our relief, he told me my symptoms were a result of iron deficiency and fluid retention. The entire episode was very traumatic, at a time when my baby, family and I were at our most vulnerable. It would have been completely avoidable if I had been able to access the specialist care that I needed during and after giving birth. When I complained afterward, I was told by the health board that my baby was healthy and fine and to get on with it. I was so relieved and grateful for my baby that I put it behind me to cherish every moment, until the next time I met with life threatening challenges to accessing specialist care.

As illustrated by my experience, the decision to have a family is often more complex for people living with an LTC. They may have to seek genetic counseling to establish any risks to the baby and themselves and must consider the impact of their condition on parenting, in the context of wider social support. Further, people with an LTC are often in medically high-risk groups during pregnancy increasing their risk of a traumatic birth experience.

Traumatic birth experiences can develop into a more serious condition known as childbirth-related post-traumatic stress disorder (CR-PTSD).[43] People with an LCT are often at increased risk of factors associated with CR-PTSD including preterm birth, stillbirth, or pre-eclampsia, depression in pregnancy, fear of childbirth, poor health or complications in pregnancy, history of trauma, or mental health problems. They may also be at heightened risk of perinatal risk factors such as a negative subjective birth experience, operative birth, obstetrical complications, and severe maternal morbidity, as well as maternal near misses, lack of support, and dissociation. Further, they may also be at risk of postpartum risk factors include depression, postpartum physical complications, and stress.

> *As an expectant mother, don't assume that if you discover my child has the same rare condition I have, that I would want to terminate. There is power in knowledge, I just wanted to be prepared. Similarly, be aware that childbirth can bring back a lot of sensory recall for someone who has had surgery as a child. Be kind, be gently, listen and please try not to categorise.*
>
> **Sally, late 50s, congenital craniofacial condition, former nurse, psychotherapist, and PhD researcher, United Kingdom**

Yet, traumatic childbirth experiences and CR-PTSD remain largely unrecognized in maternity services and are not routinely screened for during pregnancy and the postpartum period. It is estimated that 6.6 million mothers and 1.7 million fathers or coparents are affected by CR-PTSD worldwide each year.[44] Prevention efforts should include screening for antenatal risk factors, trauma-informed care, early intervention, and access to trauma-focused psychological therapies.[45]

Learning from Research and Practice: Post-Caesarean Section Shivering

By Karen Neaton, peri-operative nurse, Gold Coast University Hospital, Australia
I had been working as a Peri-operative Nurse for 28 years when I studied for my Master of Nursing. I used the assignments to study elements of my workplace where improvement was needed. The biggest area of need appeared to be the consideration of the psychological elements of a patient's presentation, and the staff's ability to meet those needs.

One of the projects was a small qualitative study on the attitudes of staff to providing trauma informed care (TIC). This project was implemented on the back of a patient letter asking us to use it. Overwhelmingly, the staff were uninformed about TIC and uncomfortable with some of its elements, especially giving power to the patient. A second project, a literature review, generated enormous interest within my study group due to its resonance and I was encouraged to take it to publication.

This review looks at the non-pharmacological treatments for shivering in women who had caesarean section under neuraxial block. The study was born out of the practice of asking women to suck their thumb as a way to mitigate the shivering. As I studied, I was learning that thumb sucking sent a safety message directly to the nervous system. It made me think that if thumb sucking stopped the shivering, then maybe, the cause was fear. When I checked the definition of shivering, it literally included the word fear.

Up until now, all shivering had been treated with warm blankets and medications, including narcotics. As I researched further, I came across the Polyvagal Theory, which explained that paralysis is experienced as a life-threatening situation. This correlated with some of the literature where patients reported paralysis being their primary fear, as well as a desire to have a good relationship with their care providers. I was concerned that we might not be seeing what was in plain sight all these years.

I was able to find and implement interventions based on contemporary knowledge of the brain and the neuroscience of safety to eliminate shivering in patients, but I had to look outside the medical/nursing/peri-operative domains.[46] From my perspective, keeping in mind the internal experience of the patient, is a more sophisticated level of situational awareness and being capable enough to respond, is the level of professional proficiency our patients deserve. To do this, we need to be more psychologically informed.

Healthcare professionals also need to be aware of health inequalities in pregnancy and childbirth. Cardiac disease is one of the leading causes of death for maternal mortality.[47] Further, there is an almost threefold difference in maternal mortality rates among women from Black ethnic backgrounds compared to white women and an almost twofold difference among women from Asian ethnic backgrounds compared to white women,[48] while women living in the most deprived areas have a maternal mortality rate more than twice as high as women living in the least deprived areas.[49]

It is also important to note the effects of maternal stress and domestic abuse on the unborn child. These are multifaceted and extensive including low birth weight, preterm birth, alteration of the HPA axis and hormonal changes, and maternal and neonatal death. Brain development begins before birth, and the emotional status of the mother impacts on the baby from conception. In the womb both the mother's diet and stress can cause epigenetic changes in the fetus.[50] Epigenetic changes are modifications of DNA that occur without any alteration in the underlying DNA sequence and can control whether a gene is turned on or off. As such, researchers call for universal screening, patient engagement in prenatal care, and targeted individualized interventions to reduce the adverse effects of intimate partner violence (IPV) and maternal stress.[51]

Further, having an unwell baby or experiencing miscarriage, stillbirth, or neonatal death is intensely painful and traumatic for many parents and is associated with substantial psychological and social costs to women and their families.[52] Yet, many of these women and their families, and those who need to undergo a medical termination, receive care in "mother and baby" units alongside pregnant mothers and families with healthy newborns (see "A Mother's Story" below). This adds further harm in an already painful situation and is far from psychologically informed healthcare.[53]

Laura and her partner were delighted when they found out that she was pregnant. Laura had been told that they would find it difficult to conceive because she had endometriosis. However, at an 8-week scan they found out that they had lost the baby. Devastated, they had to walk past expectant mothers in the waiting room on their way out of the hospital. Further, Laura had to return to the same mother and baby unit in the hospital a few days later for a dilation and curettage (D & C) procedure. She had to pass a ward full of new mums and could hear the babies. She felt numb throughout this experience and developed traumatic grief in the months afterward.

Please note sensitive content

A Mother's Story

By Liz Paul (the author's mum)

My journey into congenital heart conditions started when I was about 4 months pregnant. I attended a routine antenatal clinic with my family doctor. During an examination, the doctor fell silent and asked the nurse to check for a heartbeat. She couldn't find one either. After what seemed like an eternity, they told me that I had to make my way to the maternity hospital urgently.

I had my two-year-old son with me, and I could not drive. I walked home in a daze, trying to act normally for my son. My husband would not look after our son, so we had to take him to my parents' house before he dropped me off at the maternity hospital.

The healthcare team, at the maternity hospital, could not find a heartbeat either. But I could feel the baby move a little. I was kept in for a week, but nothing improved, it was decided to let me go full term and induce me on my due date. I was informed there was something seriously wrong and to prepare myself for the worst. I hope that in over 40 years later, a mother would not be left for five months without counselling of some kind.

When she was born, my daughter was taken away before I could see her because my womb hemorrhaged. It was late at night when they could fit me in to be induced, so the midwife rang the on-call doctor. When he finally arrived, he packed my womb, and I was taken to intensive care. I was told nothing until a doctor arrived the next morning to tell me my baby was slowly slipping away. I was transferred to a ward with three other mothers who all had their babies with them. Each night, I was woken up every few hours by the nursing staff, along with the other mothers, to feed my baby because the staff kept forgetting she was not there. I could not stand without fainting and was promised repeatedly that a nurse would take me to see my baby in a wheelchair. This never happened, so I discharged myself three days later. Before I could visit my baby, she had been taken by ambulance to the national hospital for children in Glasgow.

My baby's life was saved that day by a wonderful doctor and team in a pioneering operation to fit a pacemaker, a first in the world at the time. This involved many problems and anxious times and surgeries on my tiny baby, it was heart breaking. My daughter's journey and mine, by her side, has been long, lonely and at times painful. I would urge healthcare professionals to be more aware of the emotional and psychological impact on children with any serious lifelong condition. There is as much need

Continued

Continued

to care about their mental wellbeing as saving their lives. The two must go hand in hand.

I froze the day they told me my baby was dying, and a part of me stayed frozen. My daughter did not have counselling, so we struggled alone in the dark. I did not know the best way to help her to cope with the terrible load she had to carry. Fortunately, she was a determined child, and I muddled my way through. As a mother, psychological help would have been invaluable. I had a difficult home life, limited support and a 3-year-old son that I hated leaving. Family counselling would have been wonderful.

When my daughter had to transition from her childhood team to adult care, she went from a caring medical team, who had known her from birth to a hospital where the only other people with pacemakers were elderly. They forgot how young she was. After struggling with her health and moving to another hospital nearer home, it was found that her pacemaker had been set for an elderly person for many years. Too many problems to mention followed until a specialist adult service was finally established.

At her first appointment at this new specialist service, I remember saying to her new consultant that I could now die happy knowing she had good care. However, my bubble soon burst when we had to visit our local hospital during an emergency. The on-call consultant was adamant nothing was wrong with her pacemaker, even though her heart monitor said differently. We knew when there was a problem. But he was the cardiologist, and he discharged her, confident she had a virus. It was a Friday evening; we waited until Monday morning until the clinic was open to demand they check her device. There WAS a fault, and she was admitted and sent to the specialist service for yet another operation.

I have a great debt of gratitude to the NHS. I would not have my wonderful daughter without it. However, amongst the wonderful consultants, doctors, nurses there are some who do not listen to the patients who have a long-term condition. My journey with my daughter has involved me having to fight for her care, especially when she was too young to do so herself. To stand guard by her bed, so they did not put her through any unnecessary suffering. This often happened if they did not know her history, hadn't taken time to read her notes or had lost results from painful procedures and had to repeat them. My heartfelt message to all involved in the medical care is to remember that patients with serious lifelong conditions and their families usually know what they are talking about and to ensure that psychological help is available for patients and their families.

Childhood Illness: Medical Interruptions to Secure Attachment and Loss of a Normal Childhood

> *As a small child being in and out of hospital in the 1970s, my mum wasn't allowed to stay with me. This was extremely upsetting for me on every occasion and to my mum. I did on occasions try to escape the hospital and got into trouble from staff, obviously. Therefore, my only escape was to shut down mentally, stay still, stay quiet and wait for time to pass. All awhile being extremely lonely, afraid and sad. This I believe has had a long-lasting effect on my overall wellbeing, abandonment issues, being vulnerable in relationships. Parents and caregivers can stay with children now thank goodness, but there will still be families, for example, lone parents who maybe cannot stay over with their sickly child due to having more than one child to care for but possibly a grandparent, aunt or other close member of the family could.*
>
> —Maggie, 53 years old, congenital heart condition, United Kingdom

My mum was unable to hold me until I was 6 weeks old, already bearing scars from two thoracotomies and recovering from a stroke. She tells me she took me home to "love me better." As a young child I clung to the safety of my mum, I was shy, quiet, and at times withdrawn. I vividly remember a family member commenting that "someone needs to cut the apron strings" not long after I came home from hospital from yet more cardiac surgery. Such lack of wider understanding only made me feel shyer and more unsafe.

As a child, I did not have the words to express how I was feeling. From an early age I learned to block any distress, refusing to talk about my hospital experiences the moment we drove out of the hospital car park. But sometimes the terror leaked out in unexpected ways. Once, my mum, brother and I planted cress seeds in old ice cream containers. I was excited to grow a plant all by myself and happily slotted the containers underneath the sofa to germinate. When we retrieved our boxes, success: there were rows of neat, green stalks, each topped with two small leaves. I began to scream uncontrollably. To me, the cress protruded like the black wire stitches in my skin after surgery. I was repulsed. My mum threw the cress away.

On another occasion, my parents had bought me a Sesame Street book as part of my Christmas. When I opened the book, it said that big bird had a pacemaker. Again, I uncharacteristically responded with terror, ripping the book up and becoming very distressed.

It would have been helpful if I had been taught healthy ways to express what I was going through, but back then, no one knew about trauma or the emotional and psychological impacts of serious illness. Everyone was just muddling along, trying to do their best to keep me alive.

We now know that feeling safe, loved, and cared for is essential for healthy physical, psychological, and emotional health and social development. As mammals, we are hard-wired for extensive care, connection, and belonging from birth. These basic needs are even greater for children with a serious health condition who feel unwell and are often subject to painful medical treatments. Yet, fulfilling these needs can be more challenging because they may be incubated in intensive care or high dependency wards in the hospital. It is physically difficult to hold a baby who is attached to an array of medical drips and monitors, often unable to breastfeed, and, for some, requiring a gastrostomy tube and unable to bottle feed. Further, parents may not have been allowed to stay with them in the hospital or for invasive surgeries and procedures.[54] While the importance of early attachment is now better understood there can still, even today, be medical barriers to this. The British psychologist and psychiatrist John Bowlby proposed his widely influential work on attachment theory in *A Secure Base* (1988),[55] which built on his earlier, groundbreaking work that highlighted the detrimental impact of maternal deprivation on hospitalized and institutionalized children.[55]

Under normal circumstances the baby engages in an innate biological dance with their primary caregiver through eye contact, touch, and vocalizations. The caregiver's presence, touch, and soothing voice are essential to healthy development for babies. When this relationship is predictable and safe, a secure bond, known as a *secure attachment*—a healthy attachment to each other—develops. These early interactions shape our nervous system and provide the template on which our future relationships are built. Bowlby termed this template the *"internal working model."* When this relationship is healthy and consistent, over time, babies develop the ability to regulate their own emotions and to navigate their social world. Children with a secure attachment to their primary caregivers are more resilient to traumatic life events.[57]

The distinguished American psychiatrist Dan Siegel (2012) describes four S's of secure attachment: safe, seen, soothed, and secure.[58] *Safe* pertains to creating an environment for the child, safe from both physical and emotional harm, to explore and build trust in the world, self, and others. *Seen* means the child's experiences are acknowledged and validated, enabling them to develop a sense of self-worth and learn to trust that their needs and feelings matter. The third S, *Soothed*, is crucial in building attachments and involves providing comfort, reassurance, and support when the child is upset or distressed.

This enables them to develop emotional regulation capacities and healthy coping skills. The final S, *Secure*, relates to creating a sense of security and predictability in the child's relationships, enabling them to develop a sense of trust and confidence in others. Secure attachments in childhood positively impact emotional regulation, self-esteem, resilience, social development, and cognitive development.

As such, children have innate, basic needs for the soothing presence of warm and responsive caregivers, extensive affectionate touch, connection, a sense of belonging, consistency, validation, and the opportunity to play and learn.[59] Yet, as described, children with complex health conditions may face medical barriers to these basic needs. They may be separated from their primary caregiver at a time when they need them most. Further, parents may be less emotionally available due to their own circumstances and mental health. Studies have shown that early stress or trauma experienced by infants and children affects neural, behavioral, and psychological development, with long-lasting effects across a wide range of domains. Chronic illness during formative years can disrupt attachment, play, and learning opportunities, contributing to emotional challenges that persist into adulthood.[60] As such, developmental medical trauma can narrow the window to feeling safe as our bodies tune to meet adversity. This may negatively affect the development of self-soothing strategies that enable self-regulation of emotions in later life.[61,62]

I had a serious breakdown whilst my son was in hospital. I was suicidal most of the time. What contributed to this was how traumatic his admission was. I went to accident and emergency three times the week he went into septic shock and I was turned away. I didn't feel listened to as a parent. . . .I was transferred to a hospital far away from home, leaving my other son (4 at the time). Lockdown happened as he was on ECMO and the whole hospital went into a panic. Straight away I was told I couldn't stay at the hospital accommodation and if I wanted to sleep on the chair in my son's room, I could but I would not be allowed to leave the room or see my other son. I was allowed to wash my clothes in the sink and have a shower if escorted by staff off the ward. I was not allowed visitors. I couldn't sleep for the duration. The monitors and emergencies (both with my son and other children) were constant. I saw two children die and saw how distressed their parents were. There was a lack of consistency and frequent changes in policy. On one occasion I was told I would be allowed to see my other son, only for him to arrive at the door of the ward (I could even hear him) to be turned away by the manager. There was little empathy exerted by staff who frequently told me that everyone was disadvantaged by the COVID restrictions. What made it harder was during this time was the "eat out to help out" government

> scheme. I watched from the hospital window people enjoying their night out. My mother died whilst my son was in hospital and I was not allowed to see her or go to the funeral. I sat alone whilst he was on life support by his bedside.
>
> —Hollie, 38 years old, mother of a son with bronchitis obliterans, 11 months old at time of admission, United Kingdom

As described, infants need emotionally available and responsive caregivers for healthy development. Yet, having an unwell child can increase risk to mental health for parents.[63] Kazak et al. report that post-traumatic stress disorder and post-traumatic stress symptoms are commonly experienced in adolescent childhood cancer survivors (8–16 years old) and their parents.[64] Participants in this study included 150 adolescent survivors of childhood cancer, 146 mothers, and 103 fathers. They completed the Impact of Events Scale–Revised, the Post-traumatic Stress Disorder Reaction Index, and the PTSD module of the Structured Clinical Interview for the Diagnostic and Statistical Manual of Mental Disorders, fourth edition. The researchers found that mothers and fathers had relatively equal rates of current PTSD and levels of PTSS. Nearly 30% of mothers met diagnostic criteria since their child's diagnosis, with 13.7% currently experiencing PTSD. Further, nearly 20% of families had at least one parent with current PTSD. Ninety-nine percent of the sample had at least one family member re-experiencing symptoms.

> Hospital accommodation should not be shut down even in a pandemic as parents need to be close to their very sick children. Critically ill children need both parents and parents need each other for support. There needs to be more flexibility using a trauma-based approach.
>
> —Hollie, 38 years old, mother of a son with bronchitis obliterans, 11 months old at time of admission, United Kingdom

It is important to note that parental "visiting" of children in hospitals was widely restricted until the 1970s and even the 1980s.[65] Excluding parents from baby's care was also widespread during the COVID-19 pandemic with one study reporting that 72% parents could not parent together with their child in hospital, affecting their mental health, while 70% reported this also affected ability to bond with their baby,[66] practice that is inconsistent with psychologically informed healthcare.

Further, it has been reported that historically the medical community did not consider babies to feel pain in the same way as adults, leading to newborns sometimes not being given adequate analgesic or anesthetic agents during invasive procedures, including surgery.[67] This was due to a mistaken belief that neural pathways in neonates are not fully myelinated and therefore could not transmit pain to the brain, with no capacity for verbal self-report. Studies challenged this understanding by reporting a decrease in vagal tone, as estimated by amplitude of respiratory sinus arrhythmia and higher-pitched cries (the *pain cry*) associated with circumcision without anesthetic in newborn babies. Individual differences in resting vagal tone of neonates were also indicative of heart responses to stress.[68] Together, research challenging this misconception led to calls for same humane considerations in care of neonates and young, nonverbal infants as for children and adults in similar painful and stressful situations.[69] This legacy potentially has underrecognized implications for some survivors who underwent medical treatments prior to the mid-1980s.

Despite the development of tools to assess pain in nonverbal infants and a range of interventions to reduce pain associated with medical procedures, studies suggest that pain in children is still not always adequately addressed. A recent narrative review[70] reported that while infants who are born preterm are at an elevated risk for repeated pain exposure in early life, many infants receive little to no pain-relieving interventions. Moreover, the authors report that parents are still significantly underutilized in provision of pain-relieving interventions, despite the known benefit of their involvement.

A review of 18 studies examining pain exposure and analgesic practices[71] found that hospitalized neonates were undergoing 7–17 painful procedures per day. Procedures included heel lancing, naso- and endotracheal suctioning, venipuncture, and insertion of peripheral venous catheters. Further, more routinely performed painful procedures include intubation, chest tube placement, lumbar puncture, insertion of arterial and venous umbilical catheters and peripheral arterial catheters, intramuscular and subcutaneous injections and tape removal. Studies included in this review reported that infants went without any form of analgesia during painful procedures ranging from 42%–100% of the time, with most studies reporting no pain treatment.

Such poorly treated and or prolonged pain exposure in preterm neonates has been linked to lasting consequences during a critical time in brain development. In a recent review the authors note that reported adverse outcomes include physiologic instability, pain sensitivity, negative impacts on cognition and behavior, poor executive function and visual abilities, alterations in the HPA axis and in brain development, and epigenetic changes in infants born preterm.[72] These are important considerations both in terms of improving care for babies and also in making sense of the lived experience of adult survivors of a serious medical condition from childhood. Children in the hospital setting often also witness another children's suffering and may be aware of mortality long before their healthy peers.

It is also important to note that some congenital conditions are also associated with a greater risk of neurocognitive difficulties, for example, congenital heart conditions are associated with higher risk of a low-level developmental delay including cognitive, attention, and executive functioning difficulties and problems with motor and language skills. Further, babies with a congenital heart condition often experience problems with feeding, sleeping, settling, soothing, and autonomic and motor organization, which can also affect early attachment with the main caregiver.[73]

Historically children have been left voiceless in the medical setting. Yet, growing evidence suggests children have specific needs in preventative and pediatric care as they live with long-term illness in increasing numbers. Encouragingly, children are increasingly being involved in decision-making about their healthcare, but this is far from routine. Psychologically informed healthcare promotes healthcare that is child- and family-centered, participatory, interdisciplinary, and driven by the input of children in need of services.

Please note sensitive content

Reflective Exercise: Children in Hospital Also Witness Suffering of Other Children

Finally, I am well enough, and it is time for me to go home. I look around my ward and see a toddler, with brown hair and eyes, on his bed. His mum and dad sit by his side as the nurse cleans the tracheostomy in his throat. Many of the children on my heart ward have a tracheostomy, leaving them unable to speak.

A little girl, not yet 2 years old, lies curled up in the next bed, sucking her thumb. She has a tube going into her nose, a needle in the back of her hand and lots of leads and tubes attach to her to a heart monitor and drips by her bed. She stares into the middle distance. Her blond curls cover her face and hide her dull eyes. Her gran visits when she can.

I did not like the feeling of those tubes and leads coming out of my body. I was glad when they were taken away. Even though it hurt to have the stickers taken off and tubes pulled out. Having my stitches removed hurt even more, but having the chest drain removed was worse.

An older child lies on his bed softly crying as a physiotherapist repeatedly taps his back to free his lungs of the mucus that builds up continually because of cystic fibrosis.

We are in this together in a way that the adults who care for us will never fully understand.

Three children were taken to the theater today but only two came back to the ward.

> Mum and I fondly say goodbye to the nurses, doctors, and other staff, thank them, and hand over a box of chocolates.
> Mum tells the other families we will be thinking about them.
> I smile to the rocking horse at the end of the ward that I was allowed to sit on 2 days ago, letting me know I was almost well enough to be allowed home.
> My mum and I set off along the corridor—passing Tigger, Eeyore, Winnie the Pooh, and Mickey Mouse, who cover the walls— pass through the swing doors, and exit the ward. The constant bleep of heart monitors fades, while the smell of disinfectant lingers, as we enter the lift. I clutch my arm protectively over my tender chest and grit my teeth in pain, as the lift bumps to a halt.
> When the doors open, we walk past the toy shop to the left and the café on the right, to the exit. My legs feel wobbly, my chest aches, and butterflies dance in my stomach.
> We step outside into the sunshine. The smell of fresh air and sound of birds singing make me smile. I glance back at my hospital, a black building with distinctive pink windows. It sits on top of a hill. I turn to look out to see the city and the university of Glasgow beyond. Mum glances at me nervously, are we ready for this?
> I am happy to be going home and looking forward to seeing my friends, but I wonder what will happen to the children we have left behind.
> Adapted from author's lived experience.
> Consider:
>
> - What is the impact on children and their families of witnessing other unwell children in hospital and being exposed to their suffering and at times death?
> - How can healthcare settings better recognize, protect, and support children in this regard?

Finding Connection in an Ableist World

I am fortunate that I have always had a supportive social network. However, my health condition has undoubtedly affected all of my relationships. Living with a serious health condition and facing challenges, which the people around you often cannot fully understand, can, at times, be isolating, while fear of being pitied or stigmatized can prevent you from sharing your experiences. As a child, I sat and watched other children taking part in gym lessons, playing skipping games, and running around carefree. There were parties and holidays that I was not invited to because my friends' parents and even some relatives did not want the responsibility of having me there. Even my grandparents did not want to risk having me, without my mum, for a sleepover, only taking my older brother. There were many experiences, such as going through heart surgery, that I could not share with my friends because I did not want to seem different or weird or evoke pity. On the odd occasions when I tried, I was invariably told I was being too serious or bringing the mood down. There have always been parts of life that while normal for me are not relatable to anyone I know such as wearing a 48-heart monitor and dealing with the leads and sticky electrodes, how it feels when you think your pacemaker has malfunctioned and you are missing heart beats or how itchy a scar gets when it starts to heal. They also include bigger life issues like how to deal with repeated educational and career gaps, manage chronic fatigue and whether or not to risk having a baby. I think this contributed to me being so quiet as a child because many of my experiences were not topics of conversation. There have been countless times when someone has said to me, "but you look normal," when I tell them about my heart condition, with no insight into the fact that they have just implied that I am not. Because my condition is hidden, at times other children (and some adults) questioned why I was getting "special treatment" for example, by "getting out of" gym class, time off school, or a new toy following surgery. As an adult, there have been family, friends, and colleagues who have found it difficult to empathize with the impact of my health on my daily life and relationships strained by a lack of support, dismissal, or toxic positivity with comments such as, "I get tired too, but I just push through it, I don't allow myself to take naps during the day." Health privilege and ableism are ubiquitous often underpinned by a just world fallacy; the cognitive bias that good things happen to good people, and those who befall adversity somehow deserve their lot. Some barriers to inclusion are minor, such as the many work lunches I've spent zoning out listening to colleagues compare their personal best (PBs) for running, presumably forgetting I can't contribute, jibes about why I needed my mum's help when my son was a baby or how lucky I am to only work part time. However, some are more significant; on two occasions I have resigned from my job when staff changes led to a new team leader who questioned reasonable adjustments to my workload that had been agreed with previous management. Often it only takes one person to make inclusion unfeasible. Broader social inclusion is also affected; for example, when my husband and I bought our house we had to take out a mortgage in his name because I cannot get life insurance, every time we go abroad our holiday insurance can be prohibitively expensive while access to specialist medical care, if required, is an important consideration, and working or living abroad have never felt like an option for me.

Living with a serious medical condition has also strengthened connections by proving who has shown up for me and stayed the course during challenging times. Thankfully, I have a close circle of people who have done their best to understand, support, and unconditionally accept me. I met my husband when we were in our late teens. My mum says she knew he was a keeper when she came to visit me in hospital after surgery to find him by my bed holding a cardboard sick bowl. Few 18-year-old boys would stick around for that. He has stuck by me through countless health crises over the almost 30 years since. While it has not always been easy, we have always found a way through with humor, mutual support, and love. He kindly tells me that what I have been through has made me the person I am. There have also been teachers, lecturers, colleagues, and managers who have taken the time to try and understand how my condition affects me and worked with me to enable me to partake. For example, when I was carrying out my PhD, at a time when working from home was uncommon, my supervisor provided me with a laptop and told me he was happy for me to work from home on a Wednesday. Without this understanding and flexibility I would have had to give up my studies. On another occasion, after a prolonged health crisis and absence from work, my manager, at the time, encouraged me to return to work by offering reduced hours and adjustments to my workload while compassionately supporting me on my return. Like many living with an LTC, regardless of the circumstances, often it only takes a minor adjustment to either help, or leave me unable, to take part, but all too often this is left to the discretion of whoever is in charge, which can change. At times it can feel exhausting.

Social support is the most important protective factor for mental health for people living with an LTC, whether diagnosed in childhood or adulthood.[74] Yet, living with a health condition can present added challenges in romantic relationships, with parents, having and raising children, siblings, wider family, friends, colleagues, and peers. We are innately social beings who commonly deal with life's challenges by sharing our experiences with others. This can be challenging and isolating for anyone living with an LTC when others in our social network are not going through the same challenges.

Parenting can also be more challenging when you are living with a chronic health condition. In addition to any potential health risks to the mother and child, both men and women with an LTC can face considerations around heritability, prognosis, life expectancy, and having the energy to deal with a family while managing debilitating symptoms. The availability of wider, supportive social support is often an important consideration.

If I am to receive treatment, such as cardiac exploratory work or pacemaker replacement, I look for my wife to be by my side, but not my two kids. This puts me at ease and ensures I don't have to worry about driving home afterwards. It also allows us as parents to control the narrative to the kids.
—David, 45 years old, congenital heart condition, United Kingdom

Stigma theories assert that anyone with a perceived impairment may be devalued and mistreated by others. Stigma theories view stigma as having three separate elements that need to occur in combination:[75] attitudes (e.g., "People with illness are lesser"), emotional reactions to those attitudes (e.g., fear), and discrimination (e.g., "I'm not giving someone with a mental illness a job with me"—associated discrimination). Some stigmatized identities can be hidden or masked (for example, with a hidden condition).

People with an LTC often report *internalized stigma*, including negative beliefs and feelings about themselves. This results in feelings of shame, guilt, and diminished self-worth, feeling different and less attractive, which can also negatively affect the development of sexual confidence.[76] Self-stigma can be symptomatic of complex trauma[77] and creates barriers to help seeking associated with poor physical and mental health.[78]

Health conditions can also attract *experienced stigma* or *enacted stigma* from others such as pity, fear, avoidance, stereotyping, and even anger. With socially transmittable diseases, such as HIV/AIDS, the social stigma is even greater[79] and has been reported in healthcare settings, by people living with HIV/AIDs who report receiving poor care, being denied care, and being blamed for their illness by healthcare workers.[80] Interpersonal discrimination and daily microaggressions can contribute to poorer emotional well-being for people living with an LTC. These comments reveal stereotypes and may include microinsults (e.g., "you only got your job because of affirmative action."), microassaults (e.g., "malingerer," "faking it," "lazy," "benefit scrounger"), microinvalidation (e.g., "But you look well," "How come you managed to . . .," "She just uses her condition when it suits her"), and environmental microaggressions (such as a lack of realistic representation in books, films, or TV).

Stigma may be less obvious, for example, through "*inspiration porn*," in which people with disabilities are used to inspire able-bodied people (for example, I was once invited by a tabloid journalist, who was covering my advocacy work, to "jump in the air" for an accompanying photo, I politely declined; muttering under my breath that I was not a performing monkey!). *Anticipated stigma*, the extent to which people expect to experience stereotyping, prejudice, and discrimination, is also associated with increased psychological distress[80] and may understandably lead to avoidance for people with an LTC.

People with an LTC can face concerns about when and how to reveal their condition in a new relationship, especially if this has led to rejection or discrimination in the past. This can result in masking symptoms, finding it difficult to trust others for fear of negative judgment, concealing concerns, and overcompensating an attempt to "fit in."[82]

Body image concerns can also present a barrier to sexual health.[83] Men face cultural expectations to be strong, fit, and muscular. Women are also under pressure to have the "perfect body" and may feel anxious about, for example, showing a partner a mastectomy scar. For many people, physical changes that occur with serious illness can be devastating. This may include hair loss, living with a colostomy bag, weight loss or gain, loss of mobility, scarring, or loss of bodily parts. We need to feel psychologically safe for sexual intimacy and healthy relationships. Yet, internalized, experienced, and anticipated stigma can affect feelings of psychological safety, which may adversely impact on developing healthy relationships.

People with a disability or chronic health condition are also at increased risk of sexual violence and intimate partner violence. This increased risk is also associated with poorer health status and limited access to healthcare. Despite this, sexual health is poorly addressed for people with LTCs, in part, due to attitudinal barriers and ableism in healthcare practice.[84] Conflicting medical advice can worsen sexual health concerns, particularly about recommendations around restricting physical activity or pregnancy risk, while mental health difficulties and psychotropic medications can cause sexual dysfunction.[85]

Kathleen Bogart, a professor of psychological science at Oregon State University who specializes in disability and ableism, reports that people living with a disability often share disadvantages with other minority groups including disparities in civil rights, discrimination, income, education, employment, social representation, self-efficacy, and underrepresentation (or misrepresentation) in the media and politics.[86] Such marginalization was clear during the COVID-19 pandemic and associated media messaging, for example, around "herd immunity" or "survival of the fittest."[87]

Childhood illness can lead to school absences and exclusion from gym classes and play. There may be interruptions in education due to frequent hospitalizations and the requirement for added support in education. These interruptions may prevent individuals from completing their education or vocational training and result in them being isolated from their peer groups. Although improving, support within schools can unfortunately be inadequate. Increasing awareness and educating school staff is vital to promoting social inclusion and support. We need better recognition of children's healthcare experience, their longing for other children, and inclusive school systems that recognize them as individuals not just their medical condition.[88]

Studies have found that LTCs take a heightened psychological toll at midlife, a life stage when adults are expected to be "able-bodied."[89] Workplace discrimination, defined as being disadvantaged for a reason that relates to your disability (Equality Act, 2010) is all too common. This can be direct (e.g., missing a promotion), indirect (e.g., a rule or policy that has a worse impact on someone with a protected characteristic), harassment (being treated in a way that violates your dignity), and/ or victimization. Work and educational practices are set up by and for the "healthy" majority, often limiting the opportunity to partake if you do not fit the mold (e.g., an expectation to work for 8 hours for 5 days per week). A wider neoliberal culture that prioritizes the market economy over quality of life does not help.

While many people with an LTC can work full time, this depends on their health status. For example, Gong et al. report that compared to healthy adults, even among the healthiest adults with a congenital heart condition, there are significant decrements in life expectancy, employment, and lifetime earnings.[90] Most countries have employment laws that aim to protect workers from employment discrimination. However, the reality is there is often a shadow culture of health privilege, and living with an LTC can impact on employability, income, health and life insurance, and overall ability to live independently, while workplace bullying is a risk factor for disability retirement.[91,92,93] In the United States, and other countries with private healthcare systems, the availability of affordable health insurance can affect the ability to support oneself financially and make a successful transition to adulthood and can affect choice of career.

Ben was finding it difficult to work in construction after being diagnosed with multiple sclerosis. However, he knew that if he lost his job, he would lose his medical cover. If he stopped working, he could get government aided medical care. However, he did not want to stop working entirely because he felt like he could still fulfill a part time role, and he knew that his mood would deteriorate if he did not have a job. He felt frustrated, alone, and stuck.

Together, this paints an isolating picture. Social exclusion can have a devastating impact on mental health. Studies show that being socially excluded activates the same brain pathways as physical injury.[94] This leads to an overdeveloped threat system and pervasive feelings of shame, which can bias us toward feelings of hopelessness, disconnection, and self-criticism and increase vulnerability to anxiety and depression.[95]

The Person Beyond the Condition: Self-Esteem and Body Image

While it should not be assumed that people with an LTC have low self-esteem, as described above, such individuals are often marginalized, pitied, and even blamed for their condition. Together, this can have a devastating impact on self-esteem.

Living with a chronic health condition can also negatively affect trust in one's body. Physical activity contributes to the development of positive body image and reduces social physique anxiety.[96] Yet, people with LTCs are less likely to access and take part in sport and physical activity and report higher sedentary behaviors.[97] Such messaging often starts in childhood; in schools, disabled students still are and feel excluded from physical education classes.[98] Further, restrictions on exercise and physical activity were commonly recommended by healthcare providers for people with some childhood health conditions until recently, while guidance about physical activity can remain poor, confusing, and unsupported. Since sports are often a rite of passage, especially for adolescents, any loss of such opportunities can lead to missed opportunities to develop strong, lasting friendships while also having a negative impact on self-esteem.[99]

Melanie Fennell, consultant clinical psychologist and researcher at Oxford University, in the United Kingdom, defines self-esteem as the degree to which we accept and value ourselves, thus achieving a basic feeling of self-worth.[100] Her cognitive behavioral model proposes that low self-esteem is a negative image of oneself which is global, persistent, and enduring. Negative life experiences, particularly early in life, can lead to the development of an overall negative belief reflecting our sense of worth. Living with an LTC can negatively affect self-esteem, which in turn can lead to self-criticism and self-defeating behaviors and increase vulnerability to low mood and anxiety.

More recently, Rimes et al. have built on Fennell's model of self-esteem to include sociometer and hierometer tracking functions.[101] *Hierometer theory* suggests that self-esteem is a marker of one's perceived level of status within social hierarchies, with status defined as being respected and admired. *Sociometer theory* proposes that self-esteem reflects the individual's level of perceived relational value, namely, being liked, accepted, and included by others. It has been proposed that such monitoring processes have evolved because social inclusion and successful management of social hierarchies are important for survival. While socially disadvantaged group membership will not necessarily result in low self-esteem for everyone, it can contribute to low self-esteem for some individuals.[102]

Further, the British clinical psychologist and founder of *compassion-focused therapy* (CFT), Paul Gilbert, proposes that our emotions are controlled and regulated by three brain systems including the threat, drive, and soothing systems (see Figure 1.3).[103] The *threat system* works to keep us safe, triggering the body's alarm system when we are at risk. As social animals, being excluded from our social group can trigger this system, leading to feelings of panic, anger, and shame, and self-criticism. If we do not feel included in our social group, we can feel intense shame or anger, self-conscious, powerlessness, and the desire to disappear or hide away for our own self-protection.[104] If we feel shame regularly, it can have a detrimental impact on our self-esteem and lead to depression and self-harming behaviors. When we experience hardship during childhood, for self-protection, it is safer to assume that we are the problem. This is more tolerable, for a child, than believing that the world and/or the adults responsible for their care are unreliable or harmful. However, this coping strategy can lead to the development of deeply entrenched shame and negative core beliefs about the self, such as *I am unlovable, I am defective*, or *I am bad*.

The second system, our *drive system*, motivates us to achieve our goals and get things done by providing direction, focus, and feelings of reward. Finally, our *soothing* system has a calming influence and is linked to feelings of psychological safety, contentment, and feeling connected to others. This system is developed in our early years through a healthy attachment to our main caregivers and enables us to self-soothe and regulate our emotions.

Anna had always prided herself on being fit, strong and healthy. When she was diagnosed with arthritis in her early 40s, she decided it was mind over matter and pushed herself. However, the harder she drove herself the worse her symptoms became, until she ended up in hospital. She felt like her body had failed her and sunk into a deep depression. A nurse suggested that she join a peer support group with other people living with the same condition. She felt compassion for other members of the group and found herself recommending that they go easier on themselves. In time, this led her to being more compassionate with herself.

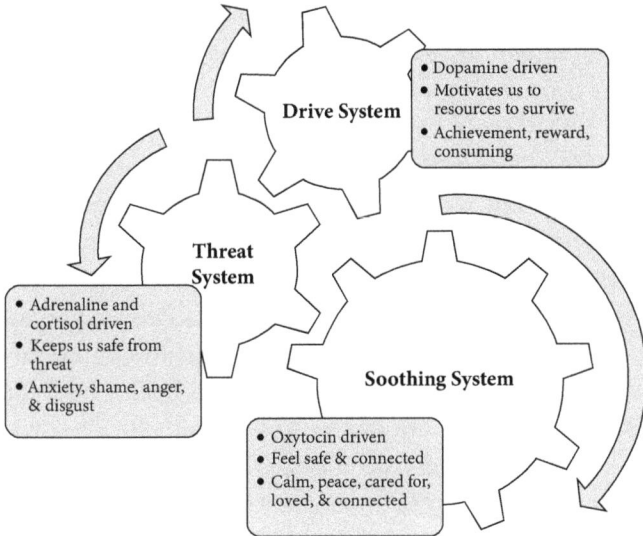

Figure 1.3 The threat, drive, and soothing systems
Source: Adapted from Gilbert, P. (2009). The compassionate mind. Robinson.

If we experience a lot of early adversity, we can develop an overactive *threat system*, while interruptions to a secure early attachment can result in an underactive *soothing* system. Gilbert notes that we tend to deal with this by overrelying on the *drive system* to feel good.[105] Otherwise, the threat system takes over, leading to persistent anxiety, depression or anger. Feelings of shame can lead people with an LTC to reject parts of themselves (such as their health condition). They may overcompensate by setting unrealistically exacting standards and engaging in self-punitive behaviors such as perfectionism, disordered eating, risk taking behaviors, or not looking after their health.

The Psychological Impact of Working in Healthcare Settings

People are commonly drawn to caring professions because they want to alleviate suffering. Yet, such individuals can be routinely exposed to patients' and their families' distress, pain, fear, and sadness. Working in an acute healthcare setting can involve witnessing serious illness, death, and dying, and workplace violence is an added occupational risk. Repeatedly being exposed to these highly stressful situations can trigger traumatic responses and have serious repercussions on health and well-being. In this situation, when there is no place to express, process, and share a normal emotional response to these demanding situations emotionally distancing yourself from patients may become the only coping strategy on offer.

Healthcare professionals can also face daily organizational challenges including competing demands, targets, waiting lists, and dissatisfied patients who have endured long waits to access care, limited resources, financial constraints, a hierarchical culture with layers of bureaucracy, clients with complex presentations and systemic limits on offering care. There can be tensions between supporting modern reforms to deliver patient-centered, compassionate, and dignified care and meeting the clinical needs of the patient in context of increasing demand. Within health and care systems, often performance problems are not addressed and so-called wicked problems, or multilayered, complex challenges, are avoided leaving individuals to navigate the impact. Over time, these challenges can result in demoralized staff. It is also important to note that many healthcare professionals are living with an LTC themselves and trying to manage this while fulfilling their role.

As a former Nurse myself, and someone who has supported student nurses through training, I understand how difficult it can be to manage the constant demands of people in your care, to give of yourself day in and day out. Staff shortages, time restraints, and long days can be difficult and draining.

—Sally, late 50s, congenital craniofacial condition, former nurse, psychotherapist, and PhD researcher, United Kingdom

As a result, healthcare professionals often experience high rates of psychological distress which can lead to burnout, compassion fatigue, vicarious trauma, and associated mental health problems such as anxiety and depression. It is important for healthcare workers to be aware of the signs and symptoms of their own stress to ensure self-care, early intervention, help-seeking, and support. Further, it is important that organizations are proactive in supporting staff to mitigate these occupational hazards (discussed in Chapter 5).

Perfect Storm: Understanding the Impact of Living with an LTC on Mental Health, Recovery and Well-being

Considering the above, it is not surprising that LTCs are associated with a heightened risk of depressive symptoms, anxiety and compromised daily mood, life satisfaction, self-esteem, and body image.[106] These outcomes are due in part to lower levels of social integration and activity, discrimination, diminished sense of self-efficacy, poorer quality employment, reduced work hours, and financial strain.[107,108] Specifically, a range of conditions including cancer, chronic pain, autoimmune disorders, arthritis, epilepsy, sickle cell disorder, heart disease, diabetes, asthma, endometriosis, and high blood pressure have been found to increase the risk of mental health difficulties such as depression, anxiety, post-traumatic stress, and suicidal ideation while negatively impacting well-being and overall quality of life.[109,110,111,112,113,114]

> *Once when I was in the hospital, I asked my care team if there was someone I could talk with to help me prepare for my upcoming surgery. That afternoon a play therapist came into my room. I was 30 years old! I couldn't believe they didn't have any mental health professionals that specialized in working with their adult patients. It only brought my stress level up even more.*
> —Alex, 57 years, congenital heart condition, United States

In short, given the profound and extensive impact that living with an LTC can have on psychological and emotional health we need a psychologically informed healthcare system that holistically acknowledges, considers, and supports well-being for patients and healthcare professionals.

2
The Cartesian Problem in Healthcare

> *Healthcare can also feel quite fragmented. Everyone doing their specialist part for the patient can be wonderful but there also needs to be a holistic view of the person. As someone with chronic health difficulties, one can feel passed around with no one really talking to each other or wondering about the whole person. One ends up repeating the story over and over and medics passing on or assuming it's someone else's remit to address that bit. It can waste time and important health factors can get missed, people get lost in the system, but it also wastes precious resources and money.*
> —Sally, late 50s, congenital craniofacial condition, former nurse, psychotherapist, and PhD researcher, United Kingdom

The 16th-century French philosopher Rene Descartes proposed the mind and body as separate entities, and *mind-body* or *Cartesian dualism* influences philosophy, epistemology, empiricism, ontology, medicine, and psychology to the current day. Yet, it is evident that physical and psychological health are entwined, indeed in his book Descartes' Error Antonio Damasio, the Portuguese neuroscientist, argues that our emotions and somatic markers serve as guides that are critical for rational decision making. As such, both reason and emotion are intertwined and necessary for making wise decisions.[1]

In his book *The Birth of the Clinic: An Archaeology of Medical Perception* the philosopher Michel Foucault (1963) describes *le regard médical* (the medical gaze, which inspired the book's title),[2] arguing that Western medicine has objectified the human body, which has become viewed as separate from personhood. In turn, the "patient" story is morphed to fit the biomedical paradigm with a focus on symptoms and test results. While this approach has been successful for acute presentations, with clear diagnostic signs and treatments, it can result in medical gaslighting, whereby parts of the patients' account are filtered out, dismissed, and at times rejected. Most commonly, it is the idiopathic and often diffuse, chronic medical symptoms that do not fit textbook cases, such as pain and fatigue, that are poorly addressed. This reductionist approach can lead to neglect of the emotional, psychological, and social aspects of illness. Arguably, in this "patient" role the individual becomes beholden to healthcare structures, often underpinned by socioeconomic drivers, when they submit their body for medical examination and treatment.

Survival-Focused Healthcare

The personal cost of this reductionist approach is evident in a 2023 *Endometriosis UK* report involving a survey of 5,500 women.[3] Endometriosis can have a significant effect on all aspects of life, including fertility, relationships, sexual health, education, career, quality of life, and mental health. Yet, the report states that women living with endometriosis describe being "dismissed, ignored and belittled" when they seek medical help, with pain and symptoms often brushed aside as normal. The report states that as of 2023, the average length of time to diagnosis across the United Kingdom for this condition is almost 9 years. This journey is often "circuitous, torturous and lengthy," with most women repeatedly seeking help on multiple occasions. Specifically, the authors found that 74% of the respondents to their survey had attended five or more appointments with their general practitioner (GP), almost half had visited their GP 10 times or more, 52% had visited emergency care at least once, and 20% reported seeing a gynecologist 10 times or more prior to diagnosis. Yet, without diagnosis treatment cannot be accessed and the disease may progress. Further, 78% of respondents who later went on to receive a diagnosis of endometriosis had experienced one or more doctor telling them they were making a "fuss about nothing" or similar comments and many had the severity of their symptoms questioned by healthcare practitioners.

Regardless of condition, being invalidated and dismissed about your lived experience can significantly add to the burden of living with a health condition. It presents a risk to physical health and barriers to accessing treatment while negatively affecting empowerment and self-management and exacerbating feelings of anxiety, low mood, helplessness, lack of control, frustration, and risk of post-traumatic stress.[4]

Further, feeling unheard can hinder people from seeking emotional and psychological support when they are living with a chronic health condition because they fear it may contribute not being taken seriously. Conversely, mental health–related stigma in the healthcare system creates barriers to access and quality of healthcare for people with a mental health diagnosis.[5,6]

My care would have been better if I did not have to retell my story again and again and again, if there had been an option to choose a female or male healthcare worker,

if professionals asked me what I needed to feel emotionally and physically safe recognising this can change, choice of music in the operating theatre, knowing in advance what day and time a consultant was going to call, especially when awaiting scan results, more sign posting for psychological support, better recognition that returning to the same hospital, scan or consulting rooms post diagnosis even years later can be triggering and difficult and personalised care tailored to my age and life stage.
—Sarah, 44 years old, undergoing breast cancer treatment, United Kingdom

We need to move beyond the medical gaze to psychologically informed healthcare by promoting a humanistic, person-centered approach that recognizes the bidirectional mind–body link and emphasizes relational safety. Not only are people with a long-term health condition (LTC) more likely to experience a mental health problem but people with a mental health problem are also more likely to experience physical health difficulties.[7] Further, some physical conditions and treatments directly contribute to mood, such as certain medications, an overactive thyroid, and hormones. For example, the relationship between asthma and psychological factors is complex. Evidence suggests that people with asthma are more vulnerable to depression, which in turn negatively influences asthma symptoms, yet psychological support is still underresourced for people living with this condition.[8]

Psychological and emotional difficulties can worsen symptoms of LTCs and increase medical nonadherence and substance abuse, while people experiencing depression or post-traumatic stress disorder (PTSD) have a higher likelihood of nonadherence to doctors' recommendations.[9] Depression among adults with LTCs is also correlated with increased "self-medicating," for example, through excessive alcohol use and cigarette smoking.[10] This suggests that untreated mental health difficulties can directly affect physical health and longevity. It is also important to recognize intersectionality and health inequalities in this multifaceted picture; for example, LTCs are more prevalent in lower socioeconomic groups and other oppressed groups.[11]

There needs to be integration or at least frequent communication between specialists. In my area there is no integration of physical and mental health and no easy route of access to support at diagnosis or a later stage.
—Yvonne, 45, psoriasis and psoriatic arthritis, United Kingdom

In short, while the success of science and medicine is clear, overreductionism and specialization can promote objectification of the human body for examination and treatment of health problems and at times inattention to the individual's embodied experience. A survival-focused approach that attends to test results and physical symptoms can lead to healthcare systems that do not adequately consider the psychological and emotional well-being of patients. At times, this may create circumstances that unnecessarily exacerbate mental health risk factors. Psychologically informed healthcare aims to acknowledge and address these factors, such as disempowering aspects of healthcare, the so-called compassion crises in healthcare, and poor sleep, with the aim of improving patient well-being.

The Doctor Is Ready for You Now: Disempowering Aspects of Medical Care

All over the wards and hospital were large posters with the mission statement of the hospital, emphasizing that patients were at the centre of all their work. During my extended stay on a transplant ward, I personally found, at times, that this wasn't the case, and that the patients had to cope or adapt to the services provided. One example was that, at one stage, we were all transferred to a different ward, since ours was being refitted. On this ward, their regime was that they would wake everyone up at 0630 am for breakfast, since it was a very short-term ward, with high patient turnover. I had been used to being awakened at 0700, with breakfast at about 0800. There was a lack of planning. I was also shocked and surprised to find copies of all our medical notes in the day room, following the regular nurse hand over in the morning. There was a lack of care and attention around this privacy. Further, we were mixed in with other short-stay patients, (often 3–4 days only) whose needs were very different. I caught COVID from one of them, meaning I had to come off the transplant list for a time, which wasn't great. There was a general lack of storage, no lockable cupboards to store our personal belongings, which built up over the months. Some of the short-stay patients were very elderly and infirm, sometimes with dementia, meaning that cleanliness wasn't always great as they weren't able to cope on their own and sleeping was made more difficult. As we used to say, "we live here" and it was annoying and stressful when our long-term environment was spoiled.
 —**Richard, 60 years old, congenital heart condition, heart transplant recipient, United Kingdom**

A biomedical approach to healthcare provision can lead to a power imbalance between those in the role of healthcare professional and those in the patient role. However, feeling powerless is a psychological risk factor, leading to increased vulnerability to anxiety, depression, and post-traumatic stress. It can negatively affect resilience and recovery, and it is inconsistent with a person-centered approach to patient care.[12] Recognizing and carefully reconsidering the aspects of patient care that worsen feelings of powerlessness and lack of agency is a vital part of psychologically informed healthcare. Disempowering aspects of care include waiting, hospital attire, disease prestige, and epistemic injustice.

Patiently Waiting Across the Healthcare Journey

Hospitals can feel like conveyor belts sometimes. Dignity is left at the front door as far as hospital gowns are concerned, waiting rooms can be makeshift and tight in space. From parking to waiting times and everything in between, only that time between patient and healthcare professional feels truly patient-centered. That has been my experience, but it must be said that the staff I encounter in the UK NHS system do their best within the constraints they have.

—David, 45 years old, congenital heart condition, United Kingdom

One of the hardest parts of my lifelong patient journey has been fostering the patience to wait, in countless ways, for the medical treatment I depend on. As a child, I sat shaking, dizzy, and nauseous, as we waited by the phone for my cardiologist to return my mum's call when I was unwell. We waited at outpatient appointments during biannual "check-ups" and frequent unscheduled ones when my pioneering pacemaker saw fit to play up—which it often did. We spent endless hours in the "waiting area" outside my consultant cardiologist's office, while I cuddled into my mum, who read to me from the least sticky book we could find from the toy corner.

We waited at each stop on the obligatory hospital tour of various departments for my height and weight to be taken, an X-ray (me in a hospital gown, cold, and self-conscious), pacemaker interrogation, ECHO, and blood tests. I lay, semidressed, during each procedure trying not to focus on what was being done to my body. We ended the appointment, back where we'd started, nervously waiting on my cardiologist calling us into his consulting room to share the results with us.

If treatment was indicated, we waited for a bed on the pediatric cardiology ward, or a date for further investigations, or surgery. Inpatient life also revolves around waiting; for the doctors' round each morning; to be collected by a porter for procedures; for results; for your slot on the surgical list (hungry, sedated, and sick to the stomach with nerves); post-surgery for the nurse to come and help you change into your pajamas from the hospital gown; to remove the cannula, stitches, and various other pieces of medical equipment;

for the doctor to write the discharge letter and for the pharmacy to prescribe the discharge medication so you can finally go home.

As a pediatric cardiology patient receiving pioneering treatment, I was able to access specialist care when I needed it, albeit after some waiting. As an adult, I've struggled to access specialist care and I have had to wait out additional steps; for the family doctor to call us back, in accident and emergency, in the assessment unit of the local hospital, to be moved to the local cardiology ward, and for a bed at the specialist center. At each stage, I must retell my colorful medical history to the nurse, the on-duty registrar, the consultant, and the trainee doctors who have heard rumors about this "novel presentation." At times, this "wait" for the specialist care I need has been life threatening, leading to my advocacy efforts to improve care provision with healthcare standards and increased funding for congenital heart disease (CHD) care in Scotland.

A few years ago, I spent over a month in my local hospital, on telemetry because the leads of the pacemaker I am completely dependent on developed an intermittent fault (again!). I had to wait for a surgical slot to have my 11th pacemaker and leads fitted at the specialist center. My mum, young son, and husband visited daily, the anxious wait a family affair. Waiting gives you time to think. Impotent, you allow fear to grow in that time. When you are in pain or feeling unwell, it can seem intolerable, the hours and days stretch before you, life is on hold. It can make you feel frustrated and unimportant, leaving loved ones feeling helpless or, as they chase the doctor down, deemed demanding (adapted from Morton, 2021).[13]

Please make communication with you easier for your patients, and work to cut down on waiting time for results.
—*Alex, 57 years, congenital heart condition, United States*

Across the patient's journey, waiting can worsen feelings of disempowerment for patients and their families. Originating from the Latin *patiens* from *patior*, the word "*patient*" means "to suffer." Patients often must develop the forbearance to endure illness, medical treatment, and dependency on others for care, doing so *patiently*. As described, waiting as a "patient" can occur in a multitude of ways. It is common for there to be delays at every step of the patient's journey, exacerbating uncertainty and frustrations. Poor communication about waiting times and cancellations can add to this burden. It is not surprising, then, that healthcare satisfaction and social attitude surveys repeatedly find that access and waiting times are a major source of dissatisfaction for patients, reason for complaint, and an indicator of poor-quality care.[14]

Six-year-old James came back from surgery mid-morning, and it is now late afternoon. He has been recovering well, but the cannula in his hand is causing him a lot of distress. His mum asked the nurse if it could be removed but he said it would have to stay in for a few hours. Even although more than a few hours have now passed, no one has come to remove it. James keeps asking his mum when it can be taken out. He is becoming increasingly distressed and tearful about it, and it is preventing him from being able to fall asleep. His mum feels bad about approaching the busy nurses again, but she is increasingly upset that while everything else has gone well, he has been left with this unnecessary discomfort.

When you are in pain or feeling unwell, waiting can seem intolerable, worsening the feeling of frustration, leaving loved ones feeling helpless or, as they chase the doctor down, considered demanding. Despite knowing that the required expertise, tests, and treatment exist, you are powerless to access them in a prompt fashion. When you have a lifelong condition, this becomes a constant stressor, and it sometimes prevents people from seeking medical care.[15]

Hospital Attire

The last time I was in the hospital awaiting surgery I was about to embark the surgical trolley when the nurse realized they had not taken my weight. I was already feeling vulnerable about facing more surgery, and I remember feeling a mixture of amusement and complete humiliation at being escorted across a remarkably busy ward, wearing only a backless hospital gown, surgical stockings, and a hairnet. I had to clutch the back of the gown to maintain some dignity on my way to and from the scales.

The backless hospital gown is symbolic embodiment of the medical gaze. Being told to strip off and put on this revealing gown can exacerbate feelings of vulnerability associated with being in the "patient role." Being escorted in this attire, often through public areas of a hospital, at times without under garments, or having to wait in a communal area (for example, for an X-ray) can make matters worse.

What we wear affects how we feel about ourselves. Clothing affects self-esteem, while getting dressed is a process of self-expression and individuality informing others of our social standing, ambitions, emotions, motivations, and even employment status. Yet, despite efforts to empower patients with patient-centered care, the institutionalized acceptance of the hospital gown persists in many healthcare settings.

It is likely that the backless hospital gown finds its roots in early public health measures to control the spread of disease. In the 1860s, Joseph Lister "the father of modern surgery" applied Louis Pasteur's "germ theory" to surgery by introducing aseptic precautions such as handwashing, masks, sterilizing surgical instruments with carbolic acid, and the use of clean surgical gowns. Prior to this, surgeons wore their own clothes, sometimes covered by a "butcher's apron" that was often covered in blood and pus. Due to this practice, around half of patients undergoing surgery died postoperatively from sepsis. The introduction of aseptic methods significantly reduced such deaths from "surgical fever."

Florence Nightingale widely promoted these new measures while nursing soldiers during the Crimean War, helping to influence healthcare culture and improve patient safety. Early modern hospitals often served the disadvantaged (with wealthier people opting to be treated at home) at a time when removal of personal clothing was promoted to prevent the spread of infection and parasites. The uniform design of the gown may have been adapted from those worn by surgeons as aseptic precautions to prevent the spread of postoperative infections. Initially, a "theatre gown" with a backless design would help with aid their application and removal from the unconscious patient and offer infection control. Given this historical context, it seems likely that the current hospital gown is a "medical relic" unchanged in design for the best part of a century.[16]

Psychologically informed healthcare aims to challenge such cultural norms, as dehumanizing aspects of care can increase a patient's risk of further episodes of hospitalization. We explored patients' experiences of wearing the hospital gown using a sequential, multimethod approach,[17] as described below.

Learning from Research: The Hospital Gown as Symbolic of the Medical Gaze

We explored patients' views and experiences of wearing the hospital gown within the UK context using a sequential, multimethod approach.[18] The first study consisted of in-depth interviews (n = 10) with adults living with a lifelong chronic health condition. The study found three themes: *embodying the sick role, relinquishing control to medical professionals,* and *enhancing physical and emotional vulnerability*. The first theme, embodying the sick role, was reflected in quotes such as these:

> *If you put on a hospital gown it sets in that something is wrong. That makes things all the more real, at least in my experience. So, I guess there would probably be an association between that feeling and the hospital gown.*
>
> *There's nothing individual about it. It's a little bit like you're just a patient, another number. They (healthcare professionals) don't even say like "do you want to put this on?" "Are you comfortable?" It's just like "you know the drill." That's what the last one said to me. It's like you've already dehumanised me before I've put the clothing on. You're like a piece of flesh; you're not a person. As soon as I get into my own clothes, I feel like my own persona again. So, you definitely just feel like a (pauses) I don't know, like a piece of packaged meat. You know, in a conveyer belt of sickness.*

The second theme, *relinquishing control to medical professionals*, was expressed in quotes such as these:

> *It's all part of the whole process of not being in control, not being able to wear your own clothes and not being able to do what you want to do and then you have to let the medical team sort of take control of everything.*
>
> *I think I'm (pauses) pretty controlled. I'd say it lowers you're mood, you know, the fact that you're gonna go somewhere and obviously to an operation and trusting a team of people who are going to look after you in a very vulnerable time, you know, obviously you think things have got to go right with the anaesthetic and the respiration and you trust that they can do that and normally I do because they're a team that have always done my operations since I was a child but I think it's just that it leads to feeling controlled. I think it's partly down to this sort of insistence on wearing something (hospital gown) which is not something that you would choose to wear.*

The third theme, enhancing physical and emotional vulnerability, was reflected in the following participants' quotes.

> *It's like a part of it is like the trigger, it actually feels like a trigger. Soon as you put it (hospital gown) on. Soon as you're handed it you get the feelings like these fears and anxieties to the point that when you get to certain stages I have to shut down, you can't cope (pauses), I can't cope. I go and shut down cause it's the only way I can get myself through certain parts and then when you're hospitalised, you don't take in information. I think the clothing is a part of that, it's just (sighs) the clothing is a trigger.*

Continued

> *Continued*
>
> *I'm not even a person anymore. So this can be really hard especially when they (exhales sharply) take your ECGs and they'll ask you to take your bra off and they go "oh put your gown on back to front so it ties at the front." You just feel exposed.*
>
> In a second study, we conducted a cross-sectional online survey exploring patients' views (n = 928) and experiences of wearing the gown. Most participants reported that they felt exposed, self-conscious, and vulnerable when wearing the gown, and that they had been asked to wear it despite feeling unsure that it was medically necessary. Over half of the participants reported that they felt uncomfortable when wearing the gown, and less than 10% reported that it made them feel "cared for," and 41% reported being offered a second gown by healthcare staff to wear the other way around to protect their dignity, termed *double gowning*.

Disease Prestige

I wandered through the medical system for years with severe pain and many different symptoms. Noone could help me. This left deep scars on my nervous system. At the age of 37, I was finally diagnosed with endometriosis. I kept hearing from doctors: "That can't be right. I've never heard that before." That made me feel deeply insecure. It was only through trauma-oriented body therapy that I learned to trust myself again. The medical system wants obedient patients who don't disrupt the process. It took years before I dared to express and assert my needs. As a patient in hospital, you feel like you're on a conveyor belt in a factory. There is little room for your own needs. Sitting in bed in a hospital gown does not make it easier to stand up for your rights. So much has happened to me as a patient that I can't put into words. A doctor once told me that she doesn't earn as much with an endometriosis patient as she does with a cancer patient. I have experienced doctors not wanting to take me into their practice because of my complex illnesses. It is necessary for medical staff to be psychologically and trauma informed.

—Lou, 48, bowel endometriosis, Germany

As described, one of my most debilitating health difficulties has been chronic fatigue. It seems likely that this symptom is a consequence of my complex medical history, the medical interventions I have needed over the years, and an interplay between the physical, psychological, and emotional impact of this. Yet, no one takes an interest in this diffuse, chronic symptom that I have had to manage lifelong. Over the years, I have variably been told by a range of consultants that there is no physical reason that I need so much sleep, that this symptom is not the concern of their medical specialty, or I am just lucky to be alive at all. Yet, having to manage chronic fatigue affects every aspect of my life. From everyday considerations like meeting a friend for lunch, to my educational and career choices and deciding whether to become a parent. As a student, when I got my new class timetable the first thing I did was anxiously check to see if my classes looked spread out enough for me to manage them; looking for a job I have to find something part-time and hope for a considerate manager; I had my son when I was young enough to have plenty of grand-parenting support around. It would help me to have this ongoing experience acknowledged, validated, and routinely explored considering new medical developments.

Interestingly, the Norwegian sociologist Dag Album found that healthcare professionals rank different diseases in a *prestige hierarchy*[19] and that diseases convey meanings that are not restricted to the "strictly medical." Album reports a comparative analysis of three survey studies conducted in 1990, 2002, and 2014. Each year, a sample of Norwegian physicians was asked to rate 38 diseases on a scale from 1 to 9 according to their prestige. The results revealed stability in ranking order over the 25 years. The top three diseases in all three surveys were leukemia, brain tumor, and myocardial infarction. The four lowest ranked were fibromyalgia, depressive neurosis, anxiety neurosis, and hepatocirrhosis.

The authors report that stability of the ranking rests on three sets of prestige criteria; the disease and its typical course, the typical treatment, and the typical patient. Diseases with high prestige were deemed "non-self-inflicted" and acute with clear diagnostic signs. According to a second group of criteria, high-ranked diseases were active, risky, with technological treatment options that lead to effective recovery. Finally, the typical patient is young and accepting of the physician's understanding of the disease, and the treatment is efficient without long-term heavy burdens.

By contrast, the categories consistently ranked at the bottom of the prestige hierarchy are not organ-specific and do not have objective diagnostic signs, and efficient therapeutic options are unavailable. Often the patient's symptoms form diffuse bodily complaints that are challenging for healthcare professionals, and it is common for patients to understand their suffering quite differently than the healthcare professionals. The authors conclude that differences in disease prestige are a significant aspect of medical culture and understanding these preconceptions is important because disease prestige may influence healthcare decision-making.

Epistemic Injustice

A few years ago, I attended a conference held at The Royal College of Surgeons in London. Fascinated by medical history, I was intrigued by their small museum. It was interesting to see the evolution of medical tools and techniques on display, alongside the names and backgrounds of their eminent inventors. I was particularly impressed by the vast collection of apothecary jars. Yet, I could not find any account of what it felt like to live with the various health conditions mentioned throughout history, nor how patients experienced the various remedies and cures. Where were the patient's stories? While several ornate medical robes adorned the wall, I could not help but contrast them with the backless hospital gown and its absence from the display.

On reflection, there are many reasons why the patient voice is quiet, these stories poorly documented. Often people with serious health problems are disempowered by the vulnerability of being in the patient role while the burden of their health condition can make it challenging to find the energy and resources to voice their experiences. Further, many do not want to seem ungrateful for lifesaving treatment by documenting the challenges, to risk being labeled a "difficult patient," or to concern other people with similar conditions and their families while social stigma and traumatic experiences can contribute to feelings of disempowerment and a "veil of silence."[20] Further, medical science has arguably been developed by white, rich, often male populations that disproportionately represent WEIRD (Western, Educated, Industrialized, Rich, and Democratic) populations; as such, healthcare inequalities can consolidate this experience since minority and socioeconomically deprived populations are more likely to experience physical health problems, yet less likely to contribute to documenting history.[21] Indeed, Holland et al. report a dearth of research studies that include patient and public involvement (PPI) from people with lived experience of health conditions.[22]

Yet, people living with an LTC need to be able to tell their stories to heal and to be represented to feel included in society. When I have worked therapeutically with clients recovering from traumatic medical experiences, repeatedly, they have reported that their distress is grounded in not feeling heard by healthcare professionals, having their experiences dismissed by others, and being left feeling disempowered and isolated. Complaints processes can further invalidate their experience and serve to entrench feelings of anger, frustration, and hopelessness, contributing to post-traumatic stress, low mood, and anxieties about accessing medical care in the future.

> *I feel there is a deep set of beliefs that many still hold about certain, poorly understood, conditions. This can sometimes present a barrier and some are not willing to listen and be open-minded, leading patients to feel disregarded and unsafe.*
> —Becky, 36, Ehlers-Danlos syndrome, postural orthostatic tachycardia syndrome (POTS), chronic fatigue, United Kingdom

Coined by Miranda Fricker the British professor of philosophy at New York University, *"epistemic injustice"* describes injustice related to knowledge.[23] *"Hermeneutical injustice,"* a type of epistemic injustice, occurs when someone's experiences are not well understood by themselves or others. Rosen notes that in healthcare this can occur through unjust ways of listening to patients, for example, by objectifying their lived experience, dismissing aspects of their *patient testimony*, and not sharing information about their care, often because of the epistemic privilege of the healthcare providers.[24]

For example, patients suffering from fibromyalgia often report that healthcare professionals do not take their testimonies and interpretations seriously. Heggen and Berg propose that epistemic injustice in healthcare settings may occur because of the gap between a patient's lived experience of illness and the professionals' conceptualization of illness as a disease.[25] Further, as described, focusing on the biomedical model can devalue individual patient stories.

Therapeutic life story work (TLSW) supports recovery for people with a traumatic history, who often have fragmented memories of what has happened to them, by offering an opportunity to explore, question, and make sense of their past experiences and by providing a safe space to feel and express emotions.[26] When we are not able to understand and make sense of the trauma we have experienced, this can prevent us from processing these feelings, leaving us preoccupied with past experiences.[27] To this end, to make sense of my own experiences, I tried to access my childhood medical records. I uncovered a greater act of hermeneutical injustice than even I expected: an act of injustice that clearly highlights the desperate need to reform patient access to our medical information, as detailed below.

Learning from Lived Experience: Epistemic Injustice and the Loss of My Childhood Story

Our medical records detail the most notable events in life; birth, early development, illness, pregnancy—all the way to our last moments. So why is it still so challenging to access this vital information in a way that supports us as patients?

Growing up, my pediatric medical notes were a source of mystery. At medical appointments, my consultant added scribbled observations to a file bursting at the seams with letters, results, and medical images, while my mum and I nervously waited. During frequent hospital stays this important folder lay at the bottom of my bed. While tempted, I knew not to touch it. A prompt for discussion between doctors and nurses, to me it was forbidden. More recently, medical information has become digitalized, but during consultations the computer screen is angled so that I still cannot see what is being written about me.

In the hope of filling the gaps about my medical experiences, I submitted a request to access my pediatric medical records. I was shocked to learn that all of the cardiology medical records detailing the first 18 years of my care had been destroyed. When I tried to find out why, I was sent around the houses. I have spoken to the service that commissions congenital cardiac care in Scotland, to the health board responsible for the national service, to the Scottish Public Services Ombudsman, and to the Information Commissions Officer, the independent body set up to uphold information rights. To date, none of them seem to want to take responsibility. In Scotland, government guidance states that childhood medical records should be retained until the patient's 25th birthday unless the illness could have potential relevance to adult conditions, in which case, they should only be destroyed based on specific clinical approval. I have found no evidence that a clinician approved the destruction of my records. What I have found, however, is that the record was not labeled with a "do not destroy" sticker. And so, an assumption was made that they could be disposed of. Nobody thought to check with me.

My health board says that an adequate clinical summary of my childhood notes was provided when I moved to adult care and that this summary means I am not at clinical risk. But I have been unable to find the summary record that the health board is referring to. From a medical perspective, as one of the longest-living survivors in the world completely dependent on a cardiac pacemaker, this has left me in a vulnerable position. My care was a first, and my healthcare needs are lifelong. It is impossible to know which parts of my medical history may become relevant.

On a personal level, I feel very sad that such a significant part of my childhood has been destroyed. I will never know how many cardiac procedures I have endured; how many hospitals stays, the story behind some of my scars, or what happened

to me. Like the child sitting in the hospital bed, my childhood medical notes and the opportunity to better understand my childhood experiences are now forever beyond my reach. My childhood medical records have been wrongfully destroyed without my knowledge or consent, and in breach of the law, my data protection, and patient rights. I have been completely silenced as a patient. This sets a precedent for children's health rights everywhere.
—Adapted from "The Injustice of Losing My Childhood Medical History," [28]

There have been recent calls within medical practice to better incorporate patient knowledge and expertise. Ashdown and Jones report an autoethnography study which explores the experiences of a physician-turned-patient during a two-and-a-half-year long hospitalization. Findings included critical reflection from the patient, medical educator, and research perspectives. The authors report 7 themes that emerged upon critical analysis of 11 scenarios that described real-life healthcare encounters of the physician-turned-patient: experiential learning, reflection, what counts as medical care, vulnerability, patient-centered care, agency, and patient expertise. The authors note that these themes are often neglected in medical education. They reflect that biomedical knowledge gleaned from medical education is different from the experiential knowledge of patients and that (re)humanization of medical education is needed, which patients can contribute to. Further, patients are experts by experience and medical education should mobilize this and partner with patients in areas like admissions, curriculum, teaching, assessment, and governance. This study highlights differences between academic and experiential knowledge, and challenges medical education to harness the expertise that patients have and actively involve patients as equal stakeholders in curricula.[29]

The Compassion Crisis in Healthcare

Throughout my life, both personally and professionally, I've encountered many different doctors and medical professionals. As a journalist, I used to find it amusing to verify or debunk stereotypes about surgeons, or ER doctors, or nurses. But eventually, as a mom, the things I overheard in rooms and hallways stopped being funny and became deeply disturbing. Every wrong approach leaves a mark, reinforcing my belief that basic communication skills should be a mandatory part of medical school curricula.

—Katarina, 42, daughter, now 6, born with a single ventricle heart, Croatian living in Belgium

While a lack of compassion is a recognized threat to patient safety, shortcomings have been reported in health systems due to a lack of compassion in healthcare delivery. In the United States, in a national survey asking 800 hospitalized patients and 510 physicians about the US healthcare system, almost half of the respondents reported that the US healthcare was not compassionate, signaling a "compassion crisis."[30]

Chaney notes that while the word "compassion" is now ubiquitous in modern healthcare, the term only became widely used in healthcare in 2009.[31] The author reflects that in the United Kingdom, a public investigation into Mid-Staffordshire National Health Service (NHS) Foundation Trust (2010–2013) led to increased attention to the emotional side of care. The investigation was prompted by several deaths after routine operations in dire conditions. Led by Robert Francis QC, the report outlined several causes of poor care, including chronic staff shortages, bad management, low morale, and poor nursing care that lacked attentiveness and compassion. The final *Francis Report* recommended "an increased focus on a culture of compassion and caring in nurse recruitment, training and education."[32] This was adopted by NHS England, which launched a 3-year strategy, "Compassion in Practice," in early 2013, outlining six values—care, compassion, competence, communication, courage, and commitment—to be upheld by nursing, midwifery, and care staff.

My chronic health conditions (psoriasis and psoriatic arthritis) first presented in my early 20s during my first university degree. I had a great GP who listened to my concerns and knew me reasonably well but ultimately had to refer me to specialists. I can vividly recall my first specialist appointment. I was given a diagnosis in a very matter of fact manner, I had very little explanation of the conditions given and was given leaflets to read at home. The interaction was very cold and I left feeling worse than when I arrived. Whilst the consultant may deal with many people throughout the day and is used to delivering this news it was all very new to me! There was no consideration given to my emotional wellbeing or the psychological impact of diagnosis. This was despite the fact that there has been significant research on the impact of my conditions on mental health and depression being a well recognised co-morbidity. Diagnosis and illness had a huge and immediate impact on my university studies and I blamed myself for that at times.

—Yvonne, 45, psoriasis and psoriatic arthritis, United Kingdom

Studies also reveal missed opportunities for offering compassion during healthcare encounters, with doctors commonly missing emotional clues from their patients. Specifically, one study reported that doctors miss 60%–90% of opportunities to respond to patients with compassion.[33]

There are many issues that may contribute to this, such as burnout, compassion fatigue, and moral injury (see Chapter 5). Depersonalization of patients can occur when healthcare professionals are stressed, underresourced, poorly supported, and working in a toxic environment with poor leadership. This may be emphasized by depersonalizing aspects of care, such as the backless hospital gown.[34]

The rise of information technology may further contribute to the problem; for example, one study found that doctors spend as much time looking at their computer screen as they do at their patient.[35] Further, Trzerciak and Mazzarelli suggest that empathy declines over the course of medical training, in part, due to a "hidden curriculum" whereby mentors' role-model a lack of compassion during their interactions with patients, teaching their trainee doctors to do the same.[36]

A recent study that aimed to scope the communication curriculum currently delivered within undergraduate children's nursing programs across the Republic of Ireland and the United Kingdom noted a gap in delivery and content of communication training within children's nursing curricula. The authors report that despite an identified need for a comprehensive and effective communication curriculum within undergraduate nursing, findings show variability in the delivery and content of communication training across higher educational institutions across the 32 program leaders who completed the survey (51% response rate). While core communication modules were featured across all nursing programs, only two program leaders reported delivering standalone child-centered communication modules. Further, communication training was not always delivered by an educator with professional experience of children and young people in healthcare. The authors call for more work on equipping undergraduate children's nurses with the unique skills needed to communicate effectively with children and young people and incorporate learnings into nursing pedagogy.[37]

> As an adult, a consultant was very flippant to me in breaking news about a diagnosis, assuming I knew about it when there is no way I could have as I had not seen a cardiologist for decades. When I asked what this meant I was met by the reply you'll need surgery, when I asked when, feeling extremely anxious, only to be told some time in the future no one knows. How is this helpful, what kind of approach is this with another human being? There was no empathy, no gentle approach and certainly no explanation. Coping with this news was so scary but

having children to care for I had to try and stay positive. This could have been approached in a much more sensitive way, asking what I understood and knew prior to breaking news like this. I understand staff especially in the NHS are under extreme stress, pressure and time constraints but please remember we are human beings.
—Maggie, 53 years old, congenital heart condition, United Kingdom

Mehta et al. (2024) report that many medical schools have failed to implement compassion training for medical students possibly because traditional medical educators assume compassion is inherently present in medical students.[38] This notion of compassion as a natural aptitude or calling has permeated contemporary healthcare[39] and for too long it has been left to the "bedside manner" of the attending healthcare professional.

Further, outdated medical training methods may be linked to a lack of compassion. Specifically, studies have found that teaching by humiliation is still common in medical training. Teaching by humiliation typically happens when an educator embarrasses a trainee in public teaching spaces such as hospital wards, operating rooms, or medical conferences. For example, senior doctors aggressively questioning medical students about medical knowledge, mocking wrong answers or making derogatory comments about a student's capabilities in front of other healthcare professionals and even patients. This type of "educational technique" is often passed on through the hidden curriculum and hierarchical medical culture, whereby senior doctors hold significant power over the education and future careers of their trainees.[40]

In a systematic review exploring the use of teaching by public humiliation in different settings, including 33 studies and more than 40,000 people, Li et al. found that, on average, 34.9% of people experience public humiliation.[41] Specifically, they found that teaching by public humiliation was very common in medical education settings. In a follow-up study, Wigg et al. analyzed 28 studies involving nearly 35,000 medical trainees across multiple countries.[42] They found that on average, 57% of medical students and junior doctors reported that they experienced teaching by humiliation.

It seems likely this practice will have a detrimental impact on feelings of psychological safety for doctors negatively affecting their mental health, patient–doctor relationships, relational safety, and well-being. Research shows that doctors who have experienced teaching by humiliation are at higher risk of developing mental health problems. Cheng and colleagues (2020) reported that doctors who experience humiliation are almost eight times more likely to report burnout and almost four times more likely to report symptoms of anxiety and depression.[43] This practice also leads doctors to become reluctant to ask questions or seek help when they are uncertain about something, which is clearly detrimental to patient outcomes. Li et al. (2024) propose more psychologically informed teaching methods including structured feedback sessions, simulation-based training, and constructive mentorship programs.[44]

An Inhospitable Environment

Whilst we know that hospitals can be noisy places, there was often a great deal of chatter from the nurse station, into the early hours of the morning. I did have words with the matron about this and she was understanding, However, if the staff were quiet for a few days more, eventually it would all start up again. I'm a light sleeper and it didn't help. As it was, I was on furosemide infusion 24/7, meaning that I didn't have a single night of unbroken sleep, needing to pass water, during my entire stay.
—Richard, 60 years old, congenital heart condition, heart transplant recipient, United Kingdom

There have been many occasions after surgery when I have juggled an oxygen mask with a sick bowl, trying not to dislodge the tubes plugged into my body or upset my broken bones as I vomited from the anesthetic. During these times, I just wanted to be left in peace to sleep. But doctors needed X-rays, pacing tests, my blood pressure, heart rate, temperature, and blood. It felt relentless. I was bundled about by nurses and doctors to a constant background beep of dozens of heart monitors and alarms, nurses talking, and babies crying. The cleaner bumped my bed with her mop. I was utterly exhausted. On one occasion, as a child, I woke up on the ward following cardiac surgery and I could not move my head. As I came to, I realized that someone had thoughtlessly used so much surgical tape to keep a drain in place that they had stuck my neck in one position. Removing the tape from the sensitive skin on my neck, just to be able to turn my head, added unnecessary pain to an already distressing situation.

Parking at hospitals is challenging, especially when you can't walk too far or are anxious about treatment or a difficult conversation. This feels like a logistical issue rather than an emotional one but it has impacted me in the past; not seeing a space, time to the appointment ticking by, the threat of a dreaded DNA.
—David, 45 years old, congenital heart condition, United Kingdom

In many ways, the hospital environment has been designed to meet the needs of medical tests and treatments with poor consideration of wider patient well-being and recovery. There can be a lack of privacy in hospitals, especially on ward bays with multiple beds. Often each bay has a paper-thin curtain that the attendant healthcare professional pulls around the bed when they come to examine you. Sound carries easily, as you are asked to provide your full medical history, symptoms, and often highly sensitive and confidential information. You may be asked to provide a urine sample and asked to leave a bedpan in a communal toilet.

Healthcare environments can be particularly challenging for people with learning disabilities and autistic people who may require specific accommodations to allow equitable access.[45] There are many ways in which the hospital environment could better support psychologically informed healthcare, not least of all by tackling poor sleep.

Poor Sleep

Never allow a patient to be waked, intentionally or accidentally, is a sine qua non of all good nursing.

—Florence Nightingale[46]

The last time that I ended up in emergency care, a very poorly man lay in the bed across from me, trying to sleep. There was a metal pedal bin beside his bed. Every ten minutes or so a nurse or doctor would press the pedal of the bin with their foot, put their rubbish in it and as they released the pedal the lid closed with a loud bang. Each time the man jumped awake, startled by the noise. None of them seemed to notice him.

Sleep in the hospital is notoriously poor. A meta-analysis examining 203 studies found that approximately 76% of the studies reported that sleep duration in hospital was below the average considered healthy.[47] Almost half of the studies showed that adults in hospital slept less than 6 hours per night. Patients also often experience nocturnal awakenings (up to 42 times per night) and prolonged awakenings.

Many lights don't turn off in the hospital rooms. Staff become frustrated if you ask for this to be fixed as it doesn't impact on them at work, but it stopped me and my son sleeping. Equally the internet rarely works, and my son's iPad is all that keeps him distracted. It's his safety object. Families need to be kept together in crisis to prevent psychological harm, my sons have no relationship now after 8 months apart and my eldest son is quite resentful since he came home.

—Hollie, 38 years old, mother of a son with bronchitis obliterans, 11 months old at time of admission, United Kingdom

There are many reasons why sleep quality is poor in the hospital setting, including feeling unwell, experiencing pain or the side effects of medication, anxiety about health problems and anticipated tests and procedures, the unfamiliar hospital environment, and disruption of routine. However, the hospital environment itself confounds this problem. The most common issues include noise, alarm bells, heart monitors, ambulances, chattering at the nursing station, sharing a room with other patients, lighting, nursing activities during nightshifts (such as taking observations, giving out medication, handing over patients during shift changes, and admitting emergency patients).[48]

World Health Organization guidelines state that the average sound level should not exceed 30 dB in general hospital areas and 35 dB in rooms where patients are kept or observed and the maximum sound level indoors should not exceed 40 dB during the night.[49] Yet, meeting these goals in practical and clinical situations can be challenging. While there are many sources of sounds in inpatient settings, medical alarms are often listed as a main source, with the number of alarms increasing in parallel with the introduction of more sophisticated technologies to monitor and support patients. Excessive sound and noise in the intensive care unit (ICU) has been linked with adverse and potentially preventable patient outcomes and with staff errors and dissatisfaction. And, it has been argued that most of these alarms are not accurate or critical and are commonly ignored by staff.[50] Studies have suggested that noise above the recommended range affects patient and staff well-being, bringing about various physiologic and psychological changes, which directly affect health. Specifically, noise enhances the release of cortisol, increases oxygen consumption, increases sleep disturbances, increases the need for analgesia and sedation, disrupts circadian rhythms, and can contribute to delirium.[51]

Psychologically Informed Healthcare: A Culture Shift

Medical providers can take time to understand my medical history, true medical needs & get a full picture of my overall health. Often, I feel medical providers are pressed for time and prescribing drugs and making decisions based on incomplete pictures & in sufficient facts and without deep analysis of the options. Medical providers can spend more time talking me through my options and potential risks or benefits of each.
—Sebastian, 55 years, coronary heart disease, United States

While some of the challenges that can contribute to negative mental health outcomes for people living with an LTC are unavoidable, there are many ways healthcare systems could mitigate their impact to promote protective factors and positive adaptation. Psychologically informed healthcare is essential to this end.[52] While some medical professionals may not consider this as part of their role or remit, an emotional and psychological response to living with an LTC is a normal and common part of the patients' presentation. Adequate support for psychological well-being significantly affects recovery, resilience, adaptive adjustment, self-management, medical adherence, and patient satisfaction and can prevent the development of more serious psychological difficulties and medically related post-traumatic stress.

When I present my work on psychologically informed healthcare it is common for people to say that while they understand, from a patient perspective, why medical care needs to become more psychologically informed, healthcare professionals could not do their job if they focused too much on "seeing the person." Of course, professional boundaries are appropriate. There is no need, for example, for a surgeon to fully immerse themselves in a child's (or adults) story as they yield a scalpel to them. But the patient must always be seen, fully as a person, by everyone entrusted with their care. Further, a psychologically informed approach to healthcare includes supporting the emotional and psychological well-being of staff too, so they can manage any understandable emotional response they have to their patients' pain and suffering.

> *I don't think it's utopian to expect health professionals everywhere to be equally trained in bedside manners and to maintain an open, positive, and inclusive attitude toward their patients and caregivers. That there are too few of them and too much work is no excuse . . . I am convinced that respect and trust are crucial for the psychophysical health of a mother who, when encouraged and self-confident, can ensure her medically complex child lives the fullest life possible. Most of the time, though, I felt resigned. I saw this resignation in other mothers too, who were often too fearful to ask questions or too respectful toward the white coat. We were taught for generations not to question what the doctor says. But there is nothing as liberating as when one of them tells you, "I'm not leaving until you've asked me everything you need to know." . . . parents need to be systematically empowered to speak their minds, no matter how silly it might feel. . . . Asking questions means learning and learning means providing better options for our children. Knowledge is power!*
> —Katarina, 42, daughter, now 6, born with a single-ventricle heart, Croatian living in Belgium

Another common query is how already financially overstretched and underresourced healthcare services can afford to add aspects of care. Besides the moral and ethical imperative to provide the best care and "do no harm," healthcare providers and systems cannot afford to neglect the psychological and emotional side of health. For example, patients commonly consult their healthcare teams about benign symptoms resulting from health anxiety or low mood, leading to increased health costs.[53] Neglecting the psychological and emotional impact of LTCs is a false economy that healthcare professionals pay with their time and that negatively affects patient recovery, satisfaction, and well-being.

Thankfully, there has been an increasing focus on patient-centered care representing a shift from disease-centered approaches to the development and practice of healthcare that integrates the patient's needs, experiences, and perspectives. Patient-centered care has been a key part of the global health agenda, with recent policy drivers promoting a person-centered culture with the World Health Organization naming it as one of the aims of Health 2020.[54] While welcome, this is far from enough, we need a culture shift. Psychologically informed healthcare needs to be embedded into healthcare training, practice, and policy to improve mental health outcomes, well-being, and quality of life for many.

PART 2
PSYCHOLOGICALLY INFORMED HEALTHCARE

3
Good Bedside Manner
Relational Safety In Healthcare

> *We need to build our own emotional literacy and capacity. Without having a tolerance for emotional issues, we cannot possibly provide the holistic care needed by our patients.*
> —Karen Neaton, peri-operative Nurse, Australia

Psychologically informed healthcare recognizes the mind–body link while proactively aiming to promote protective factors and mitigate risk factors for psychological and emotional well-being during healthcare experiences and beyond. This approach aims to compassionately support and recognize the added challenges and barriers that people living with a long-term health condition (LTC) can face. Psychologically informed healthcare complements and builds on the influential *biopsychosocial model* of health and well-being conceptualized by George Engel in 1977. Engel proposed that to understand a person's medical condition it is not enough to simply consider biological factors— social, psychological, and behavioral factors also need to be taken into account.[1,2] Further it is consistent with other calls for psychologically informed practice, for example, in physical therapy and rehabilitation.[3] As such, *psychologically informed healthcare* comprises understanding, recognition of, and support for traumatic medical experiences, medical tests and treatments, losses, any impact on self-esteem, management of physical symptoms, and limitations. Further, awareness of health inequalities, intersectionality, and the wider psychosocial impact of living with an LTC on relationships, educational, career opportunities, and finances (as discussed in Part 1) is essential. Vitally, this approach also aims to better support emotional well-being of healthcare professionals.

With a growing number of people experiencing an LTC, it is also important to promote a more sophisticated and inclusive understanding of health and well-being that gives weight to the many attributes gifted by adverse lived experiences, such as increased empathy, resilience, determination, more meaningful relationships, appreciation of life, and insight. By tipping the scales in the right direction, patient well-being can be better supported (see Figure 3.1).

Mental Health Risk Factors:	Mental Health Protective Factors:
• Acute health crisis	• Age-appropriate communication
• Decline in health	• Coping strategies
• Difficulty accessing healthcare	• Consistency of care & trust
• Discrimination, ableism, & intersectionality	• Compassionate healthcare encounters
• Disempowering aspects of healthcare	• Condition-specific peer support
• Early medial barriers to attachment	• Cultural competency
• Impact on self-esteem & body image	• Dignity & respect
• Impact on education, work, & finances	• Embedded psychological & emotional support
• Impact on relationships	• Empowerment, choice, & control
• Issues having & raising children	• Goals, meaning & purpose
• Losses	• Healing physical environment
• Medical uncertainty	• Healthcare literacy
• Medical appointments, tests, & procedures	• Pain relief & symptom control
• Pain	• Psychological safety
• Patient admin & burden	• Relational safety
• Physical symptoms	• Rest & recuperation
• Physical limitations	• Supported self-management
• Preexisting mental health condition / neurodiversity	• Social support
• Poor sleep	• Soothing presence of loved ones
• Social isolation	• Trauma informed care
• Traumatic medical experiences	• Signposting to practical support, allyship, & advocacy

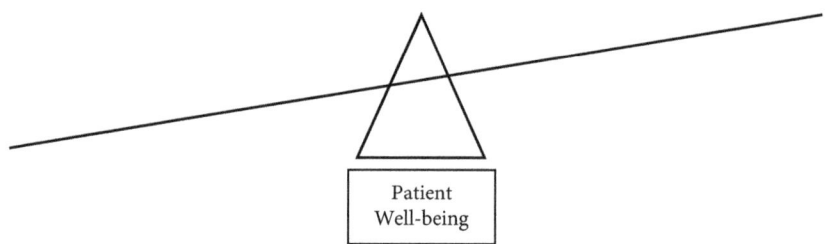

Patient Well-being

Figure 3.1 Psychologically informed healthcare involves proactively recognizing and mitigating emotional and psychological risk factors that are associated with living with an LTC and promoting protective factors across the healthcare journey to "tip the scales" and improve well-being.

> **Psychologically Informed Healthcare: R.E.S.P.E.C.T.**
>
> Psychologically Informed Healthcare aims to embed contemporary understanding in psychological and emotional health into healthcare practice grounded in the core principles of R.E.S.P.E.C.T:
>
> - **Relational safety**, providing mandatory training in and delivery of compassion-focused healthcare for all healthcare professionals.
> - **Empowerment**, supporting self-management and healthcare literacy and challenging disempowering aspects of healthcare.
> - **Soothing presence** of caregivers supported across the healthcare journey, as wanted by each individual patient.
> - **Psychological safety** (polyvagal informed) for patients and healthcare professionals, including emotional and psychological support that is preventative, embedded (not just reactive), and that acknowledges and validates a normal response to adverse circumstances. Implementing coping strategies and support throughout healthcare delivery.
> - **Environment**, healthcare settings and policies that support healing and psychological safety.
> - **Culturally sensitive**, tackling ableism and discrimination and recognizing health inequalities and intersectionality.
> - **Trauma informed healthcare**.
>
> This book draws from the latest psychological evidence, theories, and understandings and includes real-life testimonials and case studies. It also includes examples of innovative, inspiring, and good practice from across the world. Psychologically informed healthcare is a framework, and of course there are many aspects of healthcare that are compatible with this thinking. In reading this book, I hope you will be inspired to create more. This is an ongoing and changing landscape, drawing from the latest evidence, as our understanding improves, and we work together to improve psychologically informed healthcare and tip the scales toward well-being for all.

Relational Safety: Our Innate Need for Social Connection

I was referred to an Occupational Therapist (OT) who was a significant help with both my physical and mental health. The OT actively listened, she took time to get to know me and she asked how I was coping physically and mentally. The OT was professional but was also warm and engaging, which has not often been the case in my experience. The OT discussed my conditions with me and explained some of the complexities that I did not understand, she also offered ways to manage these. It was only at this stage that she backed up the information with leaflets which I could take home. This approach helped me greatly instead of just being handed some pieces of paper and feeling like I had to digest that alone. The OT helped me to accept some of the changes in my life and to recognise the impact my conditions were having on me. Due to the OT recognising the emotional/psychological impact of the conditions I was able to access Cognitive Behavioural Therapy and fatigue management sessions which were so helpful.

—Yvonne, 45, psoriasis and psoriatic arthritis, United Kingdom

We each have an innate need for safe social connections, especially when faced with adversity. When we do not feel safe, whether because of a natural disaster, loss, injury, or threat, we look to one another.[4] We communicate psychological safety with each other through compassion and building trust.[5]

Hupcey describes findings from a qualitative research study using grounded theory that explored the psychosocial needs of critically ill patients, with participants reporting an overwhelming need to feel safe.[6] The study included 45 critically ill patients in medical or surgical ICU, for a minimum of 3 days, in a rural American care center. Four categories of needs were found to affect feeling safe: knowledge, regaining control, hoping, and trusting. The first category included patients knowing what was happening to them. The second category, regaining control, marked a turning point in their recovery when they felt like they were beginning to regain some control. In contrast, before this point, the participants described feeling like they had lost control, which was frightening. Regaining control typically involved small steps such as ambulating and taking back some responsibilities for their own care. The third category, hoping, pertained to holding onto hope of recovery, for example, of getting a transplant. The final category, trusting, involved being able to trust that nursing staff were watching over them and meeting their needs. Patients who did not feel like they could trust staff became vigilant about their care, expressed concerns about the competency of staff, and described not feeling safe. Overall, feeling safe was influenced by family, friends, ICU staff, religious beliefs, feelings of knowing, regaining control, hoping, and trusting.

It helps me that my regular doctor took time so we could get to know each other (what is my/his personal history, what is important to me, what my/his family look like), it helps when healthcare professionals explain their non-verbal communication (e.g. why they are smiling, looking away or frowning etc.) when they are talking about my results or my health (heart) situation in general; when they put me at the end of their outpatient day so I don't have to stress about time to perform the outpatient consultation and when I am literally in a room with a view. Being honest in an empathic way about test outcomes and my prognosis and discussing openly the possibilities and why some cures or palliative actions are not a possibility in my situation also helps.

—Roy, 57, complex congenital heart disease, Netherlands

In Chapter 1 we explored this biological need for safe social connection[7] and considered polyvagal theory (PVT) as a framework for understanding psychological safety in healthcare settings. PVT emphasizes the role of the autonomic nervous system (ANS) in perceiving safety or threat through neuroception, a subconscious process that influences physiological and behavioral states.[8] Feeling safe involves social signals of trust, compassion, and connection, which are crucial for fostering engagement and reducing stress in patients (Chapter 1, Figure 1.2). Psychological safety is not simply the removal of threat; we constantly seek and exchange signals of safety with each other through voice tone, facial expression, body language, trust signals, and reciprocity.[9]

As such, we use our connections with others to predict and cope with challenges; a process that Sue Carter, an American biologist and behavioral neurobiologist, describes as "*sociostasis*." This need for safe social connections is linked in mammals to the evolutionary development of oxytocin, "the love hormone," which is critical for feelings of emotional safety and which plays a significant role in physical and mental health, sociality, and loving relationships.[10]

In sum, when someone is unwell and in need of medical attention, it can be incredibly stressful for them and their loved ones. In this situation, it is natural for them to look to others for support. Healthcare professionals have an important duty to care for the emotional and psychological needs of patients during these challenges. As such, in healthcare the "soft stuff" really does matter, because this is how we communicate and enhance feelings of psychological safety—through *relational safety*.

Compassion as a Cornerstone of Psychologically Informed Healthcare

I have benefited over the years from countless examples of compassionate healthcare providing me with the strength to face frightening medical experiences and to cope with pain, discomfort, and distress. My pediatric cardiologist always spoke to me with warmth and kindness. He wore a colorful bowtie or a tie featuring a cartoon character, and his approach was gentle. Compassion was clear from small acts such as warming up the cold stethoscope before placing it on my skin to advocating for my care when others saw me as a "lost cause." He was a tremendous support to my mum, carefully listening to her concerns, working collaboratively with us to battle the uncertainty of my prognosis and dependency on pioneering technology. Similarly, the pediatric electrophysiology team did their best to make uncomfortable cardiac tests easier. One electrophysiologist wore a white coat covered in colorful badges. During tests he encouraged me to focus on choosing which badge I wanted, and he would give it to me at the end of the procedure.

I also recall a theater nurse with curly brown hair and warm brown eyes. She arrived with the team in green scrubs to collect me from the children's heart ward to take me to the theater. Before they wheeled me away, she took a moment to let me know that she knew how I felt. She pulled down her top a little to reveal her own "zipper scar" from open heart surgery. At once I knew I could trust her, she was one of us, and I felt just a little bit safer. On the ward, I did not trust nurses who told me a procedure would not hurt, especially when I knew it would. Nurse H was always honest, she carefully explained to me and my mum why I needed any medical procedure and what it would involve and got it done as efficiently, painlessly, and quickly as she could with empathy, humor, and compassion. She earned my trust, and I always felt safer in her care.

As an adult, my cardiologists have taken an interest in me as a person, beyond my condition, enquiring about my studies, work, and family. Continuity of care, by having the same cardiologist and team, who are aware of my complex history, helps me to feel more comfortable and safer. The last time I went for surgery, as I lay in the pre-op room, waiting to be taken through to theater, the surgeon carefully and calmly explained to me what he was planning to do. As he walked away, he patted my foot. This simple act felt reassuring. I felt seen as a person and more trusting of the team.

There is often a sense of camaraderie in hospital, it can feel like you are all in it together. There were many occasions when we would end up laughing at the absurdity of the situations we found ourselves in. Sometimes, a bit of "gallows humor" helps, and there are many hospital characters that help to keep everyone's' spirits up, from the porters tasked with wheeling you for a medical test, to volunteers in the shop and healthcare workers.

Unfortunately, there are also medical encounters that I will never forget for the wrong reasons. As a young teenager, I had an unfortunate encounter with an anesthetist. I had not cried about my hospital experiences since I was a toddler. My mum (who was trying her best, with little guidance or support) tells me that when I was around 3 years old, I began protesting during cardiac tests in hospital. On one occasion, they were simply unable to complete the required procedure because I was crying and wriggling around so much. Tough love was needed, so she took me to the bathroom and gently but firmly explained that these tests were going to be part of my life, and no one could do anything about that. She said that I could either cry and struggle, which would mean being there for hours, or I could lie quietly and still and get it over with. Then she would take me to the little shop in the hospital lobby and buy me a treat. I understood, opting for the latter. Perhaps, I understood too well, because I did not cry again about any of my hospital experiences, in or out of hospital, until I was around 13 years old. On this occasion, I burst into tears as I met the anesthetist on my way to the theater. He scolded me, saying that I was too old to cry and to stop being a baby. I still remember the deep sense of shame I felt.

Further, as described in the preface, during my teens, I underwent a series of cardiac surgeries and investigations in the space of just a few years. It was a challenging time as I approached my teenage years and wanted to just get on with life. My education was also becoming more important, and I was keen to go to university. However, I developed debilitating chronic fatigue and was barely able to attend school.

At one point I was admitted to hospital while this "unexplained symptom" was explored extensively by my dedicated cardiac team. Eventually, because my dad had narcolepsy, they referred me to a pediatric neurologist to investigate. He clearly did not agree with the referral. I remember him coming into my cubicle with his entourage and smugly handing me a brown paper bag as he told me dismissively that my problem was simply that I was "not breathing properly." He told me that breathing into the bag should sort out my hyperventilation and marched back out. I felt utterly dismissed, disbelieved, and ashamed. Further, as much as I tried, no amount of breathing into a paper bag or abdominal breathing exercises helped. Thirty years on, I still suffer from unexplained chronic fatigue and feel angry when I think about this encounter. Recently, I found out I have restrictive ventilatory function, a recognized complication of undergoing thoracotomies, especially during infancy.[11] I'd undergone six thorocotomies and open-heart surgery by the time he gave me the paper bag. It was harmful to leave me feeling that this was a failing on my part rather explaining it was a complication of undergoing cardiothoracic surgeries. Even if this was not recognized at the time, there was no need to leave a child feeling responsible for their symptoms.

I have also experienced difficulties accessing the specialist care I need as an adult. Unfortunately, specialist care for the growing number of adults living with congenital heart disease had not developed in time for me reaching adulthood. This culminated in a life-threatening incident in my early 30s, when I was sent away from emergency care by an on-duty cardiologist who did not believe that my pacemaker was failing, even though the heart monitor kept dropping to zero. He would not listen to my lifetime of experience or my family and confidently sent me home. It was a Friday evening, and I spent the weekend worrying about what would happen if my device broke completely. My son was just 5 years old at the time. My mum took me to the cardiology department when it opened on Monday morning, and I insisted that they check my pacemaker. Sure enough, the device that I depend on for every heartbeat had developed a life-threatening intermittent fault. I never got an apology from the cardiologist who sent me home from emergency care. The team adjusted the settings on my device to compensate for the fault, sending me home with the instruction not to drive, while they organized the complex lead extraction surgery that I needed. As a young mum, awaiting yet another life-threatening surgery, the last thing I needed was to have to fight my way through the medical system and be made to feel voiceless and unsafe by those entrusted with my care. The choice was made to save my life as a baby, knowing I would need lifelong care. My difficulties accessing this as an adult left me feeling abandoned and led to my decade long campaign asking the Scottish government for national healthcare standards to improve care.

More recently, I recall sitting in my cubicle, as an adult, the night before a risky operation to remove and replace pacing leads. My husband, mum, and young son had not long left. I sat looking out of the window, trying to find the resolve to keep going despite being terrified that something might happen to me and that I would leave my son motherless. A surgeon (not mine) burst into my room with a terrified looking entourage of student doctors. Without asking my permission, he pointed to my scars and barked "diagnoses?" at them. I sat there, in my pajamas, silently as they guessed my condition. He followed this by asking "and what complications might there be during her surgery tomorrow?" I was stunned into silence as they discussed all the things that might go wrong with my forthcoming procedure. I ended up feeling sorry for the junior doctors who he enjoyed humiliating when they could not answer his questions.

Over the years, I have gone over and over these moments in my mind, wondering why I lost my voice and re-experiencing the anger and shame they evoked. Looking back, I now understand that in each of these stressful situations, when I did not receive compassion from healthcare professionals to help me cope, my threat system was activated. To deal with what was happening to me, my system went into hypoarousal. Powerless, I had no other options, I needed these life-saving procedures for survival, and I was dependent on these healthcare professionals to provide this. So, I became numb to what was happening to me. Under such circumstances, when we experience social threats, we often feel a deep sense of shame. I have no doubt the cumulative effect of these experiences contributed to the post-traumatic stress that I developed. Through my campaign work and advocacy, many others have shared similar difficult medical experiences with me.

> Over time, we got to know the staff quite well and vice versa (on the transplant ward). They got to know our preferences for eating, how we liked to spend our days and what we needed at night to rest properly. They could not have done more for us. It was obvious that they cared for us and would show emotion when one of us was whisked off for transplant or when we saw them afterwards. I could see tears in the eyes of the lovely nurse that I bumped into post my own operation, a sense of relief and happiness, I guess. It was clear also that the more senior staff, consultants etc. were also invested in me, they saw us most days and I was able to talk to them in detail about what was happening, on a very regular basis. This definitely helped with my wellbeing, that they were really on the ball when it came to knowing me as a patient. I am referring specifically to the congenital heart team here. Other patients in our cohort were not congenital and often would go for long periods of days or weeks without this depth of input.
> —Richard, 60 years old, congenital heart condition, heart transplant recipient, United Kingdom

Compassionate care lies at the foundation of Psychologically Informed Healthcare. Often considered the first principle of care, especially in nursing, compassion describes how we respond to another's pain deriving from the Latin "pati" and "cum" which mean to suffer with. Compassion drives connection. It is a deep understanding of another person's pain and willingness to relieve them.

The renowned American Psychologist Carl Rogers, founder of *humanistic psychology* and *person-centered therapy*, described empathy as being able to perceive the internal frame of reference of another person with accuracy including the emotional components and meanings.[12] Empathy involves *feeling with another* through perspective-taking, staying out of judgment, recognizing emotion in others, and communicating this to them. Empathic acceptance means valuing otherness, receiving them with openness, attuning to their experience and communicating understanding. Importantly, it also means not over identifying with those feelings and being able to recognize and hold in mind that they belong to the other.

Compassion takes this one step further by wanting to act to relieve another's suffering. Research has shown distinct neural pathways for empathy and compassion. While empathy activates the neural pathway involved with experiences of negative emotions and pain, compassion activates the pathway involved with positive affect and affiliation.[13] In other words, we are programmed to help each other and gain pleasure from doing so.

Compassion also involves humility and an understanding of the shared human condition as fragile and imperfect, and a willingness to extend that understanding to others.[14] In other words, *"There but for the grace of God go I"*—any one of us may find ourselves in the patient role in need of medical assistance.

Compassion has a positive effect on the physical, social, and psychological health of the giver and receiver.[15] Compassionate interactions help our nervous system use our social engagement system, helping us to feel calm, to relax, and to heal. During compassionate medical encounters we are more likely to remember medical instructions and better able to respond to important questions and follow recommendations.

When we do not receive compassionate care, we are more likely to go into defense mode during stressful medical situations. We may go into fight or flight, leaving us overwhelmed by feelings of anxiety or anger. This can lead to challenging encounters, frustration, and difficulty engaging with healthcare professionals or remembering key information. Some patients may go into fight mode, leading to aggressive outbursts, which is clearly detrimental to all. Alternatively, we may go into hypoarousal, where our overwhelmed systems shut down and we dissociate from harm or use fawning behaviors in an attempt to pacify perceived interpersonal threats while neglecting our own needs. This can be misperceived as coping, leaving the patient without the support they need. Over time, hypoarousal can increase the likelihood of developing longer-term mental health difficulties such as post-traumatic stress or panic attacks and may impair recovery and immunity.

As such, compassion is fundamental to relationship-based care and understanding of patients. People remember the compassion they have received during health-challenge experiences.[16] They also remember when they have not received compassionate care. Compassionate care helps patients to feel safe and increases engagement and participation in treatment and interventions. It is linked with an increase in the patient's hope for recovery, accountability, control over their health, and satisfaction while leading to the provision of safer care and enhanced resilience for healthcare professionals.[17]

Compassion is linked to health outcomes too, with survival rates increasing when doctors make eye contact and provide reassuring touch to their patients.[18] One study found that feeling safer during hospitalization increased feelings of control, calm, and hope.[19] Studies have also found that compassionate touch from a supportive other can lower blood pressure[20] and that a compassionate connection with a healthcare provider can improve pain following major surgery[21] and helps to build trust.[22]

> *I found it helpful to be given choice and the maximum amount of control over what happened to me, being signposted to accessible information in a range of formats, peer support both online and in person, clear communication from professionals before, during and after any and all procedures, recognition of my agency as a patient and right to participate in decisions regarding my care and treatment, having a named point of contact (breast cancer nurse) to help coordinate care and provide emotional and practice support outside of scheduled appointments, kindness and compassion from healthcare providers and relationship-based care and support.*
> —Sarah, 44 years old, undergoing breast cancer treatment, United Kingdom

Most people have a natural capacity for compassion, which can be honed and strengthened. Compassionate communication can be taught and incorporated into healthcare teaching and practice. When we recognize the fundamental importance of relational safety during stressful medical experiences, it is clear to see this must include all touch points for patients from receptionists to cleaning staff, porters, nurses, doctors, surgeons, and allied health professionals. Compassionate communication, within the context of a boundaried professional relationship, is an essential part of training for all healthcare professionals to facilitate mutual respect and alleviate distress; it is conveyed through tone of voice, facial expressions, body language, trust signals, and reciprocity.[23]

Delivery of compassionate healthcare is a mindset involving many aspects toward building connection and trust. Respecting our body is the basis for self-compassion which can be challenging when you have a long-term health condition. Living with a chronic health condition can negatively affect self-concept and trust in one's body. As such, it is essential to validate the patient's account of their embodied experience without dismissing symptoms (e.g., using terms such as "medically unexplained" or "you shouldn't be feeling that") and to ensure any distressing symptoms, such as pain or fatigue, are effectively managed.

Compassionate care also means consistency from familiar medical staff to help to build a trusting relationship, for example, by having a named point of contact, such as a specialist nurse and designated consultant. It is also important that patients can trust that healthcare providers understand the limits of their competencies. As such, consulting with specialist colleagues as needed, acknowledging the patient's lived experience, and taking their (and their families') concerns seriously is vital. In short, patients must feel confident in the attendant healthcare professional's clinical competency to feel psychologically safe; this includes being aware of competency limits and seeking advice and support as needed, particularly for more complex medical conditions.

> Many times, it was apparent that different nurses had different understandings of the basic regular procedures that were required. One notable procedure was the cleaning and maintenance of the PICC (peripherally inserted central catheter) line for infusions. There was considerable variation in the understanding of how this was to be done, leaving me a little bewildered and anxious about who I was going to get, when the next regular weekly process needed to happen. There was also considerable variation between staff of their ability to take bloods, which were required almost on a daily basis. Ultimately, I would always request to have a professional phlebotomist, if possible, since they were way better at it, however this wasn't always possible.
>
> —Richard, 60 years old, congenital heart condition, heart transplant recipient, United Kingdom

For people living with an LTC it is also important that healthcare professionals recognize that hospitals and medical teams are often a significant part of life and that repeated exposure to medical trauma can negatively affect feelings of psychological safety across the lifespan, especially in healthcare settings.

Compassion is also a cornerstone for palliative care, a type of healthcare or resource for individuals with a serious illness. It differs from a hospice, as it is not just for end-of-life care, and it can be helpful to anyone who is suffering in relation to their medical condition. Unlike a hospice, patients can continue to receive their curative treatments while receiving palliative care which focuses on helping individuals manage their symptoms, discomfort, and improve their quality of life. Some of the services that can be provided include pain management, the planning and coordination of care, and mental health treatment. Compassionate palliative care has been associated with improved quality of life and survival.[24]

> **How to Build Compassion**
>
> Our capacity for compassion can be strengthened. Compassion includes four components:
>
> - Bringing attention or awareness to recognizing that there is suffering (cognitive)
> - Feeling emotionally moved by that suffering (affective)
> - Wishing there to be relief from that suffering (intentional)
> - A readiness to act to relieve that suffering (motivational)

One of the most helpful things I recall as a child was when the nurses came to me after waking from surgery. The nurse would gently wash my hands and face and put me in my own nightclothes and told me to rest. At that point I felt safe again, I felt cared for. As a nurse, I remember doing that for my adult patients and it helped each patient to rest and recover. It's a shame that practice was later stopped in a bid to get patients looking after themselves as soon as awake. Kindness and compassion help such a lot in real terms with regards [to] recovery—physically and emotionally.
—**Sally, late 50s, congenital craniofacial condition, former nurse, psychotherapist, and PhD researcher, United Kingdom**

There have been several evidence-based systematic trainings for compassion. Mehta et al. report that while compassionate care is often discussed superficially in medical school curricula, it is seldom taught using a formal framework.[25] To address this gap, they developed an eight-session curriculum with a mindfulness-based approach to compassion. Seventeen fourth-year medical students completed the course, and the authors found that the students in the compassion curriculum showed a significant increase in self-compassion and total compassion and on the Toronto Mindfulness scale compared with controls. The authors conclude the course led to an enhanced ability to understand the human experience and to be motivated to alleviate human suffering.

It is important for healthcare professionals who are involved in training to remember that compassion (or a lack thereof) is taught through the hidden curriculum when trainee healthcare professionals observe mentors interacting with patients.

Further, simulated role play can develop communication skills and empathy training for medical students. One study analyzed videos of 20 students' performance playing the doctor role, using the Calgary-Cambridge Referenced Observation Guide (CCG). The authors report that both actor and student simulated role play improved empathy as measured using the Consultation and Relational Empathy (CARE) questionnaire. Although student rather than actor role play can help medical students better understand the role of the patient during medical encounters and is more cost-effective.[26]

Compassion mindfulness practices, such as the loving kindness meditation, can also help to improve compassion for self and others (see Appendix). Keeping a diary and incorporating self-reflection into practice with regular supervision can also support the development of a more compassionate stance.[27]

Virtual reality has also been proposed as a tool for empathy training in healthcare. It is suggested that by using simulations, healthcare professionals can gain a deeper understanding of their patient's perspective and experiences, aimed at fostering empathy and compassion. By wearing a VR headset, physicians can virtually "embody" patients who meet a series of socioemotional and medical challenges. For example, one study in New England adopted technology that teaches healthcare professionals to be empathetic with older adults. The VR software allows them to simulate being a patient with age-related diseases such as macular degeneration and hearing loss. The authors report this technology was successfully introduced as a new teaching modality to medical, physician assistant, physical therapy, and nursing curricula with enhanced students' understanding of age-related health problems and empathy for older adults.[28] While this is promising, it is difficult to see how VR can truly provide an embodied experience off illness and pain, and it is important this training is used mindfully and does not foster a false sense of living with an LTC.

Psychological Safety and Co-Regulation

Small kindnesses go a long way! A smile, a squeeze of the hand really helped me to feel reassured in difficult and scary times.
—Becky, 36, Ehlers-Danlos syndrome, postural orthostatic tachycardia syndrome (POTS), chronic fatigue, United Kingdom

Psychological safety is essential for healthcare workers due to its impact both on their well-being and on quality of patient care. Psychological safety is an essential characteristic of psychologically informed healthcare to facilitate social engagement, compassionate communication, understanding, and trust and to optimize the patient's ANS for rest and recovery. In other words, we need to recruit the patient's ANS in seeking health, rather than creating stressful conditions where it is further compromised. Polyvagal theory offers a way for healthcare professionals to better understand how they, their colleagues, and their patients are emotionally and physiologically responding to each other and their environment.[29]

Learning from Research and Practice: Barriers and facilitators to psychological safety during medical procedures among individuals diagnosed with chronic illness during childhood

In a recent study we explored barriers and facilitators to psychological safety during medical procedures among individuals diagnosed with chronic illnesses in childhood.[30] Using polyvagal theory as a framework, semistructured interviews were conducted with six participants (aged 20–64) who experienced chronic disease from a young age. The Neuroception of Psychological Safety Scale (NPSS) guided thematic exploration to understand participants' experiences. Thematic analysis found four key themes that reflect contributors and detractors to psychological safety during medical care: "Knowledge empowerment through information and facilitated inquiry," "Holistic acknowledgment of psychological and social impacts," "The role of parental involvement in healthcare interactions," and "Need for an individualized, patient-centered approach."

The first theme *"Knowledge empowerment through information and facilitated inquiry"* demonstrated that having access to clear information about their condition and procedures fostered a sense of control and confidence, while the lack of information often resulted in fear and helplessness highlighted in quotes such as:

"Doctors didn't actually tell you what was going on. They would ask you questions, and you were never encouraged to ask questions. They would tell you . . . and that was it."

"I'd never heard of the illness when I got it . . . it would have been great to have been informed that you know there were other people that suffer with it. . . . I think I probably didn't need to feel so ashamed."

A second theme *"Holistic acknowledgment of psychological and social impacts,"* reflected that participants felt that healthcare providers often focused solely on their physical health, neglecting the broader psychological and social impacts of chronic illness leaving them feeling unsupported in managing the full scope of their experiences. This theme included participant quotes such as:

> "I think it was crazy that there was never a psychologist in the room . . . you've just told a kid that they have a chronic illness. Their life is gonna change or had already changed."

> "I couldn't go out to play, I tired very easily. I didn't really have a lot of social interaction like with other children. I think everybody kinda had labelled you the kid with . . . the bad heart . . . You stop being a person to an extent."

A third theme *"The role of parental involvement in healthcare interactions"* reflected how participants described parental involvement as both a support and, at times, a limitation. While parents often provided a buffer against the challenges of navigating healthcare, their involvement sometimes led to difficulties when participants transitioned to managing their care independently highlighted by quotes such as:

> "I turned 18 and my mum was like 'you now need to start dealing with your own appointments' . . . I found it so overwhelming because I went from 'I just need to show up' to now 'I actually take charge of like my medication . . . it wasn't like you were kind of like phased into it. It was just like 'right you're 18 you gotta deal with it."

> "As a child I wouldn't really like to speak anyway, like my parents probably did most of speaking on my behalf. My mum anyway."

A final theme *"Need for an individualized, patient-centered approach"* emphasised the value of a personalised approach to care, with healthcare interactions tailored to individual needs and preferences. Psychological safety was enhanced when participants felt their unique perspectives were respected highlighted by quotes such as:

> "The way we did it was they held it in place but I pushed the buttons for it then to go in so I was in control . . . I've always had to be in control of the needle."

> "I was so anxious because I didn't know what he was going to tell me so he spent the first ten minutes just chatting about my family, chatting about things . . . and he just put me ease. I could feel myself kind of, you know, and breathe (mimics motion of breathing) so that I could actually then listen to what he was actually telling me."

Together the findings emphasize the importance of clear communication, psychological support, and a personalised, patient-centred approach in fostering psychological safety.

Via *co-regulation*, healthcare professionals can promote feelings of psychological safety for their patients during healthcare encounters and medical procedures. While parents and carers of children play an essential role in co-regulation with their child during medical procedures, PVT considers co-regulation as the reciprocal sending and receiving of signals of psychological safety that lies at the heart of human relationships. Co-regulation is the process by which our interactions with others help regulate emotional and physiological states of defense and safety through mutual comfort, support, and understanding, a bit like borrowing feelings from another. By applying the principles of PVT in co-regulation, healthcare professionals can better attune to their patient's (and their caregiver's) emotional and physiological state and navigate the complex challenges experienced in healthcare relationships. Safe, supportive relationships are instrumental in providing a foundation for trust during healthcare experiences. To this end, it is important for healthcare workers to feel within their window of psychological safety too.[31] As such, this is considered in more detail in Chapter 5.

We communicate cues of psychological safety and threat via our tone of voice, eye contact, facial expressions, physical proximity, language, and energy levels.[32] Nonverbal safety signaling includes pleasant facial expressions such as a smile, kind demeanor, a nod, or an interested and compassionate gaze. Gestures such as a warm and firm handshake, squeeze of the hand, or a gentle pat, thoughtful acts such as holding the door open or warming a stethoscope before using it, empathic words, a calm and warm tone of voice, orienting the body toward the other, and using the patients preferred name all convey psychological safety.

It can also be helpful for healthcare professionals to pay attention to these cues from their patients and their caregivers (e.g., whether their patient or caregiver is experiencing hyperarousal, the window of psychological safety, or hypoarousal). Defensive responses are completely natural when we are experiencing discomfort, when difficult memories are triggered, or in anticipation of hurt. All of these may be the case for a patient (and their caregiver) in the healthcare setting. As a result, the patient (and their caregiver) may be struggling to make eye contact, feel tense, and be holding themselves defensively. They may appear agitated or irritated, hypervigilant, their tone of voice may sound nervous or annoyed. They may be breathing rapidly; together these cues show they are in a fight or flight state of defense. In contrast, if they are feeling hypoaroused, they may appear "checked out" and disengaged, looking into the far distance, unable to take anything in. If they speak at all they may sound flat while eye contact may be fleeting or poor. They may passively agree to what is happening while taking little in (see Figure 3.2).

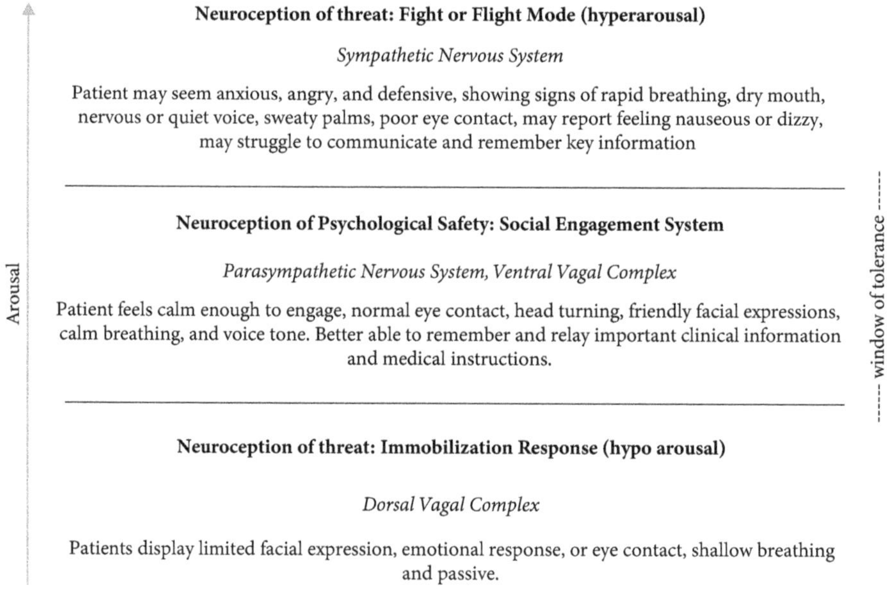

Neuroception of threat: Fight or Flight Mode (hyperarousal)

Sympathetic Nervous System

Patient may seem anxious, angry, and defensive, showing signs of rapid breathing, dry mouth, nervous or quiet voice, sweaty palms, poor eye contact, may report feeling nauseous or dizzy, may struggle to communicate and remember key information

---

Neuroception of Psychological Safety: Social Engagement System

Parasympathetic Nervous System, Ventral Vagal Complex

Patient feels calm enough to engage, normal eye contact, head turning, friendly facial expressions, calm breathing, and voice tone. Better able to remember and relay important clinical information and medical instructions.

Neuroception of threat: Immobilization Response (hypo arousal)

Dorsal Vagal Complex

Patients display limited facial expression, emotional response, or eye contact, shallow breathing and passive.

Figure 3.2 Using a polyvagal lens to improve understanding during healthcare encounters

By attuning to the patient's (and their caregiver's) emotional state and conveying psychological safety via social cues, such as a calm tone of voice, making eye contact, orienting their body toward the patient (and their caregiver), using reassuring and clear communication, and staying calm, healthcare staff can help patients (and their caregivers) to feel safer and build trust. Co-regulation and containment will enable patients (and their caregivers) to move toward their window of psychological safety. They will feel calmer and better able to socially engage, remember healthcare recommendations, and make important decisions.

To this end, for both healthcare professionals and patients (and their caregivers), it may help to build in short techniques to help to regulate ANS functioning. Deep, slow breathing can stimulate the vagus nerve, reduce anxiety, and boost the parasympathetic system. Further, mindfulness and meditation can stimulate the vagus nerve and improve vagal tone while somatic experiences, such as singing, humming, dancing, and touch, have also been linked to improved feelings of psychological safety. *Shaking it off* can help individuals soothe and calm themselves by releasing excess energy resulting from the stress response. Grounding and movement exercises are useful when we are in a state of hypo arousal. Various strategies to this end are outlined in the Appendix, which can be used as handouts for staff and patients.

Case Study: Dr. Jones

Dr. Jones has a busy clinic ahead. The day does not start well, as her childminder turns up late. When she arrives at work, her receptionist tells her that one of her patients had been on the phone and is unhappy because she was still awaiting a surgical slot. She feels herself bristling with tension. While she understands the patient's concerns, she is unable to bring the procedure forward due to a surgical backlog. She envisages a difficult conversation ahead. Her secretary breaks the news that the junior doctor has called in sick, and all his patients have been added to her clinic.

She feels stressed and overwhelmed. She steps into her clinic room. However, before calling the first patient, she takes some time to reflect on how she feels. She recognizes the stress in her body, relaxes her shoulders and takes some deep breaths. She takes a moment to ground herself in the here and now. She takes some time to plan for the day. She triages the patient list and asks her secretary to phone some of the less urgent cases, kindly explaining the situation, and to reschedule them over her next two clinics (unless their condition has changed, and they to be seen urgently). This feels more manageable, and she feels calmer. She calls her first patient into her clinic warmly and compassionately. She feels more present and can recognize and meet their distress with reassurance and her full attention.

Beyond Bravery Stickers: Providing a Safe Space for Feelings

I was a quiet child and was often told how brave and courageous I was. However, I was never sure if this was an observation, expectation, or demand. Often, I did not feel very brave, I just knew I did not have any other choice.[33] I was rewarded with a smiley sticker for keeping quiet and still while having stitches, chest drains, and pieces of medical equipment removed from my body; medical tests; and blood draws. My grandpa proudly called me his "Wee trouper," while children with congenital heart conditions are commonly called "Heart Warriors." While, as a child, these narratives fitted my experience of having to find the resolve to overcome each health crisis and they made me feel proud and strong while undoubtedly spurring me on, at times, they prevented me from expressing my distress lest I would no longer be seen as coping. Looking back, it would have helped if I had been told it was okay to cry, scream, or feel angry, even after the event, because these are normal responses to pain or threat.

War and battle metaphors are very common when you have an LTC; individuals are commonly told to keep fighting their condition and stay strong; children are rewarded for being a "good patient" with bravery stickers while some are even dressed up in superhero costumes in hospital settings and invited to ring a special bell for "beating" their condition. While most of this is done with the best of intentions and such metaphors can provide encouragement and a sense of agency, it is essential that we remain mindful of invalidating distress or creating a space where it does not feel okay to express a normal emotional response to difficult life experiences. This will only add to the burden of living with an LTC and feelings of isolation. Bravery can also mean showing vulnerability and it is important that people with LTCs are given space to do so.

A study by Hauser and Schwarz (2015)[34] reports that language of war can undermine health-promoting behavior. Specifically, metaphorically framing cancer as an enemy lessens the conceptual accessibility of and intention for self-limiting prevention behaviors. Further, if the individual experiences a decline in health and is perceived to have "lost the battle" this can negatively affect their self-worth. "Battling symptoms" may be a problematic approach for the management of an LTC, since acceptance and working with the body may lead to better health outcomes.[35]

Psychologically informed healthcare means recognizing and responding appropriately to emotions. It is understandable that anyone who is experiencing health difficulties, coping with daily symptoms, facing invasive tests and procedures, or receiving unwelcome news will at times have an emotional response to what is happening. During healthcare experiences they may feel uneasy, scared, lonely, or upset about the lack of control they have over what is happening to them. It is also common for family members to feel helpless, stressed, fatigued, and upset. Facilitating a safe space for patients and their families to process an understandable emotional reaction to their uniquely challenging life events is fundamental to supporting them, across the lifespan.

One study investigated strategies to embed emotional support from the perspectives of patients and clinicians employing focus group discussions (FGDs) and interviews from 11 patients, 2 carers, and 7 clinicians in the multidisciplinary care teams in an outpatient complex and chronic care setting in New South Wales, Australia.[36] Three main themes emerged from the experience of both the patients and clinicians: warmth and kindness, deep listening, and social connection in treatment.

Feelings convey messages about our needs. It is normal to feel anxious when we face uncertainty, pain, or threat. It is normal to feel sad if you experience a loss. Anger is a normal response to injustice or to disregard for personal boundaries. It is also common for children to express their feelings behaviorally or somatically. However, it is important to note that just because someone does not show any emotion this does not mean they are not in distress or pain; they may be in a state of hypoarousal or shock.

At times, a normal response to stress, pain, and discomfort can be discouraged in a clinical hospital environment. There can be rewards for being a "good patient" and suppressing a normal emotional response.

It is important to check in with how your patient feels. Emotional support means providing comfort, understanding, and listening to help patients and their families cope with any difficult feelings such as fear, sadness, and anxiety that may be associated with their health experiences. By empathically and calmly listening to them and providing a holding space you can validate their experience. Providing a safe space will better enable people to talk about the wider impact and raise any concerns and worries or ask tough questions they may have. This may include discussion about sexual health, exercise tolerance, pregnancy, relationships, menopause, aging, and palliative care.

> *While we encountered many shortcomings in various healthcare systems and faced numerous challenges with professionals, what helped us cope was having time to prepare and process. We had time to meet the people who would save our daughter's life, to make decisions in advance, or at least for my husband and me to get on the same page with each other and the doctors. However, the most significant source of strength came from other moms and stories of inspiration and hope. I once heard a doctor at a conference suggest that mothers should "pump the brakes" on positive stories, as they are not the norm and might paint a false reality. While I understand his point, those very stories helped me fight, not flee.*
> —Katarina, 42, daughter, now 6, born with a single-ventricle heart, Croatian living in Belgium

Active Listening: Sitting with Distress

> *Compassionate care requires honest and clear communication, active listening, considering the patients' economic and social needs, and referring patients to support services when applicable.*
> —Karla, 40 years old, congenital heart condition, United States

When we are experiencing adversity, often what we want is for someone to ask how we are feeling and to listen without judgment as we share our concerns and ask honest questions. Witnessing another person in distress can be challenging, and it is human nature to want to fix the problem. Sometimes healthcare professionals focus on medical tests and results and fixing the health problem. However, often this is not possible and there are many other aspects to living with an LTC. When we feel uncomfortable or unprepared to deal with someone expressing difficult feelings, we can try to shut down their distress to stop our own discomfort. However, the worst thing that can happen when we show vulnerability is to have our experiences invalidated. When we are experiencing difficult feelings, it is helpful to have another person provide a safe space and just listen to us express what we are feeling. When this is invalidated, we can lose trust in the other person.

Active listening involves paying close attention to what the other person is saying, through their facial expressions, body language, and spoken words. Active listening is a skill that can be learned. It is important to keep eye contact, let the person lead the conversation, avoid interruptions, and give them your full attention. Active listening involves suspending our usual ways of responding, such as giving advice, responding with clichés, quick fixes, or pity. It means concentrating on what the person is saying, and what they are not saying.

Helpful responses include using minimal prompts to encourage more speaking, reflecting back by paraphrasing or summarizing what they have said. Paraphrasing by summarizing and rephrasing the important things that are said helps develop more fluid responding. This involves concentrating on the "feeling" words, reflecting back the meaning of what has been said and picking out key words and phrases. For example, "It sounds like you are experiencing a lot of pain" while acknowledging what they are telling you and using phrases such as "This must be very difficult," "I am sorry you are going through this," "I know staying positive can be hard, how are you really?" Let them cry if they need to, avoid giving unnecessary advice or using humor unless they have used it themselves.[37]

Common obstacles to listening include, interrupting, reassuring, trying to stop someone crying, minimizing experiences, getting distracted by details, making assumptions and judgments, talking about ourselves, and offering quick fix solutions. Further, asking closed questions, generalizing, or using clichés can be unhelpful. Try and not compare your patient's experience to others by saying things like "Well, other people have it a lot worse," "Usually people with this condition don't feel this way," "This is the first time we have heard about this symptom, I don't think it is related to your condition," "You just need to get on with it now," or "Your probably just a bit anxious." When we are upset, it is often enough to feel heard. Listening to what your patient is telling you, validating their experience, acknowledging how difficult it must be, can help.

Listening can be broken down into stages: receiving, understanding, evaluating, remembering, and responding. Each stage is crucial in the healthcare setting, where missing or misinterpreting information can have significant consequences.[38]

It is okay to acknowledge that you do not have all of the answers, but it can be helpful to provide some hope by saying that you can discuss any unsolved queries with other colleagues, refer them to another specialist or by reminding them that medical science is constantly bringing new solutions (although be careful about creating false hope). If you feel that your patient would benefit from further emotional support, then referring them on to counseling or psychological therapy may be indicated. It can also be helpful to work with and direct patients to organizations that can offer further support. This may be practical (financial, help with household tasks, getting a lift to appointments, lifestyle advice, and advocacy about education, employment, finances, life insurance and travel), emotional (peer support groups, therapy, or spiritual), or advocacy (nonprofit organizations related to their condition).

It is important to note that neurodivergent individuals may communicate differently. This could manifest in less eye contact, more limited body language, and more blunt and unfiltered use of language. When in conversation with neurodivergent individuals, practice content-oriented actions like paraphrasing, summarizing, and asking questions to help the other person feel heard. Further, if someone is very anxious, they may be in hypoarousal, which may also lead to less eye contact and more limited body language.

> **Key Active Listening Skills**
>
> - Be attentive.
> - Refrain from judgment.
> - Attend to body language.
> - Ask open-ended questions.
> - Use minimal responses to encourage the speaker.
> - Request clarification.
> - Paraphrase.
> - Be attuned to and reflect feelings.
> - Summarize, share, and reflect.

Active Listening Skills Exercises

Role play is a useful way to develop active listening skills[39] and compassion. With a colleague, take turns as the patient and as the healthcare professional. This can also be done in a triad with an additional person acting as an observer to provide formative feedback to both the speaker and listener. Triad work is an effective way to develop clinical skills by transforming knowledge to practice and increasing self-efficacy.[40]

Exercise 1: Listening Without Interrupting

This exercise will help you develop attentive listening skills.

- Find a quiet place where you can speak without distractions.
- The speaker should talk about something important to them (but not too triggering) for 4 minutes.
- The listener should listen without interrupting or interjecting, focusing on the key takeaways, the main themes, what matters most to the speaker, and what interests them most.
- After 4 minutes, the listener should share what they think they heard the speaker say.
- The speaker should be given the opportunity to clarify any misunderstandings.
- If there is an observer, they can provide feedback to the speaker and listener.

Exercise 2: Active Listening

Practice active listening with a colleague. Take turns to share a story of something emotional (but not too triggering) that happened, and the listener will practice the following techniques:

- Listener should demonstrate listening through body language and nonverbal responses.
- Listener should reflect back the content of what the speaker shared.
- Listener should reflect back the emotions that the speaker shared.
- Listener should check in the speaker (and observer) for feedback.

Fiona has been attending cardiology appointments since childhood due to a single-ventricle heart condition. While she had always known that she might need a heart transplant one day she did not expect that day to come so soon. At her appointment, her cardiologist and specialist nurse recommended that she go on the transplant waiting list. They have prepared for the consultation, ensuring they have plenty of time and privacy and by establishing that she wants her partner present during difficult news. The cardiologist makes sure that they are facing Fiona and her partner, ensures that he meets their gaze and gently delivers the news. Fiona starts to cry, and the nurse lets her know that this is completely understandable, that they are all there for her and her family, and that as a team they will ensure that she gets the best care possible. They give her and her partner plenty of time to ask any questions, provide a direct number for any queries following today's meeting, and let them know about the next steps. They also organize a session with the specialist psychologist and provide information about a nonprofit organization that supports patients facing transplant and some leaflets about facing transplant.

Questions to Ask Your Patients to Support Mental Health and Well-Being

Don't sugar coat the news. Don't say it's not a big deal, because it usually is. Please don't tell me I worry too much. Please speak with me, not to me, and use kindness, compassion and honesty.
—Alex, 57 years, congenital heart condition, United States

Listed below are some questions it may be useful to use in supporting your patient's mental health and well-being. It may be useful to use patient prompt sheets and concern inventories that patients can complete and bring along to their appointment to help them to express any concerns and feel heard.

- How are you feeling generally?
- What are your biggest worries about your health and well-being?
- Does thinking about your health make you feel worried, low or afraid?
- What is important to you?
- Would you like to discuss longer term health outcomes?
- Do you have someone to talk to about your concerns?
- Would you find it useful to have someone to talk to?
- It is understandable if you feel overwhelmed, you have a lot to deal with. How can we help?

Delivering Difficult News

> *Some barriers (to good care) may include providers being poorly trained in how to communicate difficult news, overbooked schedules (needing to rush to the next patient), and a lack of awareness around the mental health impacts of living with a chronic health condition.*
> —Karla, 40 years old, congenital heart condition, United States

Delivering difficult news can be one of the most challenging parts of working as a healthcare professional. One study, conducted in the US, found that while 93% of surgeons that took part in the study perceived being able to deliver bad news as an important skill, only 43% felt they had been adequately trained to do so, and 85% felt they needed additional training.[41] The authors report that during such encounters doctors commonly fear being blamed and unable to answer questions while having to manage their own feelings about illness and death. In turn, poorly trained healthcare professionals can deliver challenging news in an insensitive manner while emotionally disengaging from their patient. This can damage the patient–doctor relationship, negatively affect the patient's adjustment to their condition (or their loved one's), and contribute to medical trauma.

> *Our daughter's heart problem was diagnosed in utero. A doctor in Beirut, Lebanon, where we lived at the time, noticed that her heart was not developing properly at my 12-week pregnancy check-up. To say I was numb from the news is an understatement. I vividly remember my heartbeat pounding in my throat, saliva filling my mouth, fear flushing my body, and my eyes burning because I forgot to blink. These memories are as vivid now as they were then as I feel it all the same now, just thinking about it. Yet, I also remember the doctor's respectfulness, the time he gave us during that and following appointments, and how he answered all our questions.*
> —Katarina, 42, daughter, now 6, born with a single-ventricle heart, Croatian living in Belgium

---

Guidance for Delivering Difficult News

A patient- and family-centered approach to delivering difficult news is recommended, including the patient's loved ones when possible (with the patient's consent). The location should be quiet, comfortable, and private without interruptions and ample time. Various protocols for delivering difficult news have been proposed which inform the following steps.[42,43]

> **Preparation**: Establish a suitable time, space, and information to be shared while being sensitive to the patient's cultural, religious, and spiritual beliefs. Establish available social support and whether the patient would prefer a family member or friend to be present.
>
> **Information Acquisition**: Establish what the patient already knows, how much they want to know, what they believe about their condition.
>
> **Information Sharing**: Preferably done in person, build rapport, ask for the patient's information preferences and any learning or communications difficulties, compassionately deliver the news in language that can be understood by the patient, consider chunking information, validate any emotions, allow emotional expression, and answer any questions. Convey some measure of hope.
>
> **Clarification/"Teach Back"**: Ensure the message is understood, provide details about a contact point for further questions, inform them about any further support, and summarize the encounter.
>
> **Self-care**: Acknowledge your own feelings about the encounter, the impact it had on you physically, emotionally, and psychologically. Take a few moments to ground yourself and reach out for support from a colleague, supervisor, or supportive manager if needed.

Establishing Trust with Children

Thestrup et al. report that while communication skills are important, they are often neglected during pediatric medical training. They conducted a study that explored children and adolescents' perceptions of healthcare professionals using narrative and play-based interviews to include the perceptions of 8 preschool children aged 3–6 years and an online questionnaire to explore those of 54 schoolchildren and adolescents aged 5–18 years. They employed thematic analysis of the qualitative interview data and open-ended questionnaire responses and found that preschool children found familiar approaches, physical contact, and their parents comforting and that healthcare professionals should use playful methods, child-friendly words, and tangible rewards.[44]

Piet Leroy, professor in procedural sedation and analgesia in children at Maastricht University, has led pioneering work combining pediatrics and medical education. In a recent review Leroy and colleagues note that establishing trust is a foundational skill for healthcare providers who care for children. Trust helps to manage the child's emotional state, elicit cooperation, and create a positive experience.[45] Yet, the authors report that there is no systematic approach or formal training for developing this skill set for healthcare professionals. They propose a framework to this end that involves a cyclical process of perceiving, accurately interpreting, and appropriately responding to the child's verbal and nonverbal cues. By assessing the child's emotional state and employing engagement methods healthcare professionals can help to alleviate fear and establish trust. Continuously observing and iteratively adapting their behavior and communication style in response to the child's emotional state is part of this process. The authors propose a range of techniques to support this approach including arousing the child's curiosity, use of appropriate vocal tone and body language, matching the child's nonverbal cues (mirroring), desensitization to any objects that may be used during the medical procedure, incorporating guided play, and distraction.[46] This approach is consistent with psychologically informed healthcare by adopting co-regulation to establish psychological safety through relational cues, empowerment, and compassion.

Dr. Smith always keeps a teddy bear and a play medical kit in her clinic room. She invites her pediatric patients to listen to the teddy's heart with the child's stethoscope when she is listening to theirs. She has noticed this helps them to feel more relaxed, trusting and in control. If they bring their own toy, she invites them to listen to its heart too. Sometimes she asks them how they think teddy is feeling and what would help him when they are struggling to describe their own feelings.

Caring for Teenagers

When I reached my teens, I started to feel self-conscious about attending a children's hospital surrounded by babies and young children. The walls of the hospital were covered in cartoon characters, when I lay on a bed for tests or procedures there was often an infant mobile hanging from the ceiling. Toys and books in waiting areas were provided to amuse young children, but there was little to entertain a teenager. There was no formal transition process back then, I just moved to an adult cardiology service in my late teens. I felt bereft at leaving my much-loved cardiology team, whom I'd known since birth, and the hospital that felt like a second home to me. Unfortunately, adult care provision had not developed in time to meet the needs of the growing population of adults with congenital heart conditions, there was no specialist congenital cardiology service to move to, leaving us as "medical orphans." Consequently, throughout my 20s, I was seen in a routine cardiology service, attending a pacing clinic with people who were mostly over the age of 60. This added to my sense of feeling different and isolated in my healthcare experiences. I have had to advocate for the specialist care I need since, leading to my campaign efforts for better care.

While WIFI access and mobile devices mean that adolescents are better able to amuse themselves in these settings, it remains the case that adolescents' needs are different from both adults and children, and it is important to consider this in hospital and healthcare settings.

The Teenage Cancer Trust recommends specialist wards for teenagers aged 13–18 years old, yet one study found that many adolescents are being admitted to children's hospitals where they are not cared for in age-appropriate environments.[47] Teenagers face different challenges to younger children including puberty, balancing increasing amounts of schoolwork and exams, and navigating relationships with friends. At a time when they want to fit in, being unwell or attending healthcare appointments can make them feel different and isolated from their peers, affecting their developing self-esteem and autonomy. Adolescents may find it harder to share their concerns, feel more self-conscious, particularly about having physical examinations, and have a greater need for privacy. It is important that healthcare providers are sensitive to these needs, particularly for individuals who have an ongoing condition. Specifically, Thestrup et al. found that schoolchildren and adolescents preferred healthcare professionals who were friendly, patient, attentive, communicated clearly, and engaged them in conversation.[48] They did not like it when healthcare professionals appeared stressed, did not keep their promises, or forced them to do something. Building trust, providing a named point of contact, and limiting the number of people who come in and out of the clinic room are all important aspects of care. Asking the patient whether they want their parent or caregiver present, especially during physical examinations or sensitive conversations is also important.

Some hospitals have created dedicated calming spaces for teenagers moving to adult care. The Bristol Heart Institute outpatients' waiting area has been enhanced with calming wall murals aiming to help young patients as they transfer from children's services to the adult setting and to support patients who present with learning disability or who are neurodiverse. These changes were developed in consultation with a learning disabilities team and young people with lived experience.[49]

Alex has needed regular scans due to a health condition from childhood. However, since reaching puberty he has become very self-conscious. His mum used to accompany him during these tests, but he no longer wants her to see him in a revealing hospital gown. A nurse notices how uncomfortable he is and discreetly asks him about his preferences. Alex tells her that while he still wants his mum to come along to appointments with him, he would prefer it if she waited for him in the waiting room during these tests and procedures. The nurse facilitates a conversation with Alex and his mum to gently ensure this happens and that as few people as possible are present during these encounters.

Seasons of Life: Transition to Adult Care

Moving from your childhood healthcare providers to an adult service can be challenging. This occurs at a time when lots of life changes are taking place and can evoke a range of feelings like anxiety, loss, and hope. Guidelines recommend that young people are involved in decision-making about their healthcare.[50] Transition to adult care should be supported in a way that is developmentally appropriate considering their maturity, cognitive abilities, psychological status, needs in terms of long-term conditions, social and personal circumstances, and communication needs. Transition should be strength based, person-centered and support the young person to make decisions and build their confidence in directing their healthcare. Healthcare professionals should work in an integrated way to ensure smooth and gradual transition, across health, social care, and education.

Key Recommendations for Communicating with Children

Attitude and Appearance
DO

- ✓ Say hello and introduce yourself
- ✓ Know the child/adolescent's name
- ✓ Smile and have a calm, kind appearance
- ✓ Be patient and avoid forcing anything
- ✓ Take time to talk
- ✓ Use humor and jokes if the child/adolescent is open to this

DON'T

- × Appear stressed, as the child/adolescent may think you are angry
- × Leave in the middle of a conversation
- × Scold or nag
- × Use humor or jokes if the child/adolescent is not open to this
- × Tell the child/adolescent that they look good/fine if they do not feel well

Participation and Understanding
DO

- ✓ Talk directly to the child/adolescent
- ✓ Talk about things other than illness or treatment
- ✓ Provide information according to age and developmental level
- ✓ Choose words carefully and provide information in appropriate doses
- ✓ Ask how the child/adolescent feels physically and mentally
- ✓ Ask the child/adolescent how much information they would like
- ✓ Prepare the child/adolescent for procedures and treatment

DON'T

- × Talk too fast
- × Talk over the child/adolescent's head and talk only to parents
- × Ask the same question over and over
- × Talk to adolescents as if they do not understand anything

Relationship and Trust
DO

- ✓ Make clear agreements
- ✓ Let the child/adolescent know what you are going to do before you do it
- ✓ Engage in play and activities
- ✓ Distract the child/adolescent during unpleasant procedures
- ✓ Acknowledge the child/adolescent (e.g., after a procedure)

DON'T

- × Do something that has not been agreed on first
- × Force the child/adolescent to do something against their will[51]

Caring for Older Adults

Older people can experience inequality of treatment when it comes to accessing healthcare services and in the standard of care provided. This can result from physical, communication, and other barriers. It is important to speak to older adults with dignity and respect, as individuals, bearing in mind their sociocultural background. They want to be listened to and supported to make their own decisions, as much as possible. Older adults may prefer more formal language and to be addressed using their title (e.g., Mr. or Mrs.). Ask patients which name they prefer. They may be more reluctant to ask questions or challenge healthcare professionals, which can leave them with unanswered queries.

It is important to be aware of any communication difficulties, cognitive impairment, or mobility issues. They may require assistance with technology, form filling, or being escorted around the healthcare setting. Making sure your patient can hear and see you, face them directly, try to match your communication style to that of the patient, take time, allow for questions; using clarification to check the patient has understood, provide a written summary of the encounter and language assistance if required.

Including family members or carers, at the discretion of the patient, may be useful, but ensure you include the patient in any conversation about their care. Ask the companion to step out of the consultation room during physical examinations and to enable some opportunity for sensitive topics. Take time to provide clear explanations about any diagnosis and medication regime and include them in their treatment plan, especially when this involves lifestyle changes.[52]

Kirsty gets to the hospital as soon as she can when she finds out that her elderly mother has been admitted, but she lives quite far away, and it is a long drive. She is shocked to find her on the ward, sitting by her bed, in a revealing hospital gown. Her mum always takes pride in her appearance and looks lost, cold and like a shadow of herself. Kirsty is terribly upset to see her like this. The first thing that Kirsty does is get her mum dressed in some nice pajamas and a dressing gown and brushes her hair.

Hidden Patients: Supporting Carers

Caring for a loved one with significant health needs can take its toll. It is important for healthcare providers to check in on caregivers and be mindful of signs of illness, stress, and burnout. Be mindful that parents may be disempowered during their child's healthcare experiences and feel obliged to comply with doctors and reluctant to voice concerns to ensure their child gets the best care. Referring or signposting carers on additional support, in addition to ensuring the patient has other support to enable respite, may be indicated.

> **Reflective Exercise: Age-Appropriate Care**
>
> Consider your healthcare service across different patient ages.
>
> - Does your organization consider the age of patients and differing needs?
> - In what ways could this be improved?
>
> What organizational facilitators and barriers are there to making these changes?

Trauma-Informed Healthcare

Trauma-informed care also underpins psychologically informed healthcare. Being trauma informed involves recognizing when someone has been affected by trauma and collaboratively adjusting your work to consider this. For example, feeling safe has also been found to improve healing and recovery during maternity care of women who have experienced childhood sexual trauma, while feeling unsafe with professionals could be experienced as retraumatization.[53]

Trauma-informed care involves responding in a way that supports recovery and does no harm while also recognizing and supporting people's resilience. Ken Epstein, licensed clinical social worker of the San Francisco Department of Public Health, proposes that being "trauma informed" is underpinned by the four 4 R's:

- Realizing how common the experience of trauma and adversity is
- Recognizing the diverse ways that trauma can affect people
- Responding by taking account of the ways that people can be affected by trauma to support recovery
- Resisting retraumatization and offering a greater sense of choice and control, empowerment, collaboration, and safety with everyone that you have contact with.

Healthcare staff are often not familiar with the impact of trauma. Professional codes of conduct need improved i.e. radiology say they have to ask if someone is breastfeeding and/or pregnant even though they have medical evidence that indicates that that would not be physically possible. Hospital systems also need improving—on admission for surgery I was asked the same questions by 4 different professionals which I found triggering/upsetting. Is it not possible to have a flag on my hospital records to remove inappropriate questions etc.?
   —Sarah, 44 years old, undergoing breast cancer treatment, United Kingdom

The San Francisco Department of Public Health (SFDPH) developed and implemented a Trauma-Informed Systems Initiative, an organizational model to address trauma at the systems level.[54] They report six core principles that underpin this approach:

1. Understanding Trauma & Stress
2. Compassion & Dependability
3. Safety & Stability
4. Collaboration & Empowerment
5. Cultural Humility & Responsiveness
6. Resilience & Recovery

Many of the aspects of care described in this book are consistent with a trauma-informed approach to healthcare delivery. As such, trauma-informed organizations embed the principles of safety, compassion, trustworthiness, choice, collaboration, and empowerment into all aspects of their work, for example, through consistency of care. They commit to ensuring that physical environments, staff behavior, and organizational policies and procedures reflect trauma-informed principles and systems. Trauma-informed healthcare organizations also consider the needs of healthcare workers in responding to people affected by trauma and aim to prevent vicarious trauma.

What has become clear to me is that it helps if the doctor, healthcare professional, actually gives shape to seeing me as a human being rather than as (only) the patient-part of that human being. And also makes himself known a little more than just as the practitioner/executor of medical-technical diagnostics and procedures. I understand that a doctor does not want to and cannot form a deep personal bond with all his patients. That's not necessary, you can't and don't have to become each other's friends. But especially in the case of people with a chronic, fairly serious condition, your regular doctor is more than just a passer-by. A substantial degree of familiarity with each other is helpful to the patient. It is good to discuss this as a doctor and patient. A conversation about how to deal with each other, how to shape the (collaborative) working relationship.

—Roy, 57, complex congenital heart disease, Netherlands

Reflective Exercise: Trauma-Informed Organizations

Consider your organization from the perspective of a patient or client with a history of medical trauma and an ongoing chronic health condition. In your mind, put yourself in their position and consider what they might experience when they try to contact your service to report distressing symptoms, when they are waiting to hear back about an appointment, when they are given details about an appointment, their travel to the healthcare setting, walking into the organization, meeting with reception staff, sitting in the waiting area, during the consultation, undergoing any examinations, tests, or procedures, and after the consultation. Consider:

- Are all touch points in your organization trauma-informed?
- What are the strengths in your organization?
- What could be done better, big, and small?
- What organizational barriers are there to improving this service, and how can they be addressed?

Recognizing Mental Health Difficulties

While psychologically informed healthcare aims to protect mental health, this approach recognizes that, for some, distress related to living with an LTC can develop into conditions such as post-traumatic stress disorder (PTSD), health anxiety, needle phobia, or depression. It is helpful to be able to aware of the symptoms of these mental health conditions to ensure referral on to a mental health professional, for assessment and treatment, when further support is indicated. As such these are outlined below. It is important to note that comorbidity of psychological conditions is common, often due to the same underlying contributing factors, for example comorbidity between eating disorders, anxiety, and depression is high while a mixed presentation of anxiety and depression is common for people with underlying low self-esteem.[55]

Recognizing Health Anxiety

A survey of over 25, 000 adults presenting to outpatient clinics (cardiology, respiratory medicine, endocrine or gastroenterology) revealed that twenty percent were experiencing significant *health anxiety*.[56] Health anxiety is when you spend so much time worrying that you are ill, or going to get ill, that it starts to take over your life.

Anxiety is a very physical emotion that affects the heart, breathing, muscle tension, and digestive system, and can lead to symptoms like headaches, a racing heartbeat, or upset stomach. These bodily feelings can understandably be misinterpreted as symptoms of a health condition, which can lead to a vicious cycle where the individual becomes hypervigilant. This can develop into "safety seeking" behaviors such as scanning the body for symptoms; frequently checking the body for signs of illness (such as lumps, tingling, or pain); finding it difficult to focus on other things; persistently asking family, friends, or healthcare providers for reassurance; worrying that a doctor or medical tests may have missed something, obsessively look at health information on the internet or in the media, and avoiding anything to do with serious illness, such as medical TV programs and physical activities.

Some people experiencing significant worry may contact their health team with great frequency, which can result in higher healthcare use and expenses. They may also present with "avoidance behaviors" such as missed clinic appointments, avoiding physical activity, or not taking medications as recommended, which can be perceived as nonadherence by healthcare professionals. Over time, health anxiety can undermine their confidence, leading to diminished social activity, missed education or work, and social isolation.

Understandably, it can be difficult for people with an LTC to distinguish between benign symptoms and more serious issues, especially if similar feelings in the past have indicated a serious health problem.[57] Further, such individuals may have experienced missed diagnosis or issues accessing appropriate care in the past, which understandably may contribute to their anxiety. Individuals with chronic illnesses often face difficult balancing acts, whereby they are asked to stay attentive to changes in health symptoms that might call for medical attention yet refrain from unnecessary health-related thoughts or behaviors. Compassionately understanding this and taking the time to validate and explore any concerns can help. Health anxiety can have a profound impact on day-to-day functioning and management of an LTC, yet it is a treatable condition. If you think a patient is experiencing this psychological condition, then referral to a practitioner psychologist for further support is indicated.

Recognizing PTSD

Trauma comes from the Greek word traûma, which means wound. People with an LTC may be exposed to medically related traumatic events. First, it is important to note that experiencing a traumatic event does not mean that someone will develop a trauma disorder, most people who experience a traumatic event fully recover.

Bearing in mind the impact of trauma on the brain, described in Chapter 1, following exposure to a traumatic event, it is normal for people to replay the event in their mind, often as nightmares and flashbacks. This helps them to make sense of what has happened, especially if they were too overwhelmed to process what was going on at the time. Following these challenging situations, it is also common and understandable to feel anxious, angry, guilty, and sad. They may have trouble sleeping, continue to feel hypervigilant after the situation is over, avoid reminders of the trauma, or block out thinking about it.

These signs are a normal response to an unusually difficult situation. Usually, they will fade in the days and weeks after the event. However, sometimes they persist and develop into the more serious anxiety disorder known as Post Traumatic Stress Disorder (PTSD).[58] Historically associated with soldiers returning from combat and initially termed "shell shock,"[59] PTSD often develops when the individual did not have the resources they needed during and after the traumatic event. Many of the symptoms of PTSD are essentially normal responses to trauma that do not "switch off." If they persist or get worse for more than one month after the traumatic incident, however, treatment may be indicated.

PTSD can include symptoms such as hypervigilance, difficulty sleeping, poor concentration, low mood, decreased interest in things, self-blame, emotional and physical reactivity after exposure to traumatic reminders (often sensory in nature, such as smells and sounds), and reliving of the traumatic event as nightmares and/or flashbacks. Flashbacks are when we respond to memories of past events as if they are happening in the here and now, rather than unpleasant memories from the past. For example, someone may smell disinfectant which takes them back to feeling like they did when they were being anesthetized in an operating theater.

Complex PTSD can develop following repeated, interpersonal, and traumatic events, often during childhood. Symptoms include pervasive shame and guilt, difficulty regulating emotions, dissociation, relationship difficulties, and engaging in risky behaviors.

Certain factors can increase the risk of developing a trauma disorder following exposure to a traumatic event including feeling helpless and hopeless during the incident, poor social support during and following the incident, perceived life-threat, an accumulation of traumatic events, other background life stressors, and preexisting physical and mental health problems. Whereas protective factors can improve mental health outcomes, mitigating the impact of psychological trauma. These may include adequate social support and help seeking, being able to control some aspects of what is happening to you, feeling like you did the best you could during the event, and being able to access psychological support.[60] PTSD is associated with adverse health outcomes and high medical utilization and cost. It is twice as common in women and is associated with increased risk for a range of diseases, chronic conditions, and reproductive-health problems.[61]

Common Symptoms of PTSD:

- Irritability or anger
- Nightmares or disturbing dreams of the traumatic event
- Tearfulness
- Anxiety
- Returning, upsetting memories about the event
- Insomnia
- Having a startle response, for instance jumping when you hear a loud noise or siren
- Going out of your way to avoid any exposure to the hospital or your care team
- Inability to concentrate

PTSD is a treatable condition. If you think a patient is experiencing this psychological condition, then referral for further support is indicated.

Recognizing Medically Related Trauma

Medical trauma is a type of PTSD. It does not have to be because of a procedure going wrong, it can also be a response to a routine diagnosis, operation, or treatment. Traumatic stress symptoms are common among individuals following medical experiences. One meta-analysis suggests approximately 1 in 5 adults admitted to intensive care experience traumatic stress symptoms 12 months after discharge.[62] Further, a systematic review of PTSD diagnosis in adults with cardiovascular disease found prevalence rates of up to 38%[63] and meta-analytic data suggest a lifetime prevalence rate of 12.6% among individuals who have had cancer.[64] Individuals with PTSD, especially when triggered by a medical trauma, are less likely to adhere to medical advice. A trauma response can often be the result of an elevated level of stress preceding, during, or following the medical procedure.

Symptoms of medical trauma can vary in intensity and may include, but are not limited to:

- Fear of medical settings or medical staff
- Physical sensations, such as pain, sweating, feeling sick, or discomfort
- Repetitive negative thoughts about the medical experience
- Avoidance or emotional numbing
- Irritability
- Associated feelings of depression and anxiety

It is interesting to note the strong link between trauma and smell.[65] The primitive olfactory system and the limbic system, which is involved in memory and emotion, are closely linked. Research has shown that memory for smells that are associated with intense emotional experiences, are more closely connected to affect than other sensory experiences and serve as potent contextual cues for memory formation and emotional conditioning. "Hospital smells" can be strong, for example of antiseptic and cleaning products, oxygen masks, and numbing creams that are used pre-injection, and may become triggers for olfactory flashbacks. Mitigating strong smells in healthcare practice may benefit patients, particularly for people who find specific smells triggering.

It is essential that anyone experiencing medically related post-traumatic stress can access prompt and appropriate psychological support, especially considering that they are likely to have to return to healthcare settings for ongoing medical monitoring and treatment.

Recognizing Phobias

Sam developed needle phobia following an unpleasant experience as a child during which she fainted when having blood taken. Since then, she has avoided getting blood work done. However, her healthcare team have requested blood samples to assess her current health. When she arrives at the appointment, the phlebotomist recognizes how anxious Sam is. After speaking to her she delays taking her bloods and speaks with her healthcare team who refer Sam to a psychologist to address her needle phobia.

A phobia is an overwhelming fear of a specific object, place, situation, feeling, or animal that is usually associated with a particular incident or trauma. For example, social phobia is a fear of social situations.

Needle phobia is common among adults and can be associated with other medical fears while traumatic childhood medical experiences can contribute to its development. A phobia of needles may develop following a difficult experience of having blood taken. Needle phobia can prevent individuals from adhering to clinical recommendations and accessing medical treatment when needed. For example, while insulin therapy is the mainstay treatment for the management of diabetes, non-adherence to insulin therapy is not uncommon, often linked to a fear of needles.[66]

For many people, fear of needles is associated with fainting or feeling faint, when something triggers their fear (such as the sight of blood or a needle). In response to the trigger their blood pressure drops, which can cause them to faint. It is important for healthcare professionals to be aware of this so they can help them to cope during the procedure. Applied tension can help patients increase their blood pressure to avoid fainting while breathing exercises can help them to relax.

It is important for healthcare professionals to recognize the difference between dislike and a clinically significant phobia. If you think a patient is experiencing this psychological condition, then referral for further support is important. Needle phobia is highly treatable, for example, by using a trauma-informed cognitive-behavioral approach with graded exposure to the feared stimulus.

Recognizing Obsessive Compulsive Disorder

Obsessive compulsive disorder is an anxiety condition dominated by obsessive thoughts or images, commonly incongruous or with the person's values (i.e., ego dystonic), followed by compulsive behaviors and rituals. Obsessive thoughts tend to center around hygiene, harming self or others, or being inappropriate, and they may cause much distress. They are often followed by compulsive behaviors to try and prevent or neutralize distressing thoughts. Behaviors can be overt such as handwashing or switching plugs on and off, or they can be mental rituals, such as counting or replaying a situation over in your mind looking for evidence of wrongdoing (sometimes called pure OCD). OCD can be debilitating and take over someone's life. Cognitive-behavioral therapy approaches have a compelling evidence base in the treatment of OCD by implementing graded exposure to the feared trigger and response prevention in combination with psychoeducation and relaxation techniques.[67] Studies have linked physical health problems with increased prevalence of OCD, particularly for females, older adults, and those experiencing longer duration of untreated illness.[68,69]

Recognizing Panic Disorder

Individuals suffering from *panic disorder* experience panic attacks. This is when the body's alarm system is triggered due to a false threat, often a traumatic reminder or an accumulation of stressors. During a panic attack, individuals may experience symptoms such as a racing heart rate, chest pain, rapid breathing, sweating, nausea, and brain fog. While these symptoms are a normal part of the *fight or flight* response, people often report that during a panic attack they believe they are at risk of dying, collapsing, suffering from a heart attack, or are making a fool of themselves. *Panic attacks* are debilitating and after experiencing one, many individuals worry about it happening again and start to avoid anything they associate as a trigger (such as the place where it happened or what they were doing at the time). This can get in the way of daily life and develop into a vicious cycle which can seriously impair functioning. Panic disorder is treatable using psychological therapy.[70] Studies have found that people with panic disorder are at higher risk of developing cardiovascular, respiratory, and gastrointestinal problems than the general population. Further, people with panic disorder commonly share other comorbidities, including OCD, social phobia, asthma, Chronic obstructive pulmonary disease (COPD), irritable bowel syndrome, hypertension, and mitral valve prolapse.[71]

Recognizing Generalized Anxiety

Feeling anxious for an extended period is termed *generalized anxiety disorder* (GAD). This debilitating condition is characterized by almost constant worry, restlessness, physical symptoms of anxiety, and difficulty sleeping. GAD is treatable using psychological therapy.[72] GAD can also lead to or worsen other physical health conditions, such as digestive or bowel problems, irritable bowel syndrome or ulcers, headaches and migraines, chronic pain, and illness.[73]

Recognizing Depression

We all experience low mood occasionally, which may include sadness, anger, frustration, and irritability. It is normal to experience these feelings at times, especially when dealing with hardship or loss. Often these feelings are a normal and understandable response to difficult life circumstances. However, if these feelings are not dealt with, they can contribute to more serious mental health problems such as depression. *Depression* is more than low mood or a normative reaction to loss. It is a serious mental health condition that indicates specialist treatment. Depression is closely linked to physical health.[74,75] Depression can also cause physical symptoms, while untreated depression can contribute to medical nonadherence.[76]

Red Flag Signs and Symptoms of Depression

- Loss of interest in activities you used to enjoy
- Withdrawing from family and friends
- Lack of concentration
- Feeling overwhelmed, indecisive
- Loss of confidence and low self-worth
- Increased alcohol and drug use
- Sleep problems (sleeping too much or too little)
- Feeling helpless, worthless, and guilty
- Increased irritability, anger, mood swings
- Feeling sad most of the time
- Inappropriate or excessive guilt
- Negative or depressed thinking
- Suicidal thoughts or self-harming behaviors

Physical health problems can be a risk factor for suicide and self-harm.[77] If you think a patient is experiencing depression, then referral for psychological support is indicated. If they are experiencing suicidal thoughts with intent, then immediate mental health and risk assessment is vital with appropriate follow-up.

Empowerment: A Seat at the Table: Working in Partnership

Learning about my health conditions has helped me feel more in control of what is happening to me and why.
 —Lene, 27 years old, congenital heart condition, clinical psychologist, Norway

Self-management (medical, behavioral, and emotional) of LTCs promotes psychological safety among those dealing with chronic illness.[78] This can be achieved by working in partnership with them, pivotal to psychologically informed healthcare.

It is important to remember that most people do not know very much about the complex way health settings work. Sharing your name and role, providing clear, honest information and treatment in respectful ways is vital. During healthcare, clearly explaining what is happening, what will be happening, and how long this will take and providing information about any delays is important. Recommending that patients prepare ahead for their healthcare appointments with a list of questions and informing and engaging them in making choices about any medical procedures (children too) while providing accessible information and avoiding medical jargon is important. Facilitating coping techniques, explaining test results and next steps, clearly discussing medication regimes and side-effects, taking concerns seriously, respecting dignity, and being available to answer questions are all essential components of supporting healthcare literacy and self-management of LTCs. It may be appropriate to involve a loved one or advocate when this helps.

Conflicting medical advice can worsen some concerns, particularly about recommendations around restricting physical activity, sexual health, or pregnancy risk. Healthcare providers can help by confirming and exploring concerns, acknowledging and updating any mixed messaging, educating individuals about red flag symptoms, and linking with allied healthcare professionals such as sexual health teams, physical therapy, or occupational health.

Undergoing medical examinations and tests or needing help bathing can be difficult for patients who often already feel very exposed and vulnerable. Dignity-focused care comforts patients through respectful behavior and ensuring personal space even when help is needed. This can be provided using dividers and curtains and by uncovering only areas of the body that are needed. Explaining ahead why these procedures are needed, asking first about physical contact, and talking privately about any sensitive issues are important aspects of dignified care. Further, talking about patients only with approved people respects privacy and ensures ethical practice.

During hospital stays, including patients in information—about handovers, explaining visiting times and other supports, ward rounds, mealtimes, what is going to be happening, and when the patient is likely to be going home—is key to empowering patients. Small things can make a significant difference, for example, waiting for an uncomfortable cannula to be removed, for help to change from a hospital gown into pajamas, or for a water jug to be refilled or for a commode can be very distressing and significantly add to the patient burden during hospital stays.

Communicating with other healthcare professionals involved in the patient's care is also important. For example, by ensuring that general practitioners or family doctors are aware of the patient's condition, that information is available in case of a medical emergency or for other allied healthcare professionals such as dentists and education providers. This is important because difficulty accessing appropriate care is more likely to happen outside of specialist care teams to whom the patient is known. Routine management of long-term conditions is often left to nonspecialists such as general practitioners (in the United Kingdom), likewise during emergency care healthcare workers who are unfamiliar with the patient are likely to become involved in their care. It is essential, for people living with an LTC, that these wider healthcare professionals are fully informed about their condition, the support they may need, and when specialist advice and input should be sought. When adequate care is difficult to access, it can be incredibly stressful, adding to the challenge and anxiety of living with an LTC. Handheld records and access to clinical information can help to alleviate this burden.

Shared Decision-Making

Not being consulted on treatment plans and medication and just being given things and being expected to be okay with it, was very difficult for me. I don't think it should be assumed that a patient should accept every suggestion that a health professional makes and if they don't that they are being "awkward"—choice is important and valid. There are times when I've not felt listened to and/or believed and that can feel very difficult and scary. When someone has rare or complex conditions that are poorly

understood, new symptoms can often be passed off as "just because of x/y/z condition" without really being considered. I think the most important thing was to feel listened to, like I was heard and that my opinion mattered.
— **Becky, 36, Ehlers-Danlos syndrome, postural orthostatic tachycardia syndrome (POTS), chronic fatigue, United Kingdom**

Shared decision-making is a collaborative process in which healthcare professionals work together with patients to reach a decision about their care, consistent with psychologically informed healthcare. It aims to choose tests and treatments based on the evidence and on the person's individual preferences, beliefs, and values. It is important that the patient clearly understands the risks, benefits, and consequences of different options through discussion and information sharing in a clear and accessible way. This approach empowers patients to make decisions about their treatment and care that is right for them. It also allows them to choose the degree to which they want to be involved in decision-making. Some people may not want to take an active role in this, while others may.

This approach can help to rebalance the power dynamic in the doctor–patient relationship by involving the patient rather than a more traditional patriarchal approach to treatment delivery. It is associated with empowerment, self-efficacy, and healthcare literacy. Tools, such as patient decision aids, can help this process.[79] For example, Steffens et al. developed a Surgical Question Prompt List (QPL) as a perioperative decision aid to improve patient engagement in surgical decision-making.[80] This QPL aims to make the consequences of surgery relevant to patient's lives while setting realistic expectations and empowering patients to ask questions so they can play a more active role in treatment decision-making.

Talk to me and listen. Try not to make assumptions. Please listen to me and don't put my concerns down to anxiety as a default answer. I am not anxious, quite the opposite in fact. Having had so many things happen to me medically there is often very little that disturbs me now, especially having been medically and psychologically trained. However, I want to know the possible origin of new and existing symptoms; I need to ask questions and know how to best manage or care for myself. My condition doesn't necessarily appear in textbooks or medical training, I also don't look the part of the typical textbook person with a craniofacial condition but that doesn't mean that I haven't had extensive surgery and now have difficulties linked to that. Please be courteous and approach with an open mind and with curiosity.
— **Sally, late 50s, congenital craniofacial condition, former nurse, psychotherapist, and PhD researcher, United Kingdom**

Facilitating Self-Management

- Listen to your patients, they know their own bodies. They may have had similar experiences before and may be able to help. Aim to work in partnership with them.
- Check your patient's understanding about what you have shared with them.
- Give your patients an easy way to communicate with the team should they have follow-up questions.
- Provide information about self-care tips for treatment side effects.
- Don't avoid or dismiss the "difficult conversations" such as sexual health, advanced care planning, genetic counseling, transplant, and getting older. Your patient may want to discuss these issues and be worrying alone about them. It is important they are sensitively addressed as part of care.
- Understand if your patient would like to seek a second opinion.
- Promote and advocate for improved awareness and social inclusion.
- Collaborate with subspecialists and partner with your patients and their family members.
- Connect them with condition-specific networking groups for advice and advocacy.

Please note sensitive content

Reflective Exercise: A Traumatic Childhood Medical Experience: A Case for Reflection and Discussion

I cannot breathe. I am not struggling to catch my breath like when you run too fast, or a mouthful of juice goes down the wrong way during a fit of laughter. I physically cannot breathe. There is no breath to hold. The unnaturalness of this feeling floods my body with cold terror. I try to grasp how I am alive without breathing. Am I alive? Shouting for help is not an option. I intensify my gaze, willing the nurse to meet it. Suddenly, she hovers over me pull, pull, pulling endless tubes from my mouth and nose, the smell and taste of plastic and blood consume me as I gasp and retch. "You're not meant to come around while you're still on the ventilator..." Finally, cold air blasts through my airways via an oxygen mask. The shock makes the room spin. I close my eyes. Inhale. The release is momentary. The heavy weight on my breastbone, broken and re-joined by the surgeon, attracts my attention. Heart monitors bleep in time to the thump in my head... sometimes extending to a single long bleep to warn an attendant nurse about another child. Wires and tubes emerge from everywhere. I cannot tell where they end, and I begin. Acid rises in the back of my throat. I nod toward the cardboard, disposable sick bowl at the foot of the bed as the nurse expertly swaps the oxygen mask for it. "There there . . . you poor thing" she soothes as I begin to retch, shivering despite the sweat dripping from my brow. When the vomiting stops, the process of recovery continues. "You shouldn't really be awake for this either" she scolds as she tugs a chest drain from under my breastbone, blood splatters over the muslin cloth she holds, as she swiftly stitches the remaining incision. With no time to recover from the intense pain she tugs at the second chest drain. I feel shame because I want my mum, but she is not allowed in intensive care. Anyway, I am now 13 years old. So, I held back the tears. Please, please no more. Everyone says I must be used to it but there is no getting used to this.

—Author's lived experience of PICU, aged 13, following open heart surgery to repair an atrial septal defect.

Consider:

- What did the ICU nurse do well in this scenario?
- What could and should have been done differently to avoid any unnecessary pain and distress?
- How does this fit with children's rights in hospitals?
- What institutional barriers contribute to this kind of situation occurring and how can we overcome them?
- How do you think this experience will affect this patient's future engagement with and feelings about healthcare services?

4
Conditions for Healing

> *Unnecessary noise, or noise that creates an expectation in the mind, is that which hurts the patient.*
>
> Florence Nightingale[1]

Environment: Healing Healthcare Spaces

Florence Nightingale understood the role that the hospital environment plays in patient well-being and recovery, promoting large windows that allowed cross-ventilation and abundant natural light in what became known as her signature style of "Nightingale Wards." This approach recognized the importance of light and air quality for patient well-being and recovery and, as such, incorporated innovative knowledge of the time.

The design of modern healthcare settings could improve, considering recent understanding about psychologically informed healthcare, to benefit patient well-being and recovery. Often the hospital environment could be designed to better promote feelings of psychological safety, for example, by ensuring aesthetically pleasing, calming waiting areas and clinic spaces and by incorporating green spaces.

One impressive illustration of a calming distraction in the hospital environment, is a 7.5-meter-tall cylindrical aquarium found at the Royal Children's hospital in Melbourne, Australia. Developed to provide children in hospital with a positive hospital experience, the aquarium hosts 530 fish with 32 distinct species including blacktip reef sharks, an epaulette shark, and a humphead Maori wrasse named Garry. The aquarium also serves an educational role and is used to inspire story writing and drawing for the children, who can watch divers feed the fish twice a day.

Further, an intricate mural has been added to the operating theater at the Royal Hospital for Children in Glasgow, Scotland, developed in a collaboration between children, environmental psychologists, architects, and artists, and spearheaded by Dr. Alyson Walker, a pediatric cardiac anesthetist at the hospital. The theater space redesign was guided by the patients themselves, consulting children from all over Scotland, with a range of conditions and backgrounds, about the things that make them feel happiest and safest. This includes soft lighting, removal of "scary" warning signs, seating that could be turned into a rocking horse or rowing boat, and replacing a visible "blood fridge," previously accessed by staff in full view of waiting families, with a mini toy museum.[2]

> *I am lucky in that I have family support for childcare that lets me attend my clinics and appointments. I notice very little support for people in less fortunate circumstances especially when it comes to having to bring young children to an appointment. Very little safe playing areas for children in adult areas of hospitals. Very different from the more welcoming pediatric units, but children may have to visit these adult spaces and the environment would do little to endear children to the hospital system. This may result in negative memories as those children mature and need to use the system themselves.*
> —David, 45 years old, congenital heart condition, United Kingdom

In addition to the environment, healthcare policies and practices could be more psychologically informed by addressing poor sleep and privacy, promoting the soothing presence of caregivers, challenging disempowering aspects of care, ensuring adequate management of pain, embedding emotional support, and facilitating coping.

Reflective Exercise: Hospital Environment

Consider your healthcare setting through the eyes of an unwell patient, think about all the touch points from reception to corridors, to finding their way to their appointment, waiting areas, wards, and clinical and surgical spaces. Consider what they will hear, see, feel, and smell and who is around to ask for directions or support.

- In what ways could the environment be improved to mitigate stress?
- In what ways does the environment help rest, recovery, and well-being?
- In what ways could the environment be improved to help rest, recovery, and well-being?
- What organizational facilitators and barriers are there to making these changes?
- Redo this exercise, considering the perspective of a young child, teenager, adult, older adult and as worried relative (e.g., parent, partner, sibling, friend).

Addressing Poor Sleep

The sensory environment (in hospital) needs careful consideration. Noise, lights etc. as this has a huge impact on sleep and distress. Staff seem indifferent to this as it's their working environment, not where they sleep.
—Hollie, 38 years old, mother of a son with bronchitis obliterans, 11 months old at time of admission, United Kingdom

Addressing poor sleep in hospitals is essential for patient well-being. Not only is sleep necessary for recovery, but poor sleep is also a risk factor for cardiovascular events, cancer, metabolic disorders, all-cause mortality, and cognitive function deterioration. It leads to a weakened immune system and a higher risk of falls. Poor sleep can also hinder recovery, increase the length of hospital stay, and negatively affect patients' well-being and is a major risk factor for delirium.[3] Reconsideration of the hospital environment including noise levels, lighting, and medical disruptions to sleep for patients is important.

Tronstad et al. suggest strategies for improving sleep in the ICU should include introducing "sound reduction bundles" to reduce sound pollution.[4] This includes staff education, since most noise comes from human behavior such as talking, movement, and taking and lifting of objects. To this end, behavioral modification and educational programs have been implemented to make healthcare professionals aware of the activities that create noise and motivate them to follow behavior modification and education consistently.[5]

Other modifications in hospital design may also help, such as moving handover stations and entrances further from the patient's room, providing each patient with a single room with daylight, sound-absorbing ceiling tiles, visual warnings when sound levels exceed the preset levels, and high-frequency oscillator ventilators. Night-time noise reduction can include switching off electronic items, silent mode phones, white noise, talking in whispers, and lowering the sound of alarms, and a streamlined alarm profile can support patient and family satisfaction in the ICU environment.[6,7]

> **Reflective Exercise: Sleep**
>
> Consider your healthcare context as a patient who feels very unwell and needs to sleep and recover. Consider what they will hear, see, feel, and smell and who is around to ask for help.
>
> - In what ways does the environment support sleep and recovery?

> - What interruptions are there (e.g., noise, taking vitals, lighting, medical tests, room sharing), and are they necessary?
> - In what ways could the environment be improved to support rest?
> - What organizational facilitators and barriers are there to making these changes?

Soothing Presence

> *Being allowed to have my parents accompany me to check-ups, even as an adult, having the option to phone a specialized nurse or even cardiologist if I experience any sudden changes and wonder if it requires a formal check-up and being involved with patient organizations has helped me cope.*
> —Lene, 27 years old, congenital heart condition, clinical psychologist, Norway

Some of my most difficult memories of being in hospital as a child are of being wheeled away by a team in green scrubs to go to the operating theater, where my mum was not allowed, and feeling very unwell, sick, and in pain during recovery. This is not just an issue for children. Recently, I went to accident and emergency with my husband (a first time for him) due to back pain. I was shocked when the nurse told me to leave, despite the fact he wanted me there, because they did not let family members in for assessment. Not only could I have been an emotional support to him, but I could have helped to answer any relevant questions at a time when he was preoccupied with acute pain.

> *As a 3-4 and an 8-10 year old boy, I had been admitted in hospital a few times. These were some research admissions and one open heart surgery admission. What helped me coping with the emotions, pain, fear, not knowing what would happen and the memory of the hardest moments when admitted was having my parents, mostly my mum, with me in the hospital a lot of the time, telling me what was going to happen, comforting me (both of my parents are nurses so they understood and... "translated" a lot of the "medical talk" to the appropriate/my child level). Also, the fact that my paediatric-cardiologist did his best to "behave" and speak child-friendly. After this period of admissions and chd-surgery, I found myself going through it all again and again in my head when lying in bed in the evenings. As a sort of adventure movie with me in it, I went through much of my experiences when admissioned again and again.*
> —Roy, 57, complex congenital heart disease, Netherlands

Like many, during hospital stays, as long as I feel well enough, one of the main things that keeps me going is visiting time. As a child, my mum stayed with me on the hospital ward (unless I was very poorly and in intensive care).

We looked forward to my aunt's visits, most days, after the morning ward round. She always brought us treats and helped us pass the time. There were other regular visitors who would bring flowers, cards, and gifts that were often the highlight of the day such as my grandparents, dad, and brother. As an adult, expecting the arrival of a visit from my family and friends is the main thing that keeps me going in hospital.

> *Being able to have my husband there when I was in hospital was the most comforting thing to me and helped me to feel safe.*
> —Becky, 36, Ehlers-Danlos syndrome, postural orthostatic tachycardia syndrome (POTS), chronic fatigue, United Kingdom

It is well established that social support is one of the most protective factors for mental health and well-being, especially during times of poor health. At the patient's discretion, supporting the presence of loved ones can provide comfort and improve outcomes.[8] Bear in mind, some patients may prefer to be alone to sleep if they are feeling very unwell or during the early stages of recovery. Further, soothing touch expresses compassion and promotes feelings of safety;[9] and preterm infants gain significantly more weight when touched and when they can hear their caregiver's soothing voice.[10] As such, it is important that there is recognition that "parents aren't visitors" with unrestricted visiting for children in hospital.[11]

> *Visiting times (on the transplant ward) were quite relaxed, especially for the long stayers like me. This enabled our families to spend quality time with us, which made a huge difference to well-being.*
> —Richard, 60 years old, congenital heart condition, heart transplant recipient, United Kingdom

---

Reflective Exercise: Soothing Presence

Consider the current policy and procedures in your organization for parents, loved ones, and visitors.

- In what ways do they promote the soothing presence of loved ones?
- What gets in the way of this?
- In what ways could this be improved?
- What organizational facilitators and barriers are there to making these changes?

Green Spaces in Healthcare Settings

You would have thought that patients waiting for transplants would be encouraged to stay as physically fit as possible. However, at this hospital, there was zero provision for support whilst waiting. There was lots of support, post-transplant, but nothing pre. To this end, our only option was to walk the corridors, to build up steps. Personally, I found this boring and whilst I did a bit, I doubt whether it added anything to my physical fitness. At one stage a few of us decided to get together in the day room, to run our own fitness session, which our consultants thought was fantastic. But it was all un-monitored by ward staff.
   —Richard, 60 years old, congenital heart condition, heart transplant recipient, United Kingdom

On reflection, throughout my many stays in hospital I don't recall being able to access green spaces. While I have been able to spend some time outside with visitors, when I have been well enough, there has never been a space for me to go myself. I am fortunate that I have family and friends who visit me daily and can take me to sit outside for some fresh air and sunlight (albeit, usually near a concrete car park, rather than a green space), particularly during prolonged hospital stays. However, this is not the case for many people who may suffer physically and mentally, as a consequence.

The biophilia hypothesis proposes that humans have an innate tendency to seek connection with nature and are attracted to the appearance of the natural world which provides a source of peace, inspiration, and spirituality.[12] There is a growing recognition of nature's role in healing and well-being. Yet, it can be challenging to access green spaces in hospital. Besides, hospitals are often found in built-up environments. There has been a recent move to incorporate green spaces within hospital environments with multiple health and well-being benefits to patients, staff, and visitors. Weerasuriya et al. conducted a systematic review of access to green spaces in healthcare facilities.[13] They found that access to green spaces was associated with experiencing a sense of control, choice, escape, privacy, and autonomy, experiencing opportunities for socialization and engagement with and stimulation by nature.

Reflective Exercise: Green Spaces

Consider your organization or service.

- Are there opportunities and green spaces for patients to get outside in nature at all?

- Is there green space outside for staff or visitors for respite?
- What are the restrictions around this, and can this be facilitated?

Empowerment: Challenge Disempowering Aspects of Healthcare

There was little or no hospital adaptation to the fact that some of [us] were long term patients (on the transplant ward). A number of us had conversations with the ward matron, who all the nurses reported to. Her view was that she was in charge of a short-term ward (the ward also catered to short term cardiac patients requiring stents, pacemakers etc., usually post cardiac arrest.) For us, this was extremely frustrating and added to our anxiety since we weren't allowed to use the kitchen to make a cup of tea or microwave our own food. This was in contrast to other wards in the hospital, which we knew had a lighter touch in these matters. Ultimately, after having had a discussion with the matron about our key requirements, word was passed back to me via a different department "to manage my expectations." At that stage I knew we weren't going to be successful in receiving some of the conditions we had asked for, which included full access to the kitchen and provision of health and fitness services.

—Richard, 60 years old, congenital heart condition, heart transplant recipient, United Kingdom

Psychologically informed healthcare aims to address and challenge disempowering aspects of care such as holding and restraint,[14] backless hospital gowns,[15,16] and waiting across the patient journey, to support health, well-being, recovery, and trust in those who care for us. For example, redesign of the backless hospital gown could promote patient dignity consistent with protocols that highlight the importance of postsurgical mobilization.[17]

Successfully negotiating the power imbalance to engender trust can be achieved through empathic and compassionate communication, within the context of a boundaried professional relationship.

Reflective Exercise: Patient Waiting

Consider your service.

- Do you ensure patients know when to expect a call, for example about test results, and let them know if this is going to be delayed?

- At outpatient clinics do you inform patients about delays, so they can, for example, go for a coffee and come back?
- Does your hospital have policies in place to ensure that inpatients do not have to wait for basic needs (e.g., for a commode, change of clothing, replenished water jug)?
- Systemic inefficiencies such as repeatedly being asked by multiple healthcare professionals for your medical history can be exhausting when you feel unwell; are there policies to read clinical notes first and avoid unnecessary duplication?
- Do you have hidden "waiting lists," for example for assessment only, to meet targets?

Learning from Research: Views of Healthcare Professionals on the Hospital Gown

Further to patient experience of wearing the hospital gown, reported earlier, we also considered the views of healthcare professionals on the hospital gown.[18] This study adopted a mixed-method analysis informed by the theoretical domains framework (TDF) of healthcare professionals' (HCPs') perspectives ($n = 2,264$) and experiences in relation to the use and utility of the gown. The study explored HCPs' perspectives in relation to the impact of wearing the hospital gown on patient well-being and suggested alternatives and/or improvements to the gown. Findings revealed that the gown was often used when it was not medically necessary. The categories of meaning and associated TDF domains were:

- Adverse impact on patient well-being (emotion)
- Lack of dignity (beliefs about consequences)
- Increased sense of dependency and vulnerability (social role and identity)
- Hinders patient autonomy and recovery (beliefs about consequences and reinforcement)
- Reduced patient mobility (beliefs about consequences)
- Feeling institutionalized (environmental context and resources)
- Positive impact (optimism)

Findings emphasized the need for alternatives and/or modifications to the gown with a focus on a person-centered approach to its design. Obstacles to staff promoting alternatives to the gown and challenges to making institutional changes were identified. Behavioral change interventions aimed at HCPs' practices associated with the use of the gown are recommended to challenge cultural norms and practices associated with the gown and to improve the patient experience.

Reflective Exercise: Patient Clothing

Consider your healthcare setting.

- Do you use a one-size-fits all, backless hospital gown?
- Is the same gown used regardless of setting, e.g., during childbirth, on admission, during medical tests and procedures?
- Is it possible to source medical clothing that provides better cover and accommodates different patients' needs, such as a Lap Over gown?
- Is use of medical clothing limited to medical necessity?

Enabling Access to Clinical Information

What prevents me from expectable nervousness (about the uncertainty of my prognosis), in a way I don't exactly understand, is having my, complete, medical files from both the hospitals who provided the care. That includes letters from the pediatrics and pediatric cardiologist to the GP in my first months to the chd-surgery journals and all research results in the 56+ years since I was born. This means I can find things about me myself. And maybe find out things to talk about with my cardiologist to see if there are possibilities we didn't think of. Knowing and saying "I can'" is enough. Enough to, for the moment, be okay with it, live on. And when I feel to, maybe dive into the files.

—*Roy, 57, complex congenital heart disease, Netherlands*

While self-management is key to living well with a long-term health condition (LTC) and is recommended in healthcare policy, this can be challenging, because people living with an LTC often lack access to their own clinical information. The Alliance, a nonprofit organization in Scotland that supports people living with LTCs, undertook a collaborative project on human rights and digital care. They spoke to people who used digital services, those who provided services, and support workers who engaged with digitally excluded groups. Following a period of public engagement, and an online survey, one of the main principles that arose was "access to and control of personal data." This principle states that people should have ready access to the data that is held about them rather than having to submit a "subject access request" to obtain medical or social care data from a public body or other agency. Rather, the data should be immediately accessible to the individual. Further, it should be up to the individual to grant access to some or all of that data to others. This could be for a family carer, to provide evidence of eligibility for a service, give information to a care provider, or for research purposes. Personal data stores aim to use human rights approaches to data collection, storage, and sharing consistent with psychologically informed healthcare. Other options include patient held passports and co-held records.

> **Reflective Exercise: Healthcare Records**
>
> Consider your healthcare setting.
>
> - Do your patients have access to their own medical records or health information?
> - If not, how can they access this information?
> - Do you copy them into letters to other healthcare professionals?
> - Do they have a handheld summary of key clinical information?
> - How can they access information about their medical history in case of emergency, if they are out of town, or in a different country?
> - Are your patients involved in decision;-making about detaining, destroying, and sharing their clinical information?

Ward Rounds

Dignity and having regard for me as a person, no matter what age I was at the time, matter. I had extensive surgery as a child, and many surgeries as an adult for a rare craniofacial condition. I was very frightened as a child. I was encouraged to "be brave" and "try not to think of it." Yet I could hear medics and family speaking in grave tones around me—my chances weren't great apparently. Yet, it wasn't until I was 11 years old when a surgeon actually sat beside me and spoke with me and explained what was going to happen in my next major surgery. That made all the difference, I was still very frightened, but I didn't feel as alone or invisible.

—Sally, late 50s, congenital craniofacial condition, former nurse, psychotherapist, and PhD researcher, United Kingdom

When I was growing up, there were many occasions when a team of doctors would stand around my hospital bed to discuss my case, often including student doctors who wanted to learn from my "interesting" history. Sometimes I felt left out of these discussions, even though they were about me. I quietly listened to what they were saying so I could know better what was going to happen to me.

The ward round is a cornerstone of medical and nursing practice. It offers an opportunity for sharing knowledge and communication between multidisciplinary teams, patients, relatives, and carers. The purpose of the ward round aims to monitor the patient's progress, clarify diagnosis, and to coordinate, document, and communicate the care plan. It is often used as an opportunity for training students.

As a patient, sometimes it can feel like the ward round happens to you, especially when the healthcare professionals are standing at the bottom of your bed, speaking about you in the third person. As a child (and adult), it can be quite scary and intimidating to be surrounded by a large team of adults talking about you. It is important for healthcare professionals to make sure that ward rounds are done sensitively, permission is sought for involving trainees, and that patients and their families are included in discussions.

> **Reflective Exercise: Ward Rounds**
>
> Consider ward rounds from the perspective of a patient lying in their hospital bed, who feels very unwell. Consider what they will hear, see, and feel.
>
> - How do you think this would feel as a patient?
> - In what ways are patients included in this?
> - What organizational facilitators and barriers are there to making changes?
> - Reconsider this from the perspective of children across the ages; a baby, toddler, young child, teenager, adult, and older adult.

Holistic Care and Embedding Psychological Support

I believe there should be a psychologist as part of every somatic team at the hospital to assist patients with disease-specific concerns, barriers to this include a lack of resources and low priority of preventative measures.
  —Lene, 27 years-old, congenital heart condition, clinical psychologist, Norway

A teenager presented a moving talk about their healthcare experience at a conference I attended, a few years ago. They reflected that their life had been saved twice, once by a surgeon and second by a psychologist that they saw who gave them a safe space to heal emotionally from their medical experiences.

Psychologically informed healthcare promotes the integration of psychologists in healthcare teams to meet the ongoing emotional and psychological needs of patients, throughout their healthcare journey, and to offer clinical supervision and support to staff while promoting psychologically informed practice.

If this is not the case, given the prevalence of mental health difficulties for people with LTCs, it is vital to routinely screen patients' mental health and to have robust referral pathways to further support or therapy as indicated. Depending on their presentation, your patient might benefit from talking to someone who is specially trained to listen and provide emotional care or for holistic support with their condition. Some relevant professions are listed below. For children and vulnerable adults, added support may be offered to wider family, including primary caregivers and siblings.

What helps me during my healthcare experiences to cope emotionally and psychologically has been clear and honest communication from my providers, having time to ask questions, being referred to mental health professionals when necessary, and given time to process disappointing news. In contrast, what could have gone better is increased transparency, especially in times of expected discomfort, and increased time to process disappointing news. Followed by guidance for peer support or professional mental health services to help me cope if needed.

—Karla, 40 years old, congenital heart condition, United States

Professional Support in Hospitals

- Chaplaincy, spiritual care specialists, and faith leaders: help patients find meaning and purpose and explore any religious beliefs.
- Complementary therapists: help with relaxation and reduce anxiety through therapies such as acupuncture or massage.
- Licensed clinical social workers or counselors: allow patients to explore their emotions in a safe, nonjudgmental space.

- Occupational therapists: evaluate people with health conditions and help people live independently by meeting goals to develop, recover, and support skills for daily life.
- Physiotherapists: help people improve movement and manage pain, often as part of preventative or rehabilitation, and treatment for people with chronic conditions.
- Applied practitioner psychologists: help patients explore, understand, and process their thoughts, behaviors, and feelings and develop ways of coping.
- Social workers: support patients and the people important to them with emotional and social issues. They can also help with accessing social care, benefits, and support from community organizations.
- Specialist palliative care services: help to manage medical problems and reduce worries about symptoms such as pain and nausea.
- Specialist nurses: offer emotional support, and advice about managing symptoms.

I'd like to see more counselling support for not only patients but family members. Having the specialist nurses helps, The Somerville Foundation (a patient support charity) and meeting other people in the same boat as me is extremely helpful. You get to share with others, who have similar experiences and struggles, realising I'm no longer that lonely, afraid and sad small child anymore. Doing Scarred for life (a photography exhibition to raise awareness) was empowering too. Even a small article with the BHF (British Heart Foundation) makes me feel like I'm giving something back, hopefully empowering those younger than me to keep moving forward even if it's just baby steps sometimes.

—Maggie, 53 years old, congenital heart condition, United Kingdom

Autistic SPACE

People with autism experience health disparities, reduced life expectancy, and barriers to accessing healthcare associated with adverse health outcomes.[19] These challenges include patient–provider communication challenges, sensory difficulties, and resource and time constraints. Worryingly, there is a reported sevenfold increase in suicide rates across the range of autistic profiles and support needs, with an up to 40-fold increase in mortality from neurological conditions such as epilepsy. Premature mortality rates from conditions unrelated to autism, such as cancer and circulatory, respiratory, digestive, and endocrine diseases, are also elevated.[20] Yet, autism training and healthcare professionals' knowledge about autism is variable and many practitioners are unclear about communication differences, access needs, or life experiences common to autistic people.[21]

Mary Doherty from Brighton and Sussex Medical School in the United Kingdom and colleagues have developed a framework to facilitate equitable healthcare for people with autism, using the acronym "SPACE."[22] This framework, outlined below, includes five core autistic needs: Sensory needs, Predictability, Acceptance, Communication, and Empathy. Three added domains are represented by physical space, processing space, and emotional space.

Considering Autistic Space

Sensory Needs: Sensory sensitivities are common to almost all autistic people. As such, considerations of all senses are recommended, including sight (e.g., bright or flickering lighting in hospitals), sounds (e.g., sudden, unexpected, or repeated noises such as alarms, auditory clutter), smells (autistic people are often highly sensitive to smell such as strong perfumes, candles, or toiletries), taste (e.g., taste and texture of food or medication), touch (tactile sensitivities range from inability to tolerate the sensation of certain fabrics to an inability to be touched, particularly by strangers, which can lead to challenges in a medical consultation where physical examination is required—avoid casual touch, promote sensory friendly clothing), temperature, proprioception, interoception and pain (e.g., difficulties with pain perception can lead to unrecognized injuries—consider the need for adapted pain scales).

Predictability: Many autistic people need predictability and may experience extreme anxiety with unexpected change. Healthcare is an unpredictable environment with unpredictable outcomes. For example, waiting may be difficult for autistic people, especially for an unknown duration in the sensory stress of a typical healthcare waiting-room, emergency department, or inpatient ward, while interacting with unknown people can also be challenging. Providing information in advance about the physical environment, staff, consultation process, and planned procedures is likely to reduce anxiety.

Acceptance: A neurodiversity-affirmative approach recognizes that neurodevelopmental differences are part of the natural range of human development. For example, while individual in nature, autistic behavior can, in some ways, be quite different from nonautistic behavior and repetitive behavior or "stimming" is common. Acceptance leads to appropriate accommodations, including understanding that so-called challenging behavior is usually a response to autistic needs not being adequately met. For example, facilitate the need for detailed information.

Communication: Autistic people may communicate differently. While many individuals use fluent speech, they may experience challenges with verbal communication at times of stress or sensory overload and nonverbal communication can be different for autistic and nonautistic people. Differences in the use of gaze, eye contact, gestures, and posture can lead to mistaken interpretation if autistic communication is not understood and accepted. It is important to understand these communication differences.

Empathy: It is a common misconception that autistic people do not feel empathy, rather a bidirectional, mutual misunderstanding can occur between autistic and nonautistic people, termed "the double empathy problem" because of differences in communication. Recognizing this challenge and making a particular effort to consider the perspective of the autistic patient is the first step toward bridging this gap. Directly asking an autistic person for their interpretation of events is preferable to making assumptions based on nonverbal communication.

Physical Space: Autistic people may need more physical space; it is important to expect and accommodate this need.

Processing Space: Autistic people may need added time to process new information and unexpected changes, to make decisions, and to respond to questions.

Emotional Space: Sensory overload or overwhelming emotions may lead to autistic meltdown or shutdown. Considering this will minimize risks, but if this occurs, the best approach is often to allow space to recover (restorative solitude).[23]

Key Tips to Help Coping in Hospital

- Bear in mind that hospitals and medical teams can be a significant and consistent part of life for people with an LTC. They may have mixed feelings about this because, despite being associated with feeling unwell, pain, and trauma, they also offer hope, treatment, safety, and sanctuary. Every medical encounter matters.

- Always see the person; whether conscious or not, in a hospital gown or bed, asking for a commode or pain medication. In a different time or place, you or yours could find themselves in this position.
- If you are not a specialist, then consult with your patient's usual specialist care providers as soon as possible.
- Words matter. Be sensitive and try not to say things like, "You must be used to this." You do not get used to pain, discomfort, and fear, If anything, difficult past experiences can make it even more challenging.
- Encourage comforting "tools" (photos, music, books) that promote feelings of safety.
- Try to keep the hospital environment peaceful and "healing"-focused; minimize loud noises such as laughter, chat, noisy shoes, doors or bins slamming shut or constant beeping monitors. Reconsider harsh lighting.
- Consider whether disruptions to a sleeping patient are essential, such as waking patients up to take early morning observations because this time fits around a change in staff shifts.
- If they are needed at all, keep the use of backless hospital gowns to medical necessity. If possible, find a more dignified alternative.
- Minimize waiting across the patient journey, which includes appointments, phone calls for surgery slots, tests, results, and discharge.
- Try not to keep patients waiting for basic needs such as a commode, refilling a water jug or pain relief.
- Systemic inefficiencies such as repeatedly being asked by multiple healthcare professionals for your medical history are exhausting when you feel unwell. Reading the patients notes first can help.
- Ensure clear communication with others involved in patient care so tests and procedures are not repeated unnecessarily.
- Incorporate stress reduction exercises and distraction, especially during tests and procedures.
- Ensure there is free hospital Wi-Fi.
- It is important to facilitate and individualize healthy coping strategies. This might be a cuddle from a parent, humor, distraction, anesthetic cream, pain medication, sedation; ask, "What helps?"
- Consider rules around the presence of loved ones in the medical setting, for example, with unrestricted access for loved ones during hospital stays.
- Offer a supportive visit from a hospital chaplain or specialist nurse.
- Help your patient set goals and make plans.

- Be sensitive about your patient's history, ask for consent before presenting them to trainees as an "interesting case" or sharing information with others, even anonymously, for example, on social media.
- Advocate for your patient's needs.
- Be aware of past medical trauma/phobias, minimize triggers (usually sensory), and increase support.
- Provide adequate sensitivity training to front-line administrative staff who answer the telephone, schedule the appointments, and greet patients as they arrive for their outpatient appointments, help with weight checks, and so forth. Keep in mind how impactful each of these touch points can be in relaying care, connection, and calm.

Emotional Preparation for Surgery

Emotional preparation for surgery has been shown to help promote a feeling of calmness, support the immune system, and reduce anxiety. It is linked to a reduction in pain medication of 23%–50%, reduced length of hospital stays, and behavioral activation. The American psychotherapist Peggy Huddleston describes five steps to prepare for surgery, as follows. This can be done with your patient remotely or in person and involves the following steps.[24]

Emotional Prep for Surgery

1. Help the patient relax. This may involve using breathing, progressive muscle relaxation, or other guided imagery. Use whatever suits your patient best—different people find different techniques more relaxing.
2. Encourage your patient to visualize healing by focusing on *a healed outcome*, not the surgery. This involves visualizing their goals of surgery: when they first come out of surgery, 1 month post op, 6–12 months post op, and so forth.
3. Suggest that your patient organizes a support group by asking their family and friends to think positively about them for half an hour before their surgery.
4. Encourage your patient to develop healing statements that they can repeat, and if they wish they can ask the theatre nurse to say during the surgical procedure.
5. Encourage your patient to meet the anesthesiologist in advance.

> **Reflective Exercise: Facilitate Coping**
>
> Consider your organization or service and the techniques and strategies used to help patients cope with distress and difficult or painful medical tests and procedures.
>
> - What strategies are currently in place to help patients?
> - How are staff trained in these strategies?
> - Who handles ensuring good practice is carried out?
> - What could be improved to help patients during stressful medical experiences?
> - How are staff supported to mitigate burnout, compassion fatigue, and moral injury?

Pain and Pain Management Programs

Management of acute and chronic pain is essential to psychologically informed healthcare, in healthcare settings and beyond. Psychologically based rehabilitative *pain management programs* for adults living with chronic pain can help to reduce the disability and distress caused by chronic pain by providing psychoeducational information and teaching physical, psychological, and practical techniques to improve overall quality of life.[25]

iSupport International Rights Based Standards to Support Children During Medical Procedures

> *Although we met some good nurses a lot are very detached and not responsive to distress. I've had to remind several doctors especially to speak to my son before starting a procedure like taking blood. They speak to me and usually ask me to hold him down. I've lost count how many times I've been told that he's not in pain he just doesn't like [being] held when I can tell he's in pain and he's distressed.*
> —Hollie, 38 years old, mother of a son with bronchitis obliterans, 11 months old at time of admission, United Kingdom

Healthcare environments often do not adequately address the psychological safety of patients. For instance, children are often restrained during procedures, which can foster fear and contribute to long-term trauma.[26] Over the last 5 years, I have been privileged to be part of iSupport, an award-winning international team of health professionals, academics, young people, parents, child rights specialists, psychologists, and youth workers making up 50 members, led by Lucy Bray, professor in child health literacy, nursing, and midwifery from Edgehill University in England, and initiated by Katie Dixon's childhood medical experiences.

> *I experienced many badly handled procedures as a child and now as an adult the trauma still affects many of my life choices. The psychological wellbeing of a child before, during and after a procedure needs to be protected.*
> **—Katie Dixon, aged 20 years, multiple procedures experienced throughout childhood, United Kingdom**

We have developed standards for supporting children and young people undergoing clinical procedures, based on internationally agreed children's rights set out by the UNCRC.[27] The standards aim to ensure that the short- and long-term physical, emotional, and psychological well-being of children and young people are of central importance in any decision-making for procedures or procedural practice.

The standards were developed in a three-stage process, involving ongoing and extensive consultation within a collaborative group and with established youth and parent forums. We also sought wider feedback, input, and consensus through two rounds of international online surveys. At all stages we have valued the opinions and views of children, parents, and professionals who work with children.

This work has led to academic publications,[28,29] the development of a website and child-friendly resources, including comic-strips and preparation sheets to support children, parents and healthcare professionals, during medical procedures. These standards were developed in response to previous studies which found that 81% of medical professionals report children being forcefully held, often by parents, for medical procedures "frequently" or "very frequently" to get the procedure done quickly despite potentially causing them to become scared of having future procedures and contributing to post-traumatic stress,[30] and causing distress to parents.[31]

By working with the European Association for Children in Hospital (EACH) the hope is to reach as many organizations as possible, with several hospitals and healthcare organizations already signed up to adopt the standards.

Professor Lucy Bray adds,

> *Children can feel uncertain and fearful in healthcare environments and during interactions with professionals. They can feel overwhelmed and upset when having tests and treatments and can feel excluded from decisions about their care. When the provision of care does not consider the psychological and emotional impact of such experiences, this can have long-term consequences, effecting the trust children have with professionals and services and making them less likely to engage in the future. Children are more likely to have positive experiences if health professionals invest time in building trust, if children know what is going to happen and if they have some sense of control. The short and long-term impact of investing in delivering psychologically informed healthcare cannot be underestimated. Through the process of developing the iSupport standards, we have heard from many children, young people and parents who live with trauma due to experiencing fear, harm and restraint during a clinical procedure. We also heard from health professionals who were working to mitigate these harms, to inform and involve children in their care to develop psychologically informed care practices. The aim of the iSupport rights-based standards is to ensure that the short and long-term physical, emotional and psychological well-being of children and young people are of central importance in any decision-making for procedures or procedural practice.*

A copy of the complete standards for healthcare professionals, and a child-friendly version, can be found in the Appendix.

Ongoing work aims to raise awareness of these standards and to implement them across different healthcare settings. To date this has involved, for example, individual hospitals setting up a working group, organizing awareness events with promotional materials, linking with allies such as clinical health psychology teams and play specialists, auditing current practice, providing a report with feedback, and training on the standards and psychologically informed procedural practice.

This work is consistent with other commitments to improve children's healthcare experiences, such as the University of California's "Comfort Promise" to "to do everything possible to prevent and treat needle pain. For every child. Every time,"[32] which details a "Comfort Tool Kit" including numbing cream, comfort positions, distractions, choice and memory shaping, and sedative options by developmental age. Prep sheets for patients and children with information about easing procedures and space to provide more information about what may be helpful are also available.

> **Reflective Exercise: Holding and Restraint**
>
> Consider your healthcare context and current practice of holding and restraint for children undergoing medical procedures.
>
> - Are children forcefully held during medical tests and procedures?
> - Are parents asked to become involved in this?
> - What emotional and psychological impact do you think this has on the child and their parents in the short and long term?
> - How will this impact on their future healthcare expectations, needs, and relationship with healthcare professionals?
> - What organizational facilitators and barriers are there to making changes?

Managing Pediatric Pain

In addition to pharmacological pain relief, which is beyond the remit of this book, there are many recognized nonpharmacological practices that have been incorporated into the medical setting to manage distress in babies and children. In a recent review, researchers report on a variety of strategies for managing pain in neonates.[33] Breastfeeding and skin-to-skin contact, or kangaroo care, between an infant and caregiver have been found to support temperature regulation, neonatal survival, time in quiet sleep state, and decreasing crying time. Facilitated tucking, a physical containment intervention that involves placing hands on the head and limbs of an infant undergoing a painful procedure to keep them in a side-lying flexed fetal position can also help. Non-nutritive sucking, oral stimulation through sucking on a pacifier, has similarly proven pain-reducing properties in newborns.

Campbell et al. recommend that modern neonatal care be family-centered and should aim to support parental presence in the neonatal unit and involvement in care procedures, including pain management, with proper counseling and information.[34] They note that historically, the parent's role in pain care has been significantly underutilized, and there has been a lack of focus on ensuring families have the resources they need to best help manage their infant's pain. The authors further recommend that parents best perform these pain-relieving methods, with guidance from healthcare professionals and provision of knowledge and resources. This will empower families to advocate for their baby and become active participants in their care.

Piet Leroy, professor in procedural sedation and analgesia in children at Maastricht University, advocates for procedural care for children that is trauma-informed, child-friendly and conducted in a nonthreatening environment in which well-being, confidence, and self-efficacy are supported.[35] He further recommends reconsideration of medical spaces to reduce sensory stimulation, comfort-directed and age-appropriate verbal and nonverbal communication by all healthcare professionals, inclusion of age-appropriate distraction techniques or hypnosis, and family-centered, care-directed policy.

Holistic Support

My care from the Rheumatology team was amazing, especially in the acute phase, which for me was about 6 months . . . in a practical way and everyone showed compassion but no one prepared me for life with a chronic disease. No one told prepared me for the grief I would feel, the changed friendships, retirement at 40yrs old or how life would never be the same again. I was given some leaflets, which in my view were woefully inadequate. . . . I was told repeatedly that I am a disabled person now and there is absolutely nothing I can do to make improve my health in any way. This left me feeling very disempowered, frustrated, and sad. What helped me the most was my husband and my family the Rheumatology team were great with the practical stuff but I was left to navigate the psychological impact of RA by myself.
—**Connie, 48, living with rheumatoid arthritis, nurse, United Kingdom**

Holistic support can further be supported by integrating a practitioner psychologist into healthcare teams, and also specialist nurses and other allied healthcare professionals specially trained to this end, such as child life specialists, play therapists, and music therapists. There are a range of ways healthcare teams can help coping in hospital, outlined below.

Child Life Specialists and Play Therapists

Pioneering children's nurse June Jolly (1928–2016) understood that the emotional well-being of children in hospital was just as important as their physical care. In England, she introduced toys and playrooms into wards and brightly colored aprons for nurses. Challenging hidebound practice, she transformed care by rejecting restrictive visiting for parents and promoting a family-centered model. Her book *The Other Side of Paediatrics: A Guide to the Everyday Care of Sick Children* was published in 1981.[36] It is now recognized that children have the right to access play and recreation according to Article 31, United Nations Convention on the Rights of a Child (UNCRC).

In North America, *child life specialists* are pediatric healthcare professionals who work with children and their families in hospitals and other settings to help them cope with the challenges of hospitalization, illness, and disability. They focus on psychosocial development and provide children with age-appropriate preparation for medical procedures, pain management and coping strategies, and play and self-expression activities. They also provide information, support, and guidance to parents, siblings, and other family members. Child life specialists are trained to consider the cognitive, emotional, and physical development of each child.

Child life specialists collaborate with parents and other healthcare professionals to meet the distinct needs of children in managing the effects of stress and trauma. Because children may feel overwhelmed, child life professionals help children gain a sense of familiarity and control of their environment through play and exploration inside the healthcare facility. Child life specialists can help the child's siblings understand what is happening and work through any concerns they have about their brother's or sister's treatment.

Child life specialists can also work with children of adults in hospital. They can provide medical play activities to help the child become more comfortable with the medical environment and ease their discomfort with any medical equipment they may see. They can teach the child about a new medical diagnosis, provide age-appropriate information about an adult's illness and treatment, and help them cope with changes they may see—such as changes with an adult's physical appearance or their abilities, and prepare them for visiting an adult in the hospital. They can help with challenging conversations related to an adult's hospitalization, illness, or prognosis. They can also use therapeutic activities and interventions to help children cope with their feelings and help them articulate any questions they have because of an adult's medical condition. Further, they can provide support with end-of-life and grief issues in partnership with supportive services and bereavement care.

> *The play therapist that spent 1hr Monday to Friday playing with my son helped us cope. She was the only one who came in the room that didn't hurt him and I didn't have to contain his distress. I saw him smile.*
>
> **—Hollie, 38 years old, mother of a son with bronchitis obliterans, 11 months old at time of admission, United Kingdom**

Health play specialists support children through therapeutic play, which reduces anxiety and the risk of psychological trauma. In the United Kingdom, the National Association of Health Play Staff promote the physical and mental well-being of children and young people who are patients in hospital or community settings. The charity aims to promote high professional standards for health play specialists and ensure that therapeutic play interventions are embedded in the child's care plan. Play is accepted as vital to healthy growth and development and a natural part of childhood that enables children to explore and make sense of the world they live in. For children and young people who undergo medical and surgical procedures, access to play carries greater significance.

Virtual Reality

Virtual reality distraction therapy (VRDT) is reportedly transforming healthcare with the potential to improve hospital experiences through a range of recent innovative developments. In hospital settings adults have been offered a VR headset prior to and during medical procedures that transports them to somewhere with calming surroundings to help them relax.

VR has been employed during childbirth with users providing positive feedback. Specifically, in a recent controlled trial involving 21 women in childbirth, participants reported that the experience diverted their focus from a painful delivery. And 95% said that they would be open to using VR again in future labor, showing a high level of patient satisfaction.[37]

VRDT has also been used by health play specialists to reduce pain, stress, and anxiety in children and young people before, during, and after painful medical and surgical procedures.[38] Clinical studies conducted in France showed a significant reduction in preoperative anxiety (−57%) in children waiting for surgery under general anesthesia and a significant decrease in postoperative morphine consumption (−80%) for children after scoliosis surgery.[39]

The Christie, NHS Foundation Trust, a specialist cancer center in Manchester in the United Kingdom, have been using VRDT for children and young people during radiotherapy.[40] A headset, specifically designed for children and young people aged between 7 and 16, is being used with patients when they are having clinical procedures including cannulation, injections, blood tests, and dressing changes, as well as with those having radiotherapy or proton beam therapy for cancer.

The project is being delivered by the team of health play specialists at The Christie who have been collecting data to better understand the difference distraction therapy is making to the patient's journey. Before having treatment, the child chooses from a sliding scale of face emojis, each associated with a word describing how they feel. The first face on the scale represents "happy" with the last representing "scared." They then ask again after the procedure and use of the headset and compare the difference. To date, data the team has been collecting so far has been encouraging, with patients reporting a 45% reduction in anxiety after using the device.

VR can also be used in the treatment of medically related phobias using immersion-based settings customized to meet the individual's needs. For example, exposure therapy can be offered in the virtual environment to enable the client to gradually confront needle phobia.[41]

Healing Power of Music

The effect of music upon the sick has been scarcely at all noticed. . . . I will only remark here that wind instruments, including the human voice, and stringed instruments, capable of continuous sounds, have a generally beneficial effect.
—**Florence Nightingale**[42]

The healing power of music has been recognized since antiquity. Recent neuroscientific research has substantiated music's therapeutic properties, which include emotional regulation and brain re-engagement. As a result, music has been incorporated into healthcare settings as a type of "medicine." *Music therapy* is increasingly being used to help patients cope with stress and to promote healing, for example, to help co-regulation with babies in pediatric intensive care. This work involves parents by providing them with information about prenatal listening experiences and encourages them to choose a song for their child from their favorite repertoire and culture to sing or hum to them. The music therapist can then accompany parents and child in the Neonatal intensive care unit (NICU), adapting their suggestions to the child's development (e.g., autonomic nervous system and hearing). The music therapist may play music and hum for the parent and child during kangaroo care, adapting this humming to the breathing rhythm of the parent to relax them and help co-regulation with the baby.[43,44]

In the absence of the parents, music therapists can work with the baby on their own to regulate their condition, especially during or after care, during painful processes, and during physiotherapy. This also allows doctors, nurses, and therapists to work in a calmer and more relaxed manner. The possibilities for intervention are remarkably diverse.

Music has also been found to have beneficial impact on adult patients. A systematic review led by Dr. Catherine Meadsteam at Brunel University in the United Kingdom suggested that music can reduce anxiety, pain, and the need for pain killers for patients who have undergone surgery.[45] By analyzing 72 randomized controlled trials involving more than 7,000 patients who received surgery, researchers found those who were played music after their procedure reported feeling less pain and anxiety than those who did not listen to music, and they were also less likely to need pain medication. This effect was even stronger for patients who got to choose the music they listened to.

Further Harper et al. report from a randomized control study, including 750 patients, that patients who listened to self-selected music during chemotherapy infusion showed significant benefit in mood.[46] Patients could self-select an iPod shuffle programmed with up to 500 minutes from a single genre (e.g., Motown, '70s, '80s, classical, and country). The authors concluded that music medicine is a low-touch, low-risk, and cost-effective way to enhance patients' psychological well-being in the often-stressful context of cancer treatment.

Learning from Practice: Music Therapy in the NICU

By Ruth Stakemann, Dipl., Music Therapist, German Music Therapy Society, Soltau, Germany

I work in the Neonatal Intensive Care Unit (NICU) and Premature Intermediate Care (IMC) at a large children's hospital in northern Germany, with 12 ventilator equipped cots in the intensive care unit and 10 beds in the IMC.

The clinic follows a holistic approach. Immediately after birth, the children are usually supported on the Concord Birth Trolley. The Concord Birth Trolley enables the newborn to receive initial care close to the mother without the umbilical cord being cut immediately. There are many rooms on the ward where parents can stay during their child's stay. Rooming in is also possible before discharge. Parents are involved in the care of their children as early as possible and encouraged to kangaroo regularly. There is close contact and regular exchange with the obstetric ward for high-risk pregnancies. In addition to the pediatricians, members of the psychosocial team consist of a social midwife, parent counseling, breastfeeding counseling, two psychologists, pastoral care, an art therapist and a music therapist who contacts the parents before birth and continues to care for parents and child after birth in the neonatology unit.

Music therapy has been available in the clinic for over 25 years. One goal of music therapy interventions in neonatology is to create an atmosphere that supports parents and child in their respective challenges. Music therapy interventions also target children's need for rhythm and predictability, for regulating their physiological state through interaction with another person,[47] for intimacy and—as M. Sanders puts it— "loving synchrony."[48,49] In addition, music therapy supports the stabilization of vital functions and sucking.[50] It is important to maintain a balance between the acoustic stimulation necessary for development and overstimulation.[51] The physical and psychological state of the parents, some of whom are highly stressed or traumatized, cannot be separated from the physical and psychological state of the child and must be considered in music therapy interventions.[52,53]

In individual cases, the parents, with the support of the music therapist, record their voices, which are played to the children in the absence of the parents. Apart from that there are no music boxes or other playback devices on the ward.

Case Vignette
Ben S. was born in the 29th week of pregnancy and was the family's second child; his brother was 4 years old. Ben and his mother enjoyed music therapy, which took place several times a week. At the beginning, the focus was on the shared experience of intimacy and relaxation. During kangarooing, I played the monochord for mother and child, a 25-string vibratory therapy instrument that creates a feeling of security and relaxation. I had tuned the monochord so that it harmoniously embeds any monitor alarms. I also hummed little melodies in the rhythm of the mother's breathing, on the one hand to give Ben a feeling of synchronicity and multimodal perception, and on the other hand to deepen the mother's breathing. In terms of intensity and melody of my voice, I took into account Ben's body tension and his gestures and facial expressions. Ben's mother had chosen "Twinkle Twinkle" as a song that she liked to sing and hum for Ben. Sometimes we sang it together, or I sang the German version "Funkel Funkel kleiner Stern, Mama hat Dich ja so gern" ("Twinkle, twinkle, little star, Mom loves you so much") for mother and son, which moved her to tears. Ben's mother noticed that she could no longer do justice to her older son Felix and tried very hard not to let Ben sense her tension and conflict. She told me that music therapy helps her with that. When Ben was moved from the intensive care unit to the IMC, she brought Felix with her from time to time and tried to do justice to both of them at the same time by reading aloud and playing music that Felix could listen to on headphones.

When I arrived with the guitar in my hand, the mood in the room was tense. Mrs. S. tried to breastfeed Ben, while Felix was very upset because his mother had forgotten both the reading book and the headphones at home. Ben was not drinking, which increased his mother's tension. I got the monochord, told Felix that I needed his help and showed him the instrument. He plucked a few notes and the full sound surprised and fascinated him. He immediately agreed to make music together for Ben and his mother. I took the guitar, and we first played an improvised song about the situation and then "Twinkle Twinkle" in the German version, including Felix and the father in the lyrics. Felix's enthusiasm was expressed in several quite loud notes. My concern that it might be too much for Ben subsided when I saw the values on

Continued

> *Continued*
>
> the monitor and Ben's mother smiling. When I said goodbye after about 20 minutes, Felix told me to come back next time and bring the monochord. The result of this relatively lively situation for a premature baby ward was not only Felix's composure but also the fact that Ben drank well from his mother's breast the whole time.

Listening Therapy

In polyvagal theory, Professor Stephen Porges proposes our bodies are constantly looking for signals of threat and safety via neuroception. More specifically, we have evolved to respond to rhythms that enable our bodies to be entrained for co-regulation, self-regulation, recovery, and restoration. Building on this, Stephen Porges's *Safe & Sound Protocol* aims to repattern the nervous system by making ventral–vagal activation, therefore the social engagement system, more accessible. This aims to tap into our body's way of co-regulating and is currently being trialed at the Children's Hospital of Wisconsin for individuals with Ehlers-Danlos syndrome.

Further, *polyvagal music* (PVM), recently developed by Stephen Porges and Anthony Gorry, music and audio innovator, may also be useful in the medical setting. PVM signals the nervous system to support homeostatic functions through underlying algorithms that signal healing functions of the autonomic nervous system. Specifically, PVM uses biological rhythms embedded in unique musical themes to promote self-regulation. PVM is informed by decades of research studying physiological rhythms in the body, including heart rate, heart rate variability, respiration, and blood pressure. PVM is designed to supplement treatment strategies for healthcare providers when treating clients with mental and physical illness including chronic stress and functional disorders and is currently being trialed in a variety of medical and therapeutic settings.

Therapy Animals

A small pet is often an excellent companion for the sick.

—Florence Nightingale[54]

I have always found great comfort in animals. As a child we had a beautiful Alsatian named Carbonyl who had wonderful black and tan coloring and a very gentle loving nature. Home life could be difficult, my dad had serious mental health problems, and when things were particularly challenging Carbonyl and I snuggled together. Since then, I have always had a dog and that has comforted me, particularly at times of poor health and recovery. A few years ago, when the leads of my pacemaker developed a fault, I had to stay in hospital for a month during an unusually warm summer in Scotland. My husband and son were able to take me to a hospital cafe by the hospital door and often they brought our little Scottish terrier Lass, which brightened my day. Walking back to the ward, I passed a painting of a nurse with a Scottish terrier titled *Matron Dick and Roddy* by Alix Dick in 1954. An accompanying sign detailed that Matron Dick had presided over Falkirk Royal Infirmary, having started there as a nurse in 1930. Her faithful Scottie dog Roddy went with her on her hospital rounds. Each time I passed, I wished we had a Scottie dog on our ward.

Florence Nightingale introduced Jimmy the tortoise as a ward mascot for wounded soldiers during the Crimean War. In the 1970s, children's nurse June Jolly organized a circus animal visit for her patients, including a baby elephant and a lion. These early forms of *pet therapy* are now widespread practice in adult and children's wards (albeit with more domesticated animals!). Animals can support patients with unconditional acceptance, touch, physical affection, and play, and by triggering feelings of empathy, connection, and calm. I know I would have loved nothing more than a visit from a dog on my heart ward as a child.

The use of therapy dogs has a positive effect on patients' pain level and satisfaction, for example, for adults during a hospital stay after total joint replacement.[55] Studies have also found a positive effect of therapy dogs on anxiety in hospitalized children. Children who received a visit from a therapy dog and handler experienced a significantly greater decrease in anxiety than control groups.[56]

Art Therapy in Hospitals

During one of my stays in hospital as a child, when I had started to feel better, I made my own collection of animal drawings that the nurses kindly hung on a stretch of wall in the ward. I was proud of my scribbly child drawings being displayed and it gave me something positive to focus on and show my visitors.

Drawing, coloring books, painting, and crafting were pleasurable activities that I could do, even from a hospital bed.

Back in 2015, I co-created a "heart to art" photography exhibition with friends, who also happen to have been born with a heart condition. Jenny Kumar and Caroline Wilson and I created our *Scarred FOR Life* project on behalf of a charity, The Somerville Heart Foundation, which supports young people and adults with congenital heart conditions across the United Kingdom. A fashion and portrait photographer, Kirsty Anderson captured portraits of eight adults (including Caroline and me), each born with a heart condition, to help change the perception that scars should be hidden away. The story of each model's journey navigating the complexity of living with this condition, in their own words, was written on the reverse of eight-foot-high photo banners. The exhibition was launched in February 2015 at Glasgow's Kelvingrove Art Gallery and Museum, where it sat in the central hall for a month before touring several venues including hospitals and the Scottish Parliament. The exhibition received national media attention, helping to raise awareness of the unique needs of the growing population of adults with congenital heart conditions. As well as telling the story of a population hidden in plain sight, the exhibition aimed to empower survivors. Visitors' comments included "*Inspiring exhibition. Viewed while waiting as our 3-week-old son is having open heart surgery at Yorkhill*"; "*I am 11 and I have a heart condition were I only have half a heart, and I also have a scar for life*"; and "*Here with a 2-year-old CHD boy. Great to see images out for all to see. 2-year-old enjoyed spotting 'zip lines,' like his own.*"

Art therapy is a growing trend in hospitals. This evidence-based practice supports the emotional, physical, social, and spiritual well-being of patients of all ages. A wide range of mediums can be used, such as drawing, painting, sculpting, collage, and photography. This practice, guided by an art therapist, offers patients an opportunity to process their feelings and express themselves creatively, for example, about a new diagnosis, to rebuild self-esteem, to help manage pain, and to find peer support with others with a similar condition. Art therapy has also been employed to support siblings and family members. Exhibitions and displays of art allow patients to share their work and experiences.[57]

Cinemas

Cinemas have been built inside hospitals to improve the quality of life for patients and their families through the shared cinema experience of film. For example, MediCinema opened in 1999 at St Thomas' hospital in London and has since provided hundreds of thousands of cinematic experiences with specially created cinema spaces that can accommodate beds, wheelchairs, and medical equipment. This promotes social inclusion, positive experiences, and helps with hospital boredom.

Giving Back: Volunteers

In a long-established tradition, many people provide invaluable voluntary support in hospital and healthcare settings. Often this includes people with personal experience who want to "give back." Originally known as "candy stripers" in the United States, this includes a wide range of roles that support patient well-being throughout the healthcare journey, such as, running the hospital café, shop, or trolley, spending time gaming with children in hospital, organizations that make bespoke hospital clothing and condition specific toys for children, volunteers who provide patient transport, bedside, home from hospital, and end-of-life support. Other roles include "baby cuddlers," people that help to keep attractive hospital grounds, run the hospital radio, provide patient-care liaison and advocacy and advice, raise funds, support art and music groups, provide pet therapy, provide hairdressing, and work as NHS cadets and peer mentors. These roles provide much needed human contact, compassion, and access to life's normalities for people when they need it most. Often they are offered through organizations such as the Royal Voluntary Service and St John's Ambulance in the United Kingdom and the American Red Cross, which provide training and support. Volunteers need to go through a formal background screening check prior to working in these settings for safeguarding of patients.

5
Healing the Healer

You Cannot Pour from an Empty Cup

> *Paediatric cardiac anaesthesia is a wonderful specialty to work in and I know that I have made a positive impact on many children and families by helping them through these difficult days. I have been that professional, that guardian, to keep them safe during surgery . . . to deliver them back to intensive care and see the relief and thanks on the parents' faces. And that is a wonderful feeling. But the psychological impact of being an anaesthetist for children with heart problems is not to be underestimated. It is without a doubt a job that comes with enormous responsibility and stress. Most outcomes are positive. But we do experience difficult situations. I have been deeply affected by patient deaths that still upset me, years later. I remember the child whose hand I held as they died and cry every time I hear their favourite song on the radio. I remember the desperate face of the father in intensive care as he was told his baby would not survive. I remember the toddler who laughed as he went to sleep, but didn't survive the surgery. Nobody remembers the anaesthetist, but we remember them.*
> —Anon, pediatric anesthesiologist, United Kingdom

Overview

Many years ago, I was invited to present my work at a conference, where I shared the stage with an eminent, retired pediatric surgeon. Afterward, he told me that my talk was the first time he had heard someone mention that healthcare professionals were entitled to an emotional and psychological response to their challenging work. He revealed this was a lightbulb moment and that looking back on his career there had been times when, for example, a child had died on the operating table, and the loss had significantly affected both the team members involved and dynamics between them. Yet, he reflected there was no recognition, training, or opportunity to reflect, share, or process these understandable feelings, individually or as a team. I felt moved by this honesty, humanity, and our conversation, especially as someone who has benefited from pediatric surgery.

Psychologically informed healthcare recognizes that healthcare professionals also need to be supported emotionally and psychologically. Healthcare professionals experience high rates of psychological distress, which can lead to burnout, compassion fatigue, vicarious trauma, and associated mental health problems such as anxiety and depression. It is important for healthcare workers to be aware of the signs and symptoms of their own stress to ensure early intervention, help-seeking, and support. Further, it is important that organizations be proactive in supporting staff to mitigate these occupational hazards.

Establishing Healthy Boundaries

Working in a healthcare profession can be incredibly stressful, with staff often giving of themselves. This can be encouraged by social expectations to act as "heroes" called to a vocation rather than a job. However, while healthcare roles are clearly of great benefit to society, it is important for healthcare professionals to recognize their personal limits. A career in healthcare is a marathon, not a sprint, and self-care is vital.

Self-care involves establishing professional boundaries with patients and their families, by being clear about your role, avoiding dual relationships, respecting confidentiality, being careful about self-disclosure, reviewing privacy settings, and being mindful about social media use, not accepting personal gifts, and directing patients and their families to relevant further support if needed.

It is also important to keep strong boundaries about work and personal life by being assertive with colleagues and managers about time off, self-care, having a manageable workload, and seeking support and supervision.

If your feelings are affecting your work or personal life, it is important to seek support. You could consider:

- talking to your manager
- talking to other colleagues who might have had similar experiences
- seeing a counselor or psychologist
- accessing clinical supervision

You may also benefit from the exercises in the Appendix, including grounding techniques and mindfulness, dealing with emotions, somatic exercises, and self-compassion.

Organizational Responsibilities

> *It appears that our healthcare systems are so target and guidelines driven these days that it can be a struggle to take time to consider the unique person needing your help or care. Perhaps there is precious little time for staff to fully absorb, reflect on and talk about how to fully embed and implement such care. For example, it is easy to believe and acknowledge the need for compassionate and/or trauma-informed care, but as a patient, compassionate care is not often experienced. The authentic voice of lived-experience is important to learn from.*
> —Sally, late 50s, congenital craniofacial condition, former nurse, psychotherapist, and PhD researcher, United Kingdom

While self-care strategies can place responsibility on the healthcare professional, organizations must take responsibility for ensuring the well-being of staff. Organizations that encourage psychological safety have been found to cultivate adaptive learning, creativity, and nourishing relationships, with measurable improvements in people's health and well-being. Organizational responsibilities include providing appropriate workloads, safety supports, opportunities for self-care, adequate resourcing, safeguarding annual leave, valuing staff, setting reasonable and realistic expectations, encouraging social support, and providing breaks.

Burnout, Compassion Fatigue, and Vicarious Trauma

Burnout is a gradual decrease in work engagement because of chronic exposure to stressful situations, such as having a high caseload or limited resources (e.g., lack of job control, availability of feedback, or learning opportunities). It can lead to disengagement in work duties. Burnout develops gradually over time, and it is characterized by the presence of three primary types of problems:

- Physical, mental, and emotional exhaustion
- Cynicism and decreased job satisfaction
- Inefficiency at work

Burnout is associated with low energy, tiredness and sleep disturbance, decreased feelings of personal accomplishment, depersonalization, and physical symptoms (e.g., hypertension and headaches). It can also result in behavioral and mood disturbances, impaired relationships, and feelings of helplessness, hopelessness, and decreased empathy.

Often, those who experience burnout feel they lack professional support from their supervisors, coworkers, and organizations. Burnout reduces the capability to deliver high-quality care, and it is detrimental to patients and healthcare professionals. It is associated with medical error, physician suicide, and substance abuse and contributes to healthcare instability through increased sick leave and high staff turnover.[1]

While burnout was common among healthcare professionals before the pandemic, the legacy of COVID-19 includes elevated rates of burnout, vicarious trauma, moral injury, and compassion fatigue in health and social care workers.[2] It can affect fitness to practice and it is also associated with health, mental health, and well-being indicators including anxiety, depression, sleep and memory problems, and neck and back pain.[3] Severe burnout can result in self-medication with alcohol and drugs.

Compassion fatigue has been found at higher rates in healthcare settings because of high rates of witnessing suffering. Described as the "cost of caring,"[4] compassion fatigue consists of symptoms like those associated with direct trauma exposure. However, it differs from vicarious trauma because it does not require exposure to a traumatic event. Symptoms may develop either gradually or rapidly and can include the experience of intrusion symptoms, negative emotional arousal (e.g., experiencing higher levels of anger and frustration), difficulty separating work and home life, lower levels of distress tolerance, emotional outbursts, decreased work satisfaction, negative self-soothing behaviors (e.g., drinking or social isolation), and decreased general functioning and productivity at work and home.[5] Further symptoms include the inability to process emotional distress related to caring for others' suffering, poor clinical decision-making, and the avoidance of, and inability to establish, relationships with patients.[6]

Risk factors for developing compassion fatigue include a high desire to end others' suffering, an unresolved trauma history, working with traumatized children, and experiencing high natural empathy.[7] Protective factors include emotional intelligence, healthy emotion regulation and adaptive, problem-focused coping (as opposed to avoidance-based coping strategies), age and experience' setting firm professional boundaries and engaging in additional training, consultation, and supervision with experienced professionals, self-care, self-compassion, maintaining work–life balance, working within a supportive team, group cohesion, and organizational commitment to supporting staff.[8]

Vicarious trauma can develop when a healthcare professional is exposed to the traumatic content experienced by a patient. Much like the experience of a direct trauma, it can affect their worldview or belief system, cognitions, and emotional needs. Symptoms can mirror those of direct trauma exposure, such as disturbances in mood, self-identity, spirituality, and cognitive frame of reference as well as intrusion symptoms. Vicarious trauma is associated with feelings of anger, rage, and sadness; hypervigilance; preoccupation with thoughts of patients outside of work; nightmares; a sense of detachment or numbing; and withdrawal.[9]

The Cost of COVID-19

Healthcare workers were faced with a number of unprecedented occupational hazards during the COVID-19 pandemic, including a lack of preparedness or training, lack of established priorities for COVID-19 triaging, lack of access to personal protective equipment and ventilators, having to quickly learn new ways of working, redeployment, limited communication about what was happening, witnessing unusually high rates of death, dealing with restrictions to patient visiting, and growing waiting lists. Further challenges included concerns about exposure to infection for self and others and limited access to childcare in a context of being unable to access usual social support and outlets. This legacy of the pandemic includes a detrimental impact on health and well-being for healthcare professionals, as detailed in our study below.

Learning from Research: The ENACT Study

A growing body of research has highlighted the adverse impact of COVID-19 stressors on health and social care workers' (HSCWs) mental health. Complementing this work, we explored the psychosocial factors that have had both a positive and negative impact on the mental well-being of HSCWs during the third lockdown period in Scotland, using a cross-sectional design. Participants (n = 1,364) completed an online survey providing quantitative data and free open-text responses. A multimethod approach to analysis was used.[10]

The majority of HSCWs were found to have low well-being scores and elevated levels of COVID-19 stress, worry, burnout, and risk perception scores; and almost half of HSCWs met the clinical cut-off for acute stress (indicative of PTSD).

HSCWs with higher scores on adaptive coping strategies and team resilience reported higher scores on mental well-being. HSCWs were significantly more likely to seek informal support for dealing with personal or emotional problems compared to formal support. Barriers to formal help-seeking were found, including stigma and

Continued

> *Continued*
>
> fear of the consequences of disclosure. HSCWs mostly value peer support, workplace support, visible leadership, and teamwork in supporting their mental well-being.
>
> Our findings illuminate the complexity of the effects of the COVID-19 pandemic on HSCWs' well-being and will inform future intervention development seeking to increase positive adaptation and improve staff well-being. Addressing barriers to mental health help-seeking among HSCWs is essential. The implications emphasize the importance of lessons learned across health and social care contexts, planning, and preparedness for future pandemics.
>
> Reflection:
> - How did the COVID-19 pandemic affect you, personally and professionally?
> - What has been the aftermath of the pandemic on staff well-being in the organization where you work?
> - What lessons have been learned?
> - How prepared is your organization for similar scenarios in the future?

Building Self-Care and Resilience at Work

It is in the interests of healthcare organizations to promote well-being and workplace resilience because excessive stress in the workplace can lead to significant costs, not only for individuals but also the wider economy in lost working days. It is important that both individual and system-based strategies support the well-being of healthcare professionals.

One qualitative study explored occupational and psychological protective factors in the workplace for junior doctors working within the NHS in the United Kingdom. The authors found three main themes: support from work colleagues, such as help with managing workloads and emotional support; supportive leadership strategies, including feeling valued and accepted, trust and communication, supportive learning environments, challenging stigma, and normalizing vulnerability; and access to professional support such as counseling, cognitive-behavioral therapy, and medication through general practitioners, specialist support services for doctors, and private therapy.[11]

Other studies have reported that protective factors in the workplace include social support, emotional support, training in effective coping strategies, reducing high levels of work pace and conflicting demands and promoting individual and team resilience.[12] Micro practices that help to manage work stress for healthcare workers include mindfulness practice, gratitude practice, sleep hygiene, and breathing and relaxation exercises.[13] For example, based on improvements in psychological well-being and self-compassion, one narrative review concluded that mindfulness-based toolkits are beneficial for medical students' well-being.[14]

Proactive Burnout Tips

- Good coworker support
- Reducing home–work life conflict
- Job autonomy
- Relaxing activities
- Good social support
- Work tasks that energize and motivate
- Supervisor support
- Feedback seeking
- Reducing hindering job demands
- Maintaining physical health
- Setting boundaries
- Help seeking as needed[15]

Psychologically Safe Working Environments

From a polyvagal perspective, when healthcare professionals feel psychologically safe, their autonomic nervous system perceives minimal threat, optimizing their "social engagement system." This enables them to be fully engaged in social interactions and professional duties without being in a constant state of defense or hypervigilance. As such, psychological safety promotes open discussion and consideration of diverse viewpoints, ensuring that ethical dilemmas and complex decisions are made with integrity and sensitivity.[16] Healthcare professionals who feel psychologically safe are better able to communicate openly, collaborate effectively, seek support without fear of repercussions, and perform their roles more effectively. Within healthcare settings psychological safety leads to improved teamwork, communication, employee retainment, and correspondingly improved patient outcomes, as care is delivered more efficiently and with fewer errors.[17,18] Psychological safety also supports student learning and ongoing professional development by creating an environment where constructive feedback is valued and learning opportunities are embraced.[19] An inclusive, psychologically safe workplace values diversity, supporting team members to contribute creatively to team performance.

Conversely, from a polyvagal perspective, healthcare environments that lack psychological safety may trigger defensive responses, such as activation of the sympathetic nervous system (fight or flight response) or even shutdown responses (dorsal vagal complex). Such an environment can hinder effective teamwork, communication, and decision-making among healthcare teams and compromise delivery of compassion-centered care. Integrating principles of the polyvagal theory into healthcare settings can offer valuable insights into fostering psychological safety.

Compassionate Leadership

As explored in Chapter 3, compassion communicates relational safety. *Compassionate leadership* can help leaders effectively manage the performance of individuals, teams, organizations, and systems and improve feelings of psychological safety in staff. Compassionate leadership involves a focus on relationships by empathically listening to those you lead, aiming to understand any challenges they face, and acting to support them to do their job more effectively, so they feel cared for, trusted, and respected. It is associated with higher job satisfaction, engagement, well-being, creativity, motivation, and enhanced performance.

Professor of organizational psychology at Lancaster University, Michael West describes compassionate leadership as inclusive, promoting empathy, curiosity, and listening.[20] This approach welcomes difference and focuses on shared purpose and conditions that build trust. West reports that people who work in supportive teams with good leadership report much lower levels of stress.[21] Staff members are more engaged, produce better results, and demonstrate improved financial performance. In healthcare settings where staff report the absence of compassionate leadership, staff tend to report higher levels of work overload and less influence over decision-making and organizations report poorer outcomes. Further, staff treated with compassion can better support and care for their patients, resulting in higher quality of care and patient satisfaction. When this is not the case, there are lower levels of patient satisfaction, poorer quality of care, and higher patient mortality.

Compassionate leaders aim to meet the core needs of the people they work with. Compassionate leadership involves four behaviors:[22]

Compassionate Leadership

- **Attending**: This is the most important leadership skill. It means being present with and focusing on others, taking the time to listen to the challenges, obstacles, and frustrations that colleagues face as well as their successes. It involves noticing suffering at work and taking the time to ask people about difficulties and challenges.
- **Understanding**: This involves taking time to explore and understand the situations that people are struggling with, by exploring conflicting perspectives rather than imposing your own understanding or perspective. It involves withholding blame and focusing on what can be learned.
- **Empathizing**: This involves mirroring and feeling colleagues' distress, frustrations, hopes, and fears without being overwhelmed and becoming unable to help.
- **Helping**: This involves taking thoughtful and informed action to support people and teams in doing their jobs. This may involve removing obstacles, such as excessive workloads, and providing the resources people and services need, such as more training and equipment.

Recent studies on well-being in doctors, nurses, and midwives, including those in training, found that staff well-being is affected by eight key factors that can be organized into three core needs:[23]

- **Autonomy**: Describes the need to have control over one's work life, and to be able to act consistently with one' values, this includes:
  - Authority, empowerment, and influence
  - Justice and fairness
  - Work conditions and working schedules

- **Belonging**: This describes a need to be connected to, cared for by and caring of colleagues, and to feel valued, respected, and supported via:
  - Teamwork
  - Culture and leadership

Continued

Continued

- **Contribution**: Refers to the need to experience effectiveness in work and deliver valued outcomes, across:
  - Workload
  - Management and supervision
  - Education, learning, and development

Reflective Exercise: Polyvagal-Informed Wellness Action Plan (WAPs)

Wellness action plans (WAPs) are a practical tool to support well-being at work. WAPs typically focus on ways to support mental health in the workplace. WAPs can provide a structure for conversations around what support would help the individual. When used well, this can open a dialogue between managers and employers so that well-being needs are better met, which can in turn lead to increased engagement, improved performance, and enhanced job satisfaction. WAPs cover the following information (adapted through a polyvagal lens), although this can be adapted to suit the individual, their role, and the organizational context:

- How does stress affect you in the workplace? How does your body feel when you are hyperaroused, hypoaroused, or fawning? (e.g., sleep difficulties, headaches, rapid breathing, racing heart, nausea, disengagement from work, feeling emotional, overwhelmed or panicky, overeating or loss of appetite, hypervigilant, less tolerance, exhausted by trying to please everyone, diminished confidence).
- What work situations trigger you?
  (e.g., balancing work and home life, tight deadlines, things not going to plan, lack of support, challenging colleagues, difficult conversations, criticism, high caseload, authoritarian management).
- What helps you feel psychologically safe when you are working?
  (e.g., regular breaks, time for reflection, respite in green spaces, peer support from colleagues, supervision, manageable workload, feeling heard, being respected, adequate resources, positive outcomes).
- How might stress impact on your work?
  (e.g., find it hard to make decisions, difficulty concentrating, irritable, less empathy, self-criticism, social withdrawal, checking behaviors, trying too hard to please).

- What can your manager do to proactively support you in the workplace?
  (e.g., flexible work patterns, regular reviews, supervision, facilitate peer support, regular breaks, listening, compassionate approach, adequate resourcing, appreciation).
- What are the early warning signs for you, personally?
  (e.g., withdrawing from colleagues, absences, physical symptoms of stress, irritability, less empathy).
- What steps can you take if you start to feel like your well-being is affected?
  (ask for a break, speak to a supportive colleague, speak to supervisor about reducing workload, delegating, regular breaks, accessing emotional support, and a safe reflective space).

Please note sensitive content

Case Study: Nurse Thomas

Thomas is a pediatric nurse in a busy, pediatric cardiology ward. He has been nursing on the ward for 10 years. He takes pride in his work, in building relationships and providing consistency of care for the patients and their families. He has known many of the children who come to stay on the ward since they were babies. He is popular with his colleagues, his patients, and their families for his warm, caring manner and humor.

Unfortunately, during a shift when he is in charge, one of the young patients' conditions unexpectedly declines and they pass away on the ward. Everyone is in a state of shock. There is an investigation about what happened and even though he knows it is routine practice, he feels like he is being interrogated. Over the coming weeks, Thomas is unable to stop thinking about what happened. He ruminates over the events in detail, questioning everything. He has flashbacks to the girl's mum screaming and nightmares about other children on the ward dying and not being able to save them. He feels low most of the time, is tearful, cannot sleep, and has lost his appetite. He no longer enjoys spending time with his family and friends and has increasingly withdrawn from life. He starts drinking more to try and get off to sleep in the evenings. His daughter is the same age as the girl that died, and he has been checking her heart rate when she is asleep. He has become overprotective of her, leading to arguments with his wife. He dreads going into work and is hypervigilant all the time, waiting for the next bad thing to happen. He has started double and triple checking everything he does at work. His colleagues have started to notice that he takes too long during medical rounds, because of his checking behaviors. On a couple of occasions, he has been snappy with them.

In clinical supervision, he uncharacteristically bursts into tears and explains that he feels totally overwhelmed and that he does not know who he is anymore. He reveals that he is considering changing career. His supervisor and line manager work with him to temporarily adjust his work responsibilities. He is referred to the team psychologist, who helps him process the traumatic loss. With the psychologist he discusses other cases and challenges during his nursing career, which he did not have the opportunity to process at the time. Together they develop strategies to help him process and manage his feelings, reduce his checking behaviors, and gradually increase his activities. Over time he regains his confidence at work and returns to his duties. He develops a wellness action plan on his return and discusses it with his supervisor. His home life improves too, and he gradually reengages with his family and friends and feels more like his old self. With the support of his manager, he starts a peer support group so that nursing staff can meet regularly in a confidential, supportive, and safe space to share and process emotional challenges at work.

6
Culturally Sensitive Healthcare

Then I go to my brother
And I say brother help me please
But he winds up knockin' me
Back down to my knees, oh
There have been times that I thought I couldn't last for long
But now I think I'm able to carry on
It's been a long, a long time coming
But I know a change's gonna come, oh yes it will
From "A Change Is Gonna Come." Sam Cooke © June 19, 1964;
RCA Victor.

Overview

Cultural sensitivity in healthcare practice involves recognizing, respecting, and responding to the cultural needs of individuals. Researchers have recognized the value of culturally sensitive and competent healthcare as a vehicle for decreasing health disparities.[1] *Patient-centered culturally sensitive healthcare*[2] entails not making assumptions based on a patient's race, ethnicity, sexuality, gender expression, or English-language proficiency, instead approaching each patient as a unique individual with their own set of beliefs, values, and practices. Within the healthcare setting this involves respecting any cultural differences in communication, diet, health beliefs and approaches to treatment, religious beliefs and customs, and family roles. Studies have shown that cultural sensitivity, which is responsive to what the patient wants, needs, perceives, and feels, improves relationships between healthcare professionals and patients, treatment adherence, and patient satisfaction.[3]

> **Culturally Competent Healthcare—Campinha-Bacote Model**
>
> Campinha-Bacote proposes a culturally competent model of healthcare represented by the mnemonic ASKED, which stands for cultural Awareness, Skills, Knowledge, Encounter, and Desire:[4]
>
> ***Cultural awareness*** is the process by which the healthcare professional becomes aware of, appreciates, and becomes sensitive to the values, beliefs, life ways, practices, and problem-solving strategies of other cultures. This involves examining their own biases and prejudices toward other cultures and exploring their own cultural background.
>
> ***Cultural knowledge*** is the process by which we seek out and obtain education about various worldviews of different cultures. The goal of cultural knowledge is to become familiar with culturally/ethnically diverse groups, worldviews, beliefs, practices, lifestyles, and problem-solving strategies. This may involve reading about different cultures and attending continuing education courses on cultural competence.
>
> ***Cultural skill*** involves learning how to carry out competent cultural assessments. This involves assessing each patient's unique cultural values, beliefs, and practices without depending solely on written facts about specific cultural groups. Cultural assessments should not be limited to specific ethnic groups but conducted with each individual patient.
>
> ***Cultural encounter*** involves taking part in cross-cultural interactions with people from culturally diverse backgrounds such as attending religious services or ceremonies and taking part in important family events. It's important to have as many cultural encounters as possible to avoid cultural stereotyping.
>
> ***Cultural desire*** is the development of interest to engage in culturally competent behaviors.

Social Inequalities and Intersectionality

Psychologically informed healthcare promotes cultural sensitivity and awareness of the intersectionality between living with a long-term health condition or disability and belonging to other minority or disadvantaged groups such as gender, sexuality, class, and ethnic biases, which can further compound the detrimental impact of minority stress on physical and mental health. To this end it is helpful to have a deeper understanding of the links between social inequalities and health, ableism, and patient rights, as outlined below.

People with a serious health condition often face discrimination, stigma, and social exclusion, adding to the burden of living with a long-term health condition (LTC). In turn, people who face discrimination, stigma, and social exclusion are more likely to develop an LTC, while these factors can worsen the severity of any health condition. Loneliness and social disconnection negatively impact on mental and physical health.[5] Lower socioeconomic status is associated with poorer health and reduced lifespan, and many complex interacting factors contribute to these disparities in health risk and disease burden, including unequal access to healthcare and availability of social support, employment, food availability, finances, and discrimination.[6] To illustrate, Dale et al. found that individuals with prior mental health and medical adversities were more vulnerable to the COVID-19 infection.[7]

Such individuals also face disparities in income, education, and employment, and underrepresentation in the media and politics.[8] Often people with an LTC are marginalized, finding it harder to access the 5 Rs of "Citizenship" that society offers. Defined by Michael Rowe, professor of psychiatry at Yale University, citizenship refers to the Rights, Responsibilities, Roles, Resources, and Relationships that are usually offered by public and social institutions and local communities.[9] Further, people with LTCs often face the "Four I's of oppression" described below.

The Four I's of Oppression

- **Ideological Oppression**: idea that one group is better than another, "othering" (e.g., healthy versus sick, survival of the fittest).
- **Institutional Oppression**: the idea that one group is better than another group and has the right to control the other becomes embedded in social institutions (the legal system, policing, education system, media, political power, etc.).
- **Interpersonal Oppression**: The idea that one group is better than another, and has the right to control the other, becomes structured into institutions and gives permission and reinforcement for individual members of the dominant group to personally disrespect or mistreat individuals in the oppressed group (stereotypes, harassment, threats).
- **Internalized Oppression**: Oppressed people internalize the ideology of inferiority, as reflected in institutions, interpersonally from the dominant group and come to internalize the negative messages about themselves, associated with shame, for example:
  - Someone not identifying as having a disability because they worry about being "reduced to their condition."
  - Hiding or minimizing aspects of their condition to fit in.
  - Feeling shame and being self-critical about their condition.

Cultural sensitivity involves healthcare providers being aware of and tackling systemic stigma within healthcare systems, which can be transmitted through role-modeling and the *hidden curriculum*. For example, most mental health outcome measures and medical interventions have been developed for white, often male populations and are neither designed for nor tested on black populations. Critical race theory (CRT) encourages a decolonizing approach to education, science, and healthcare practice since racism has the potential to seriously effect health outcomes.[10]

For example, one qualitative study exploring health literacy when engaging people with a migrant background found that some participants described the so-called *morbus mediterraneus*, a stereotype that labels people from southern European countries as expressing physical pain intensely. As a result, their pain intensity was doubted by some healthcare professionals.[11] Further, one study explored medical students' perspectives on racism in medicine in Germany. Online semistructured focus groups were conducted with 32 medical students from 13 different medical schools across Germany. Using thematic analysis, the authors found that medical students perceive racism in healthcare in Germany as a ubiquitous phenomenon, they have problems identifying racist behavior and structures due to conceptual knowledge gaps, and they are insecure in how to deal with racism on a situational level. The authors conclude that antiracist training needs to be better addressed in medical education.[12]

Further, research studies that aim to explore the impact of living with an LTC seldom include patient and public involvement (PPI) from people with lived experience despite guidance from the National Institute for Health and Care Research (NIHR).[13,14] It is also important to acknowledge that historically women have also been underrepresented in medical science and have encountered difficulties being heard and taken seriously.[15] Dr. Kate Young notes that for much of documented history, women have been excluded from medical and science knowledge production.[16] For example, gender biases have been found toward the underestimation of pain in women.[17] A recent article in the Lancet[18] reported that female health has been historically understudied, with research neglecting widespread sex differences in prevalence and presentation of illnesses affecting the human brain. Most preclinical studies have focused on males, ignoring relevant differences between the sexes and risk for diseases more prevalent in females, such as depression.

Ageism in healthcare leads to negative health outcomes for older adults. While it is often implicit, the COVID-19 pandemic threw explicit age discrimination in healthcare into sharp relief globally. In healthcare, age discrimination affects the provision of ethical care and ranges from "micro" issues such as paternalistic medicine to "macro" system issues including barriers to prompt and effective healthcare or exclusion from research trials. Strategies to combat ageism and provide ethical healthcare include intergenerational learning, educational programs, and strong leadership from organizations to enact policy and practice changes.[19]

While 'reverse' agism has received less research attention infantiliaing stereotypes may be experienced by young people in healthcare settings. A scoping review on ageism against younger populations described social assumptions that younger people are inexperienced, incompetent and that adults know better and are entitled to act upon them without their agreement.[20] Further research is needed to explore how such social assumptions manifest in healthcare settings, particularly for people young people living with an LTC.

A Long Time Coming: History of Discrimination and Stigma

Please note sensitive content

When I was growing up, I refused "special treatment," determined to prove myself at a time when needing any additional support, for example at school or university, was highly stigmatized and support itself was scarcely available. My condition is hidden, I wanted to fit in, and it was possible to minimize my condition. I caught up with missed schooling and university lectures by myself. I found creative ways to forge a career in psychology, despite only being able to work part-time, taking a long and convoluted path. At times, this has been incredibly challenging, and I have been fortunate to have the support of my mum and husband. However, recently, I started wondering how many of the challenges that I have faced have been caused by the limitations of my condition and how many have been created by systemic societal barriers. As it happens, people with an LTC are underrepresented across most professions, including academic and practitioner psychology groups.[21] Living with an LTC can negatively affect educational achievement, career development, and financial stability—particularly when this experience is poorly understood or unsupported by rigid institutional practices and prevailing attitudinal barriers. For individuals with an LTC, employment and professional training may be affected by the need to manage symptoms, take medical leave, and navigate energy limitations.

Even in recent history people with a disability or serious health condition have experienced social exclusion and segregation. The deeply moving film The Elephant Man, directed by David Lynch, depicts the harrowing life of Joseph Merrick (1862–1890) an English man who was known for his severe physical deformities. During his short life, he was brutally treated, exhibited at a "freak show" under the stage name "The Elephant Man" and went on to live at the London Hospital as a medical curiosity.[22]

Historically, disability has been used to shape public health behaviors by blaming "poor behavior" or parenting for disability. For example, smallpox vaccination campaigns often played on fear of scarring and other disabilities, while an American poster from 1937 describes syphilis as "the Great Crippler" and an anti-tobacco video from 2016 shows the face of a man disfigured by mouth cancer as a warning against chewing tobacco. These narratives arguably reinforce stigma and ascribe shame and guilt to being disabled, contributing to social exclusion.[23]

Not a hundred years have passed since Hitler ordered widespread "mercy-killing" of the "sick and disabled." In 1933 the "Law for the Prevention of Hereditarily Diseased Offspring" was passed in Germany, allowing forced sterilization of anyone regarded "unfit," including people with conditions such as epilepsy, schizophrenia, and alcoholism. It is estimated that 360,000 individuals were subjected to forced sterilization. In 1939 the killing of disabled children and adults across Germany began. All children under the age of 3 who had illnesses or a disability, such as Down's syndrome or cerebral palsy, were targeted under the "Tiergartenstrasse 4" (T4) program, where a panel of medical experts had to give their approval for the "euthanasia," or supposed "mercy-killing," of each child. Following the outbreak of World War II in 1939, the program was expanded. It is estimated that 200,000 people with disabilities were murdered between 1940 and 1945 as part of Hitler's euthanasia program, the systematic killing of Germans whom the Nazis considered "unworthy of life."[24]

As part of his research into the causes of the Holocaust, Gordon Allport, a psychologist, created *Allport's Scale* in 1954, to measure the manifestation of prejudice in a society. The scale contains five stages of prejudice, ranked by the increasing harm they produce, a useful tool for recognizing and responding to discrimination:

1. Negative talk (jokes, rumors, offensive talk)
2. Avoidance (overlooking, neglect, refusal to interact)
3. Discrimination (exclusion, segregation, harassment)
4. Physical Attack (intimidation, physical attacks)
5. Extermination (lynching, ethnic cleansing, genocide)[25]

Just 50 years ago, many feared that cancer was contagious, leaving cancer patients battling both social isolation and a sense of shame. Thankfully this is no longer the case, as our understanding of cancer has developed. HIV/AIDS was a highly stigmatized disease throughout the 1980s, leading sufferers to be shunned and ostracized. This stigma has decreased with a better understanding of the illness. Social justice campaigns, allyship, and high-profile sufferers, such as NBA superstar Magic Johnson, have helped to destigmatize diseases such as HIV/AIDS with organizations such as the Magic Johnson Foundation helping to educate people about the disease, and empowering young people to decrease their HIV risk factors. Such efforts can lead to greater understanding of serious and chronic illnesses, and greater acceptance of those who suffer with such conditions. As society becomes more accepting, those with serious and chronic conditions may come to internalize such attitudes, leading them to a more positive relationship with their own bodies.[26,27,28,29] Indeed, Albrecht and Devlieger report the contradiction that disabled people often report a higher quality of life than able-bodied people assume, termed the "*disability paradox.*"[30]

While society has become more inclusive, it is important to remember this legacy. Stigma about health conditions stay barely hidden beneath the fabric of society. People with an LTC are often the "canary in the coal mine," as revealed during the COVID-19 pandemic (see "Learning from Research" below). The COVID-19 pandemic intensified health inequalities, with the most vulnerable facing the greatest impact physically, psychologically, economically, and socially. In the United Kingdom, 50% of adults with underlying health conditions reported that the pandemic affected their well-being and increased their anxiety levels and that they were more concerned about the future. The pandemic widened the income gap for people with LTCs.[31] Further, the report *A Disability-Inclusive Response to COVID-19*, produced by Inclusive Futures, found that during humanitarian efforts in supporting the most marginalized communities in Bangladesh, Kenya, Nepal, Nigeria, and Tanzania during the COVID-19 pandemic, people with disabilities were unable to access food, medicine, and other necessities that crisis relief efforts made available to the wider population during the pandemic.[32] Lorraine Wapling of Inclusive Futures noted, "*We knew this situation was bad for people with disabilities, but when we looked into the detail, it was even worse than we imagined. I was in shock. Despite all the hard work by organisations of people with disabilities, the right to be included in times of crisis still seems far from being achieved.*" One man, with a physical disability in Kenya commented, "*Before COVID, people with disabilities were struggling. Now with COVID, this is worse. Those I have tried to talk to see this as the end of their lives.*"

Learning from Research: An Exploration of Psychological Trauma and Positive Adaptation in Adults with an LTC During the COVID-19 Pandemic

The COVID-19 pandemic presented added challenges for people living with preexisting health conditions including increased risk of health complications, shielding and strict social distancing, changes to medical care provision, and social stigma.[33] We conducted a cross-sectional, anonymous, online study exploring psychosocial measures of traumatic experiences as well as protective factors that mitigate the risks to the mental health of adults with congenital heart disease (CHD) (n = 236) during the pandemic. Closed and open-ended questions and a series of standardized psychosocial measures of traumatic experiences, coping mechanisms, emotional regulation, and post-traumatic growth were used.

Findings from the study suggest the CHD population are at increased risk of post-traumatic stress, which may have been worsened by the COVID-19 pandemic, while emotional regulation was associated with post-traumatic growth.

One hundred and forty-four participants provided responses to a question asking them to detail their thoughts about the impact of the COVID-19 pandemic on their mental health. Most participants referred to factors that reflected their anxieties and CHD-specific concerns about the COVID-19 pandemic. These responses generated the following seven categories of meaning. (Note, 18 [14%] of comments submitted were categorized as miscellaneous as they were too broad or fragmented to categorize.)

- Anxieties (32%) (e.g., "*Potential to lose my job and life*")
- Condition-specific concerns (23%) (e.g., "*Made me more aware of my condition and the measures I should take to mitigate risk and stay safe.*")
- Social isolation (10%) (e.g., "*The virus has caused me to become socially isolated as I am off work and cannot work from home.*")
- Frustrations with the media and government handling (9%) (e.g., "*I feel this situation has been badly managed by the media and I think everyone with a severe condition should have received personal guidance on what to do and how to stay safe.*")
- Opportunity for reflection and recuperation (7%) (e.g., "*For the most part it's been better as I've been able to take a breather and focus on me.*"),
- Safety seeking (3%) (e.g., "*When case numbers were high, I just wanted all my family to stay home and be safe in our little bubble. My husband took time off work on sick leave to alleviate my anxieties.*")

- Stiff upper lip (3%) (e.g., *"No affect whatsoever it is what it is and just get on the best I can."*).

Participants (*n* = 211) provided 221 responses to a second question, "How do you feel about the way the media have portrayed the increased risk to people with 'underlying health conditions'(UHCs)?" Responses generated the following three categories of meaning.

- Unfair to people with UHCs (79%) (e.g., *"I felt like people with underlying health conditions were assumed to be frail or have a lower quality of life, and like it wasn't as bad if we died of COVID compared to the rest of the population."*)
- Balanced and fair (13%) (e.g., *"We need to know these risks"*)
- Avoidance (3%) (e.g., *"It has scared me so much that I stopped reading it."*)

We recommend a growth-focused, psychologically and trauma-informed approach to medicine and public health, recognizing the importance of supporting mental health and promoting living well with their condition. These findings are generalizable to other lifelong health conditions and shielding populations.[34]

Abuse in Hospitals

Please note sensitive content

Psychologically informed healthcare also recognizes that healthcare professionals hold a position of power over patients.[35] When we are unwell and in a healthcare setting, we are often at our most vulnerable. Whenever there is a power imbalance in a relationship there is also a risk of abuse, and it is important for all healthcare professionals to be aware that abuse can and does happen in the healthcare setting. Further, institutional abuse, defined as poor care practices within an organizational setting, including neglect, systemic abuse of power, or unfair ways of changing behavior, is a further risk factor for patients in healthcare settings.

Alzyoud et al. report that patient abuse, regardless of gender, disease, and medical treatment, is an international problem reported by researchers across the globe, and can take different forms including physical, verbal, and sexual abuse and neglect.[36] Specifically, Vedam et al. reported that in the United States, one in six women experience one or more types of mistreatment by a healthcare professional during pregnancy and childbirth.[37] In Sweden, 20% of female and 8% of male patients reported lifetime experiences of abuse across healthcare settings,[38] and in Jordan, 32.2% of women reported feeling neglected by healthcare professionals during their last childbirth, while 37.7% of women were exposed to verbal abuse.[39]

In the United Kingdom, The Stoke Mandeville Report[40] found that between 1968 and 1992, the children's TV presenter and now notorious sexual predator and pedophile Jimmy Savile abused 63 people connected to Stoke Mandeville Hospital in England. The report found that Savile's reputation as a "sex pest" was an "open secret" among some staff. One formal complaint, made in 1977 by an 11-year-old girl's father, was not reported to the police. The victims, aged from 8 to 40, were subjected to sexual abuse ranging from inappropriate touching to rape. Savile had virtually unrestricted access to clinical areas, patients, and the mortuary during the 1970s and 1980s. The report also found that over the past 40 years Stoke Mandeville had employed three doctors who had later been convicted of sex crimes against patients.

Recently, the British Medical Journal[41] published a report into the scandal of sexual abuse in NHS hospitals over the previous 5 years. The investigation found that 200 NHS trusts in England had recorded 35,000 incidents of sexual violence and misconduct between 2017 and 2022. Further, 37 police forces recorded almost 12,000 sexual crimes allegedly committed on NHS premises during this period, including almost 4,800 sexual assaults and more than 2,800 rapes. Yet, only 8% of sexual offenses committed on NHS premises had resulted in charges. Staggeringly, only 17 of 200 trusts in England have a dedicated sexual safety policy. The authors conclude that patients who are sexually abused in the NHS face an uphill battle to achieve justice, against a backdrop of overlapping investigation processes that can last years, including criminal investigations and regulatory processes before the General Medical Council or the Nursing and Midwifery Council. Further, each NHS Trust may also conduct its own safeguarding investigation or look to take disciplinary action if the perpetrator was a member of staff. The authors caution that a lack of clear policies and procedures for dealing with reports of sexual harm across the NHS discourages patients from disclosing traumatic incidents of sexual abuse and that patient victims may also struggle to understand what happened to them and come to terms with the fact they were subjected to a sexual assault, particularly when it occurs under the guise of a legitimate medical procedure. The authors report that the impact of being sexually assaulted in hospital cannot be understated including a range of psychological effects, post-traumatic stress symptoms, anxiety, depression, and feeling unable trust healthcare professionals again.

It is essential that all healthcare professionals be aware of abuse in hospitals to ensure safeguarding and, when appropriate, whistle-blowing.

Medical culture is traditionally hierarchical, which can make it difficult for less senior staff to speak up and be heard. It is vital that robust clinical governance policies and procedures are in place to ensure risk assessment and management. The described cases highlight that the system of safeguarding of staff and patients' needs to be improved.

Change Is Gonna Come: Strategic Action

Psychologically informed healthcare involves developing healthcare systems that enable the growing numbers of people living with an LTC to reach their full potential, and that embraces and supports diversity. This calls for strategic actions in addressing racism, ableism, sexism, classism, homophobia, discrimination, and structural disparities in healthcare. *Affirmative action* may include a move to improved coproduction of healthcare, working with rather than on people and communities, and inclusion of positionally and reflexive statements in research publications with clearer inclusion about the ethnicity of participants. Consistent with this approach this end the American Medical Association (AMA) Organizational Strategic Plan to Advance Health Equity 2024–2025 proposes to:

- Embed Equity: Infuse racial equity and social justice into the fabric of the AMA's culture, systems, policies, and practices [. . .]
- Build Alliances and Share Power: Acknowledge and learn from the voices and experiences of historically marginalized and minoritized physicians and stakeholders [. . .]
- Ensure Equity in Innovation: Integrate racial justice and health equity into healthcare innovation efforts, while amplifying the voices of historically marginalized individuals in the innovation sector [. . .]
- Push Upstream: Address all determinants of health and the underlying causes of inequities across the healthcare ecosystem [. . .]
- Foster pathways: Amplify marginalized narratives, quantify past harms, and embark on a healing journey to pave the way for transformative change [. . .].[42]

Further, the AMA proposes to right the injustices of the past, challenge dominant or malignant narratives, center voices and ideas of those most marginalized in any space, adopt antiracist and intersectional approaches, embrace public health frameworks of health, and act upstream and implement an "inside-outside" strategy to organizational transformation.

Safeguarding in Healthcare

Safeguarding is entrenched in healthcare practices and has long been part the mandatory training programs for anyone working in a healthcare profession. Healthcare workers meet the most vulnerable people in society, often when they are at most in need of support. For some, this is the result of abuse or neglect—either self-neglect or neglect by those who are meant to be caring for them.

As such, healthcare professionals meeting people in vulnerable situations need to be able to recognize problems, to mount a proportionate response, and to report and record the facts through a culturally sensitive lens. This may involve sharing the information with other agencies, or a more rapid response to an at-risk situation. Local and national policies in healthcare services reflect legislation designed to identify and protect at-risk adults and children.

For example, in the United Kingdom, the Care Act 2014 describes six key principles for safeguarding adults: empowerment, prevention, proportionality, protection, partnership, and accountability. These principles are designed to ensure that safeguarding practice is person-centered, proactive, and appropriate. This act is designed to ensure that there is integration between different agencies involved in a person's care, with a multidisciplinary approach. A robust grounding in relevant legislation and options for response to safeguarding concerns empowers workers to manage these situations with confidence.

Patient Rights

Patient rights and healthcare standards are integral to empowerment, safeguarding, and addressing inequalities in healthcare. In the 1940s and 1950s, rights-based organizations emerged in response to the range of injuries and disabilities from World War II. This led to the establishment of government-funded and charitable programs that focused on rehabilitation rather than institutionalization of people with health difficulties. In the United Kingdom, the National Health Service (NHS) a public health service, offering free healthcare for all, was founded in 1948. Aneurin Bevan, the Labour Party's minister for health, at the time, is popularly considered the founder of the NHS.

In 1973, The American Hospital Association (AHA) created the first patient bill of rights, specifying aspects of patient relationships with healthcare professionals, although it had little enforceability. This bill emerged from the civil rights movement, partly attributed to the civil rights activist Afeni Shakur (mother of the American rapper, activist, poet, and songwriter, Tupac Shakur).

More rights for people with health conditions followed including the UN Declaration on Rights of Disabled People (UN-CDPR) in 1975. The UN-CRPD is an international human rights treaty of the United Nations intended to protect the rights and dignity of people with a disability, first adopted by the UN General Assembly in 2006. Parties to the CRPD must promote and protect the human rights of anyone with a disability as entitled to equality by law.

In the United Kingdom, the Equality Act (2010) defines disability as a physical or mental condition that has a substantial and long-term impact on an individual's ability to do normal day to day activities. Many counties also embed patient rights into healthcare policy and practice. Typically these include items such as the following:

Example Patient Rights

- The right to access health services
- The right to access good quality of care
- The right to receive treatment from appropriately qualified and experienced staff
- The right to be involved in making decisions about your medications and treatments
- The right to be protected from abuse and neglect
- The right to be treated by all staff with respect and confidentiality
- The right to access your medical records
- The right to informed consent
- The right to complain if you are not happy or if things go wrong.
- The right to make decisions about end-of-life care

Learning from Experience: A Win for Patient Involvement

Living with a lifelong heart condition can be challenging enough without having to fight through the medical system. As such, the publication of National Healthcare Standards in Scotland for Congenital Heart Disease (CHD) marked a significant step forward for this growing population. The most common congenital condition, CHD

Continued

Continued

accounts for nearly one-third of all congenital birth defects. Incidence rates are estimated at around 1.8%, and include a wide range of heart conditions present from birth. Thanks to medical advances, in high-income countries, over 90% of babies born with CHD will survive to adulthood; an increase of more than 70% since the mid-20th century. However, 90% of the world's children born with congenital heart disease live in locations with little to no care and where mortality remains high. Over 12 million people live with CHD globally, with a population of 20,000 in Scotland.[43]

Like many people with CHD, since reaching adulthood, I have found it challenging to access the specialist care I need, particularly during pregnancy and medical emergencies which prompted me to petition the Scottish Parliament, Holyrood for healthcare standards in 2012. I was invited to present evidence in parliament, and ended up on the national news.

Little did I know how consuming this journey would be, lasting over a decade. Initially I was delighted when, in response to the petition, the NHS in Scotland commissioned a specialist *Scottish Congenital Cardiac Network* (SCCN). Disappointingly, the network was decommissioned two years later, but the *Scottish Congenital Cardiac Advisory Board* was formed to complete the standard-development work. However, in 2018, the finish line in sight, our efforts were pulled and another branch of the NHS in Scotland, Healthcare Improvement Scotland (HIS), was tasked with restarting this work. It was hard to keep the momentum going. Voluntarily committing my time, as a patient representative throughout these changes, required me to draw from traumatic personal experience while dealing with health politics in a context of ever-changing faces. Throughout, my family, friends, the CHD community, and late Michael Cumper, past chair of The Somerville Heart Foundation, provided support. I was also encouraged by the healthcare professionals who showed unwavering commitment to this work. Despite the challenges, we had to keep our hard-earned seats at the table, else CHD risked falling off the health agenda.

We kept voicing the facts; CHD is vastly different from acquired/coronary heart problems, yet public health messaging and healthcare policy consistently neglects this. CHD is incurable, and lifelong specialist care is internationally recommended. Yet, almost half of the Scottish CHD population are "lost to care," leaving them at risk of developing more serious cardiac problems and premature death. All too often GPs, medical staff in emergency care, and allied health professionals do not know what to do with us. Although CHD is the most common congenital condition, with a quarter of babies with CHD requiring medical intervention in the first year of life, newborn babies are not routinely screened for CHD. In addition to normal life challenges, CHD can impact on education, relationships, parenting, body image, social inclusion, work, and finances and involve physical symptoms and limitations, medical tests, and invasive procedures. Lifetime prevalence of anxiety, depression and post-traumatic stress is two to three times higher than the general population, yet psychosocial support remains poor.

Standards were finally published by NHS Scotland in December 2024 which aim to ensure that consistently high levels of care are offered to everyone with CHD. Some key recommendations include enhanced detection rates in unborn babies, improvements during transition from pediatric to adult care, better emergency and pregnancy care, and education of nonspecialist healthcare professionals. I was particularly passionate about including a standard on mental health and emotional wellbeing to promote provision of psychologically informed healthcare. These standards were a long time coming. The odds are that someone you know is living with CHD. My hope is that the standards will improve care by engendering trust, safety, and patient empowerment to enable people with a lifelong heart condition to live as normal a life as possible.
—Adapted from "A Win for Patient Involvement: Congenital Heart Disease Standards in Scotland"[44]

Children's Rights

Once, when I was a teenager, a family friend told me how lucky I was that my parents had brought me home from hospital as a baby because in her day many would not have. This hint at Victorian values was shocking to hear. Yet, it is true that, if they survived, children like me were abandoned in schools and institutions for the "crippled, blind and deaf" throughout most of the 20th century. In many countries children with physical health problems are still hidden away due to stigma.

In the United Kingdom, the Children's Charter was published in 1889. This was the first act of parliament for the prevention of cruelty to children. Before 1852 few hospitals admitted children, yet disease was common. Families often looked beyond medicine to cure their sick child, turning to healers who would come to the child's bedside in the family home. However, some of these healers were accused of witchcraft. Children's hospitals were founded in response with the first inpatient children's hospital *Hôpital des Enfants Malades*, opening in Paris in 1802. In the United Kingdom, the Great Ormond Street Hospital for Children opened in 1852 in England, followed by Edinburgh Hospital for Sick Children in Scotland in 1860. The first hospital for children in the United States was established in Philadelphia in 1855. The aim for these hospitals was for children to access age-appropriate care from experienced staff. In 1882, Glasgow became one of the last major cities in the United Kingdom to open a children's hospital.[45]

Approximately one in every three children born in the United Kingdom in 1800 did not make it to their fifth birthday. Thanks to modern medicine and improved hygiene, over the next 220 years, this number dropped drastically. In the first half of the 20th century medical advances were rapid. In developed countries infant mortality is now at its lowest point in history, at just four deaths per thousand births.

Not so long ago, children were separated from their parents during hospital stays, with visiting only allowed once a week.[46] By the early 20th century, "visiting hours" for parents with children in hospital were limited to just 30 minutes per week. Children were often upset after these short visits, which nursing staff considered disruptive. At the time, doctors thought that children's memories were short, and their distress would soon be forgotten. During the 1950s, James Robertson, a Scottish psychiatric social worker and psychoanalyst, and Joyce Robertson, a British psychiatric social worker, child behavioral researcher, and colleague of Anna Freud, were based at the Tavistock Clinic in London working with John Bowlby in the development of attachment theory. Using a 16-mm hand-held movie camera, the couple captured the reactions of young children to hospital admissions and parental separation. In 1952, their harrowing films *A Two-Year-Old Goes to Hospital* and *Going to Hospital with Mother* revolutionized thinking about the emotional impact of separation on the child's emotional well-being during hospital stays. Their work led to the *Platt Report* by the United Kingdom's Ministry of Health, which was published in 1959. The report recommended open visiting for parents with children in hospital and that they should be cared for by specially trained children's nurses. However, it was not until the 1970s and beyond that unrestricted visiting became adopted across the United Kingdom.

The European Association for Children in Hospital (EACH) is an international umbrella organization advocating for the welfare of children in hospitals. It developed in response to concerns about the emotional and psychological impact of care children were receiving in hospitals. Initially developed at the Leiden Conference in 1988, the "Leiden Charter" has since developed into the "*EACH Charter*" (see Appendix).

The *UN Convention on the Rights of the Child* (UNCRC) was adopted in New York in 1989 and thereafter ratified by all European countries. Many of the requirements of the EACH Charter are mentioned in the UNCRC, assisting its implementation. The UNCRC is a human rights treaty setting out the civil, political, economic, social, health, and cultural rights of children. Nations that ratify this convention are bound to it by international law. Compliance is monitored by the UN Committee on the Rights of the Child, composed of member countries worldwide. UNCRC stresses that the survival, protection, growth, and development of children in good physical and emotional health are the foundations of human dignity and human rights. The right of the child to health is also informed by the Constitution of the World Health Organization, in which health is defined as a state of complete physical, mental, and social well-being, rather than merely the absence of disease or infirmity.

The European Children's Hospitals Organization (ECHO) is a new organization representing leading pediatric hospitals across Europe, many of which helped to lead the COVID-19 response locally or regionally. ECHO members provide acute and long-term disease management, caring for some of the most complex and vulnerable patients. They call on children's hospitals and public health systems to ensure that the rights of children are central in response to pandemics such as COVID-19.

Narrative Humility, Unconscious Bias and Bridging the Empathy Gap

Healthcare providers have a responsibility to take proactive, antidiscriminatory approach to healthcare delivery. We all have our own frame of reference, this window on the world can lead us to use unconscious biases to take shortcuts to make sense of the world. While this enables the brain to work efficiently, sometimes it means that we get it wrong. We can make snap judgments, deciding who is "in group" versus "out group," especially if we are stressed or under pressure. It is important to recognize that social power and privilege is based on membership of social groups whereby advantaged groups have more of both.

Psychologically informed healthcare aims to recognize these biases and privileges and acknowledges the many factors that contribute to differences. *Cultural humility* involves valuing difference, recognizing the impact of ableism, seeing people's strengths, showing openness to learn and grow, and understanding that good practice applies to us all. Challenging unconscious bias involves slowing down decision-making, reconsidering reasons for decisions, questioning cultural stereotypes, and looking out for each other. Within healthcare practice this can involve understanding cultural differences in communication, diet, health beliefs and approaches to treatment, religious beliefs and customs, and family roles. Tucker et al. describe the *Tucker Culturally Sensitive Health Care Clinic Environment Inventory–Patient Form (T-CSHCCEI-PF)*, a psychometrically validated instrument designed to assess the cultural sensitivity of healthcare center policies and environment as perceived by adult, racially/ethnically diverse patients, which may be useful to this end.[47]

As previously described, hermeneutical injustice occurs when we or others do not understand our experiences; for example, through unjust ways of listening to patients, by objectifying them, dismissing their "patient's testimony," or not sharing information about them.[48] Rosen proposes that healthcare providers should be trained in *narrative humility*—a self-reflective approach that aims to challenge testimonial injustice and unconscious bias by keeping an openness to each patient's story.[49] Heggen and Berg argue that improved recognition of epistemic injustice is important to prevent ignoring patients' testimonies and interpretations.[50] They state that the education of healthcare professionals is needed to improve students' reflective awareness of the knowledge and attitudes guiding their clinical practice and that patient values and preferences should guide all clinical decisions. Coproduction of research and healthcare policy with people with lived experience of LTCs, and their families and carers, is recommended NIHR guidance.[51,52]

Further, practicing allyship by strategically recognizing and challenging injustice and promoting equity through public acts of solidarity and advocacy are part of this approach. Allyship requires us to become aware of our own privilege, even within a marginalized community, and to make conscious efforts to undo our own biases, champion causes that matter, and act fairly as colleagues and leaders.

Adopting a social model of disability, described in the 1980s by Mike Oliver, a British disability rights activist and the first professor of disability studies, can facilitate this approach. This model challenges the dominant medical model of disability, which views the body as needing to be fixed to conform with normative values. The social model of disability considers impairment to be the actual attributes (or lack of attributes) that affect a person, (e.g., inability to walk or breathe independently). In this model disability refers to social restrictions that do not give equivalent attention and accommodation to the needs of individuals with impairments.[53,54] Ableism describes the assumption that such individuals need to be "fixed," treating able-bodied people as the norm, and leading to a society organized to accommodate the majority (e.g., an expectation to be able to work 9–5, full-time).

The Social Graces Model

Burnham's social graces model is a mnemonic that aims to identify the key features that influence personal and social identity.[55] One of the aims of the graces is to "name" power differentials so as to identify (and work on) our own prejudice and privilege. Naming power differences can invite us to share the social graces which we feel can cloud our judgment of others. The graces do not aim to be an exhaustive list, and can be adapted depending on place, time, and culture.

The social graces include:

- G: Gender, Gender Identity, Geography, Generation
- R: Race, Religion
- A: Age, Ability, Appearance
- C: Class, Culture, Caste
- E: Education, Ethnicity, Economics
- S: Spirituality, Sexuality, Sexual Orientation

Reflective Exercise

Reflect on your own practice, in relation to clients with health difficulties:

- Are you aware of your own health privilege and biases and how they may create blind spots to promote inclusive practice (it may help to consider the social graces model)?
- Are you aware of your own relationship with ableism, health problems, and disability?
- Do you embrace inclusive practice (consider the Campinha-Bacote model)?
- What have you done to avoid oppression for your patients or clients?
- What might you do differently, in this regard, looking back?

PART 3
EMOTIONAL HEALING

7
Working with Clients Therapeutically

> *Psychological services were easily available and most of us used the psych team in house. For me, the best thing about that was that it gave you access to the hospital wellbeing support. There was a staff member who provided massage, reiki, aromatherapy and again, another opportunity to take time out from the noise of the ward to relax for an hour in her lovely therapy room. She also came to our beds when we couldn't get out. We also established a weekly mindfulness session, which I found helpful and was organised by the psych dept, at our request. In these sessions we did guided meditation.*
> —Richard, 60 years old, congenital heart condition, heart transplant recipient, United Kingdom

Please note there is sensitive content throughout this chapter

Overview

During my training as a counseling psychologist, I attended a meeting where the subject of institutionalized sexual abuse of children (CSA) in care was raised, a growing national concern at the time. After the meeting, in clinical supervision, I became very distressed about the content of the discussion. While I always feel great empathy for the suffering of others, my response was stronger than usual. My supervisor gently explored with me why I had been so triggered. I told her that I had not been sexually abused or grown up in care, and did not understand why it had resonated so viscerally. I recall feeling overwhelmed with unspeakable horror and on the brink of a very dark and terrifying place, yet I could not articulate why. My supervisor wisely recommended a body psychotherapist, whom I ended up seeing for two years. Throughout this therapeutic work, we were able to piece together that I had spent my childhood in and out of an institution (hospital) where, although I was not sexually abused, I had to frequently strip off and subject my body to often painful, distressing procedures that I had no control over with my survival not guaranteed. Of course, there are many significant differences between CSA and medical trauma but there were enough parallels for my body to become triggered before my mind understood why.

While this therapeutic process was challenging, it was life-changing to find a safe space to recognize and process the trauma, the losses, the compromises, and the injustices associated with my health condition. I was able to grieve the loss of a normal childhood, express anger at the unfairness of it and for feeling silenced and marginalized, and feel sad for little me.

I also felt empowered as I found my voice. I used to give myself a tough time for feeling tired and took criticism, for example, about needing naps or working part-time, hard. I pushed myself to function "normally" and ended up exhausted. I learned to let this go and to accept myself, trust my body, be more open with trusting others about my health situation, and take better care of the little girl with the heart condition, fundamental to who I am.

One of the hardest things for me about living with a lifelong medical condition is that I need to go through the same traumatic experiences throughout my life, from cradle to grave. Even now, as an adult, each time I go to get my pacemaker checked, or for an appointment with a cardiologist or when I need to go back to theater, I can momentarily flit back to being a child again. In those moments, I find it hard to assert myself and I feel butterflies in my stomach and catch my breath as my body numbs. I still have regular nightmares where I am back in hospital, often as a child, attached to medical equipment and surrounded by doctors discussing what to do with me as I await surgery. I can be triggered by smells and sounds; I get a fright easily and automatically flinch if someone throws something my way. But now I can make sense of these experiences and manage my body's response compassionately, as part of my condition.

This chapter provides an overview of the relevant difficulties, evidence-based treatment modalities and approaches for psychologists and therapists working therapeutically with people living with an LTC to help them overcome any medical trauma, self-manage their condition, and find social connection while recognizing and validating the challenges they face. It may also be of interest to other healthcare professionals and for people with lived experience to better understand the psychological impact of living with an LTC and the therapeutic treatment approaches, tools, and techniques available.

Ideally, a psychologist should be embedded within all physical health teams to support patients throughout their health journey and to promote psychologically informed healthcare. Further, regular clinical supervision for healthcare professionals from a team psychologist could prevent vicarious trauma, moral injury, compassion fatigue, and burnout and enable healthcare professionals to better meet the psychological and emotional needs of patients. By embedding psychological and emotional support we can take a preventive approach to mitigate risk and promote protective factors upstream rather than waiting until harm has been done.

When seeking psychological therapy, it is important for individuals to seek support from an appropriately qualified professional with relevant training and expertise. In the United States, insurance companies may provide a list of their in-network providers. Other referral sources include psychological training institutes and counseling centers. Most countries have professional organizations that list licensed practitioners, such as the American Psychological Association (APA) in the United States and The British Psychological Society (BPS) and the Health and Social Care Professions Council (HCPC), who regulate healthcare professionals across the United Kingdom. In the United States you can call the state licensing board to ensure a providers' license is in good standing. Therapy is typically provided by different healthcare professionals including psychologists, clinical social workers, and psychiatrists. In the United States, if you do not have or want to use private insurance, you will then need to pay the therapist directly. If this is the case, sometimes therapists will slide their fee scale if you don't have any insurance reimbursement. This is a conversation that is best to have before starting therapy with that individual. Another possibility is to contact a local university, professional training institution, or local clinic. Often these organizations can help to find an experienced provider.

Evidence-Based Treatment Modalities

Clearly the chosen therapeutic modality will inform the development of a robust, collaborative, and culturally sensitive psychological assessment and formulation, which will inform the treatment plan. To this end, an overview of the evidence base for different therapeutic modalities in relation to LTCs is detailed below. Risk assessment is an important part of the assessment process and ongoing throughout therapeutic contact, since physical health problems can be a risk factor for suicide and self-harm, with the development of safety planning as indicated.[1,2]

Given the complex range of challenges and difficulties that people with a long-term health condition can face, an integrative approach to therapy may be useful, grounded in a *humanistic* stance. Ensuring Rogers's *person-centered*, core conditions of empathy, congruence, and unconditional positive regard, with a focus on developing a strong therapeutic alliance, will enable the client to move toward therapeutic change.[3] This will lead to the realization of their full potential (termed by Rogers as "self-actualization"), enhanced acceptance and trust in their feelings, openness to experience, and psychological flexibility.[4]

A range of evidence-based therapeutic modalities are effective when working with people who are living with an LTC. Developing a *toolkit* of techniques and strategies to help clients manage any distressing feelings is important to help them deal with stress, challenges, and difficult emotions related to their health condition. Different clients may benefit from different approaches, depending on their presenting problems, personal preference, the therapist's skills, and timing (for example, what else is going on in their life and where they are in their healthcare journey). Specifically, if someone is going through a health crisis then a person-centered approach may be beneficial. Whereas, if their health has recently declined, they may benefit from a focus on adjusting to their situation and grieving any losses. Someone who has reached a more stable point in their health may wish to focus on processing any medical trauma or managing ongoing symptoms.

Acceptance and commitment therapy (ACT)[5] has a robust evidence base for managing chronic health difficulties, including chronic pain, through *acceptance and mindfulness*, employing *cognitive defusion* techniques and *committed action* (discussed in more detail later in the chapter). A systematic review and meta-analysis found that ACT was more clinically effective than control conditions (no alternative intervention or treatment as usual) for pain management in adults.[6] Another study found that ACT was successful in improving daily functioning in children with chronic pain.[7] *Loving kindness meditation* can support increased self-compassion, helping individuals manage stress, anxiety, and chronic pain (see Appendix).[8]

Mindfulness-based cognitive-behavioral therapy (MCBT)[9] may also be useful for this client group. Strategies such as polyvagal-informed *mindfulness-based movement practices* can help patients cope with, for example, cancer.[10] Mindfulness can also support people living with chronic illness by reducing symptoms of anxiety, depression, and pain while improving emotional regulation and well-being.[11] One study reported that brief mindfulness meditation-based stress reduction during ultraviolet light therapy can increase resolution of psoriatic lesions in patients with psoriasis.[12]

To date, medical trauma has been neglected in therapeutic practice. For client's presenting with medical trauma, evidence-based trauma treatments are indicated, including *trauma-informed cognitive-behavioral therapy* (CBT)[13] and *prolonged exposure*.[14] If your client has difficulty remembering and narrating their traumatic experiences, then *eye movement desensitization and reprocessing* (EMDR),[15] *somatic approaches*[16,17,18] including a *polyvagal-informed approach*,[19,20] and *arts-based therapies*[21] may be beneficial. For example, a recent systematic review including 34 papers, with 1,254 participants, investigated the impact of movement therapy for individuals with chronic pain conditions. The researchers found that 74% of the included studies found reduced pain through quantitative pain measures or qualitative themes for dance movement therapies including aerobic dance and Biodanza.[22]

Clients who report a high degree of self-criticism, shame, and internalized stigma may find a *compassion-focused therapy* approach helpful. Compassion-focused therapy for pain management can improve depression, self-compassion, pain-related anxiety, and pain self-efficacy.[23,24]

Living with a chronic health condition can negatively affect relationships and the development of a supportive social network. *Interpersonal psychotherapy*, with a focus on *role transition* or *interpersonal disputes*, that aims to develop a supportive social network that better meets the client's psychological and emotional needs, could be useful for clients with an impoverished social support system.[25] Further, considering the links between living with an LTC and increased vulnerability to loneliness and social disconnection, which in turn can further negatively impact on physical and mental health, authors have proposed that *emotional focused therapy* may enhance the quality of people's emotional connections with significant others.[26]

Incorporating a *strengths-based approach* that validates how much your client has come through while acknowledging a normal emotional response to any unusually difficult life events, discrimination, and barriers, and working collaboratively with them to reduce background stress and enhance feelings of calm, can also help. A focus on empowering your client to self-advocate, set boundaries, and develop meaningful life goals is important.

Clients who have a serious LTC may benefit from *existential psychotherapy*, which focuses on the anxieties and uncertainties that are part of life and existence, including death and the meaning of life.[27] Existential therapy has four key themes, often known as pillars: death, meaning, isolation, and freedom, which often cause people anxiety. In therapy, the client works through their anxieties toward a point of acceptance. This therapeutic approach aims to help clients make sense of their lives, and many therapists use it integratively.

Regardless of therapeutic orientation, it may be useful to consider the following areas in development of the clinical formulation, treatment plan and interventions.

Respecting Diversity, Recognize and Validate the Wider Impact

I was required to have a psychological assessment prior to mastectomy but it felt like a tick box exercise and was traumatic in itself—the psychologist had not been told that I had a genetic mutation and questioned why I would want to remove my unaffected breast, even though I have an 80% chance of my cancer returning if I chose not to have the surgery.
  —Sarah, 44 years old, undergoing breast cancer treatment, United Kingdom

Of course, everyone's experience of living with a health condition is unique. Even two people with the same condition will have different experiences, support networks, medical interventions, commitments, health complications, personal strengths, beliefs, finances, attributes, and life goals. As such, therapists working in physical health commonly educate themselves about their client's condition while being curious and asking questions to better understand what living with a chronic condition means for them. While medical trauma may be part of your client's presentation this is certainly not ubiquitous, many people with an LTC will not have experienced medically related trauma. Rather, they may benefit from support with managing chronic symptoms, adjusting to a decline in their health, or processing associated losses.

Some of the issues that may be relevant include any medical barriers to early attachment, impact on identity and body image, trauma, impact on functioning, losses (e.g., decline in health, ability to have children, normal childhood), sexual health, preparation for medical interventions, managing chronic symptoms, living with a medical device, facing transplant, facing discrimination, intersectionality, health anxiety, impact on life choices, relationships, career, finances, parenting, palliative care, and positive adaptation.

Sometimes it can be helpful to have a mental health diagnosis, but only when the person does not become lost behind the label. If your client welcomes the diagnosis and it leads to improved understanding, empowerment, and access to a safe space to explore and process the meaning behind their suffering then it has served a purpose. If it leads to their symptoms being pathologized, to their experience misunderstood, and to them being marginalized then it only causes further harm. People who have experienced LTCs have often already undergone extensive medical scrutiny, which can at times be dehumanizing. It is essential that we are mindful of this, do not replicate it in the therapy room and ensure *affirmative practice*.[28]

Mental Health Disparities

Throughout my early childhood, my father was a Church of Scotland minister at a church on the outskirt of Glasgow in one of the poorest areas of Scotland, decimated by deindustrialization. Scotland has a strong and stoic Calvinist culture of "just getting on with it" in the face of intergenerational poverty. Growing up, we were surrounded by social and economic hardship. Health outcomes vary widely by social class with higher rates of chronic life stressors, death by suicide, and lower psychological help seeking for those in lower socioeconomic communities.[29]

The social circumstances of many children in my hospital, the direct impact of poverty on their health laid bare, haunts me still, providing an early education in human suffering and humility.

It is important to recognize such disparities in access to and use of health services.[30] The drivers of disparities in physical and mental health access and service quality are multifaceted. Unfortunately, inequalities often mean that those who are most likely to benefit from healthcare and therapy can find it hardest to access.

It is important for therapists to acknowledge, often intergenerational, social determinants of physical and mental health, structural and systemic inequalities, systems of oppression, and power–oppression relational dynamics.[31] Miyira Khan proposes that antioppressive therapeutic practice supports an understanding of how each person is shaped by their experiences, and the underlying systemic and structural context of lived experiences, while offering a relational dynamic of equality in practice to flatten the power–oppression hierarchy. Khan promotes "working within diversity" rather than "working with diversity" to acknowledge both the therapist and client differences and the impact of each on the therapeutic dynamic.[32]

This is important because, for example, racialized people are less likely to seek out and receive psychotherapy compared to white people and are more reliant on their natural support systems such as family, friends, and spiritual/religious leaders, while higher rates of mental health stigma in racialized communities have also been identified as barriers to help-seeking.[33] Further, a shortage of racially and ethnically diverse clinicians and lack of culturally competent clinicians may fuel mental health disparities and racialized people often receive a lower quality of care than white people.[34] Clinician racial biases can lead to errors in clinician decision-making, resulting in the overdiagnosis or underdiagnosis of certain disorders in racialized clients.[35,36] Further, as discussed in Chapter 6, lower socioeconomic status is associated with poorer physical and mental health and reduced lifespan with many complex interacting factors contributing to these disparities in health risk and disease burden.[37,38]

Meyer proposed the minority stress model as a conceptual framework to account for the increased prevalence of mental health conditions in lesbians, gay men, and bisexuals, explaining that stigma, prejudice, and discrimination create a hostile and stressful social environment that contributes to mental and physical health difficulties.[39] The model describes unique stress processes, including the experience of prejudice events, expectations of rejection, hiding and concealing, internalized homophobia, and ameliorative coping processes. The model outlines "distal" and "proximal" stressors that are unique and chronic for minority populations. Distal stressors may form experiences like discrimination, while proximal stressors are more internally based processes like internalized homonegativity.

Naeem et al. propose that cultural adaptation of therapeutic practice can include:

- **Skills-based models**: emphasize the provider's ability to develop cultural knowledge of the self and others and to apply this knowledge to clinical contexts.
- **Adaptation models**: emphasize the use of systematic modifications to make conventional treatments more congruent with cultural beliefs and practices.
- **Process models**: emphasize the dynamic processes underlying therapy, particularly as they relate to client–therapist interactions and cultural meanings ascribed to behaviors.[40]

For example, cultural adaptation of CBT can be defined as adjusting how therapy is delivered, through the acquisition of awareness, knowledge, and skills related to a given culture, without compromising on the theoretical underpinning of CBT.[41] Naeem et al. state that to effectively adapt CBT for a given culture, the following areas of cultural competence (the triple-A principle) must be covered:

- awareness of relevant issues and preparation for therapy
- assessment and engagement
- adjustments in therapy techniques ("technical adjustments").[42]

Naeem et al. further proposed that adjustments to therapeutic practice include greater use of stories and a more directive style and that clients from non-Western cultures often find behavioral methods (behavioral activation, behavioral experiments) and problem-solving particularly useful. As such, muscle relaxation and breathing may be beneficial since breathing exercises are part of many religious and spiritual traditions and are commonly practiced in non-Western cultures. Patients from non-Western cultures are also much more likely than Western patients to want to be informed of the number of sessions and the structure and focus of the therapy, and to want some information on what will happen in sessions in advance.[43]

Promote Self-Care

Self-care is fundamental to your client reducing their baseline stress levels, managing their health condition, and building resilience. This includes keeping a healthy sleep routine, eating well, and moving their body (as possible) daily. Self-care also involves your client being self-compassionate, especially about any limitations or difficulties they face because of their health condition; communicating their needs; and setting boundaries in relationships.

What we eat and our physical activity can make an enormous difference to how we feel physically, emotionally, and psychologically. It may be useful to get your client to speak to their medical team to check to see if there are any dietary modifications that would benefit them. Gut health is also increasingly being linked to mood. If your client has been prescribed antibiotics for infection or post-surgery, they may benefit from taking a course of probiotics to support a healthy gut (with the advice of their healthcare team).

Some people with an LTC may have had to sit out during gym classes at school or struggle to keep up with their peers. Recommendations around physical activity for people with an LTC have changed significantly over the years, and the importance of physical activity for general health has been recognized. Likewise, the damaging effect of physical inactivity and obesity on health means that exercising, within your client's personal safety limits and advice from their health team, is recommended.

Exercise may be a challenge for clients who are feeling fearful of "pushing" themselves physically or have missed the experience of learning their physical limits. This is completely understandable and if this is the case it might take some time to build up their confidence. It might help them to start small, for example, by going for walks, and working with them to build themselves up (as agreed with their medical team).

It is important to note that recommendations about graded exercise therapy for people with chronic fatigue syndrome (CFS) have recently been debated. Revised recommendations emphasize the potential harms of exercise, based on qualitative evidence provided by a small number of service users, and the balance has shifted toward helping patients to adjust to the long-term debilitating effects of CFS.[44]

Encouraging your clients to following good hygiene such as regularly washing their hands and using hand gel; staying away from people who have a virus, a cough, or runny nose; keeping warm; and making sure they get the annual flu vaccine can also help with management of their condition.

Processing Medically Related Trauma

Trauma destroys the social systems of care, protection, and meaning that support human life. The recovery process requires the reconstruction of these systems. The essential features of psychological trauma are disempowerment and disconnection from others. The recovery process therefore is based upon empowerment of the survivor and restoration of relationships. The recovery process may be conceptualized in three stages: establishing safety, retelling the story of the traumatic event, and reconnecting with others. Treatment of post-traumatic disorders must be appropriate to the survivor's stage of recovery. Caregivers require a strong professional support system to manage the psychological consequences of working with survivors.

—Judith Herman[45]

In one of my first sessions with my body psychotherapist, she asked me how I coped with all the health problems I had been through. I replied that I was "fine" and "just got on with it," after all there was no other choice. She looked at me attentively then asked me to imagine taking my head off and putting it on the adjacent chair. I found this a bit odd but went with it. She asked me how my body was feeling. To my surprise, I became emotional. From somewhere, I replied that my body was exhausted, I wanted to be left alone, I was horrified at the thought of needing more things done to it. I felt a deep urge to protect myself and push away anyone or anything that came close to me. I could feel my scars. Half a dozen deep lines from thoracotomies etched horizontally from the middle of my chest all the way around my back, another scored vertically down my chest bone and several leaving their mark where my pacemaker now sits below my left collarbone. I drew my left arm up protectively over my body, my hand placed on my chest, a gesture I have since realized that I often make subconsciously. A habit developed as a child when my ribcage and scars were healing from thoracotomies. Paying attention to my body in this way was the start of my long journey toward recognizing and healing from extensive medical trauma. This was the first time that I had experienced someone validating the embodied impact of my healthcare experiences while being given permission to share my experiences without feeling that I needed to be brave, protect them, or be "normal."

Traditional trauma therapies involve narration in a safe space using a phased approach; safety and stabilization, remembrance and mourning, and finally reconnection.[46] Judith Herman, the leading American professor of psychiatry at Harvard Medical School proposes that clients presenting with more complex trauma benefit from this *phased intervention model of psychological treatment*[47] to ensure safety and stabilization, psychoeducation, a safe space to process traumatic experiences and any losses and to develop self-care and skills to manage stress and medical treatments. Bessel van der Kolk proposes that overcoming trauma involves (re)establishing community, effective action, emotional regulation, knowing oneself, and processing traumatic memories.[48]

Talking therapies require the brain's frontal lobe, yet trauma can leave a sensory imprint rather than a story, especially if the trauma occurred when your client was preverbal (prior to age 3). When we experience trauma, the limbic system takes over, affecting our sleep, arousal, breathing, appetite, emotional regulation, memory, language, and relationship between self and our environment.[49,50,51,52,53] This can result in *speechless terror*, whereby the parts of the brain responsible for language and memory are affected by the traumatic experience leaving the person unable to find the words to share their account. It is postulated that when self-regulation is not available, trauma symptoms arise from unregulated threat preoccupation, which affects our biology, social interaction, and maturation.[54] In this case, trauma-based EMDR, somatic approaches, and arts-based therapies can help clients process and make sense of their experiences without having to find the words.

When the Mind Feels Safer than the Body

The human mind is incredibly powerful, and it can protect us at times of extreme adversity. I have overcome periods of immense pain and distress by focusing my mind and somehow floating outside my body. Your mind can take you anywhere when your body cannot. Using my mind has also helped me to find purpose, joy, and hope. Like many, I have depended on learning, reading, writing, music, drawing, a vivid imagination, and humor to distract from and diffuse challenging situations.

It is important to note that people who are experiencing chronic health difficulties may come to rely on cognitive defense strategies, such as intellectualization, humor, perfectionism, or dissociation from their body, to manage their difficulties. They may perceive their health condition as a source of threat and feel chronically unsafe in their own body. For such individuals, working with and becoming more aware of the body can be challenging—especially if they feel like their body has let them down and is the source of pain and discomfort—and to cope with distressing symptoms and medical treatments they have learned to dissociate from the body or go into battle with it. Further, feeling psychologically safe and vulnerable can be triggering for people who have been highly traumatized.[55]

As such, in therapy clients may default to intellectualizing or joking about their difficulties while avoiding feelings, because staying "in their head" has helped them distance themselves from bodily pain and discomfort in the past. However, rigid overreliance on cognitive defense strategies, while completely understandable, may present a barrier to sharing, understanding, and processing more difficult feelings. Further, while dissociation can be a necessary survival response, and sometimes it is our only choice, longer-term it can lead to significant physical and mental health costs, especially if our autonomic nervous system is unnecessarily triggered into states of hyperarousal or hypoarousal.

Respecting and showing gratitude for these coping strategies while gently challenging them, by reflecting on this therapeutic process (rather than content) can help your client to become more aware of these defenses. In turn this can lead them gradually to let go of these defenses and better recognize and attend to their embodied experience and emotions. In time, this will enable them to process their feelings and develop strategies to move their autonomic nervous system back to a state of psychological safety allowing greater psychological flexibility. This approach must be collaborative, gradual, and nuanced and within the context of a strong therapeutic alliance.

A Polyvagal Approach to Dealing with Medical Trauma

I prepared for and followed up my operations with the help of Somatic Experiencing, a body-oriented approach. Before every operation, I listened to preparatory meditations that prepared me and my body for the operation. It was very important for me to understand the state of my nervous system. Every patient should have access to this knowledge. For a long time, I only dealt with my physical diagnoses. The knowledge of polyvagal theory was crucial to understand the effects on and in my body. This knowledge should be made available to people with chronic complex illnesses.

—Lou, 48, bowel endometriosis, Germany

Therapy informed by polyvagal theory (PVT) advocates for working with the client to help them become more aware of their body and connecting with their senses with the goal of restoring regulation of their autonomic nervous system and emotions. As previously explored, unresolved medical trauma may contribute to client's responding to past threats as if they are current, while an adverse history may narrow their window for feeling safe.[56] In this case, homeostatic rhythms become disrupted, impacting on well-being. As previously discussed, psychological safety is central to mental health and well-being and people often seek therapy because they are struggling to feel safe. Together, this can negatively affect mental health, trust in relationships, and sense of self for people living with an LTC.

Prioritizing a phase of safety and stabilization in treatment and supporting people to feel safe before traumatic memories are addressed is important. By applying the principles of PVT, through safe therapeutic presence, co-regulation, and recognition of client's nonverbal safety signaling, therapists can better attune to their client's emotional and physiological state.[57] By paying attention to the client's voice tone, facial expressions, and body language the therapist can better understand the client's autonomic nervous system and help to shift this through containment and co-regulation. PVT considers co-regulation as the reciprocal sending and receiving of signals of psychological safety. As such, via co-regulation, therapists can promote feelings of psychological safety by providing signals of safety, including intonation of voice, body language, and compassion, for their clients during the therapeutic encounter. This entrainment will help the client develop skills to self-regulate emotional and physiological states of defense and safety in a safe and supportive space.

Stephen Porges's *Safe & Sound Protocol* aims to repattern the nervous system by making ventral-vagal activation, therefore the social engagement system and co-regulation, more accessible. Embedding this into therapeutic work, for example prior to a session, may help to enhance the autonomic nervous system platform for therapy.

Sensitively working with your client toward better understanding their autonomic, physiological, and emotional responses will also help them to better self-regulate and process their emotional experiences (for example, by mapping the nervous system, see below). Our physiological state serves as the platform for our narrative state, therefore, by helping your client regulate their physiological state you can help them feel safer beyond the therapy setting. Physical and emotional healing is promoted as they become more aware of their inner experiences and befriend what is going on inside themselves.[58] Again, this must be collaborative and sensitive using a paced approach.

Client Exercise: Deb Dana's Mapping the Nervous System

Deb Dana, the American licensed clinical social worker, clinician, author, and cofounder of The Polyvagal Institute, proposes mapping the nervous system with clients.[59] To do this you can work through this exercise with your client to help them better understand their embodied threat response and how to facilitate feelings of psychological safety. Encourage them to think about their autonomic nervous system as a ladder; at the top of the ladder is "safe and social," the middle of the ladder is when they are in sympathetic activation and the last step of the ladder is dorsal vagal activation. Ask your client to identify each state for them.

Sympathetic Nervous System (Hyperarousal): For the middle of the ladder, recall a time when you felt mobilized, like there was too much going on for you and you felt worried, anxious, or scared. Consider this experience only long enough to let your body taste it so that you can map it.

- Find a word for this state that works for you.
- Identify what this feels like for you (e.g., racing heart rate, breathless, feeling nauseous).
- Identify your triggers (what triggers you into hyperarousal)?

Dorsal vagal (Hypoarousal): Now go to the bottom of your ladder. Recall a time you felt disconnected, or a sense of collapse. A time when your system does not have enough energy to function and might be shutting down. You might feel hopeless, distant, unmotivated, or lacking interest. "Dip your toe" into this feeling just a bit and then begin to map it.

- Find a word for this state that works for you.
- Identify what this feels like for you (e.g., spaced out, numb).
- Identify your triggers (what triggers you into hyperarousal)?

Ventral vagal (social engagement system): Now move to the top of your ladder. Remember a time you felt a warm feeling of well-being. Perhaps it was just a moment, or a prolonged experience. The world feels safe enough, you feel ok enough, and are generally safe to connect to yourself and others. Let this feeling fill you now and begin to map it.

- Find a word for this state that works for you.
- Identify what this feels like for you (e.g., steady breathing, calm, connected).

> - Identify your glimmers, (what helps you to feel grounded, safe, and calm) what glimmers bring you into this optimal state?

Neuroception of Psychological Safety Scale (NPSS)

Considering the relevance of psychological safety in preventing, mitigating, and treating trauma-related conditions, we developed a standardized measure of psychological safety in partnership with an international team of psychologists and researchers with expertise in trauma and scale development.[60] The Neuroception of Psychological Safety Scale (NPSS), grounded in PVT, is the first psychometric tool that aims to measure psychological safety for the individual. This scale incorporates three key factors—compassion, social engagement, and bodily sensation—which are integral to understanding the neurobiological foundations of psychological safety.

Specifically, the scale comprises 29 statement items with three key subscales: Social Engagement (e.g., "I felt accepted by others"), Compassion (e.g., "I felt like I could comfort a loved one"), and Bodily Sensations (e.g., "My stomach felt settled"). Compassion reflects the ability to engage with others in a supportive and nonjudgmental manner, promoting trust and connection. Social engagement refers to the capacity for meaningful social interactions, which are essential for fostering a sense of safety and belonging. Bodily sensation, linked to the body's physiological responses, highlights the importance of autonomic regulation and bodily awareness in feeling safe and grounded. These dimensions collectively support the prevention, mitigation, and treatment of trauma-related conditions by facilitating an environment where the autonomic nervous system can shift into a state of safety and regulation. The three-factor structure of the NPSS showed adequate fit, and good reliability.[61]

The NPSS has been widely adopted across a range of settings including evaluation of EMDR in dissociative disorders; exploring the reintegration of children and youth experiencing homelessness and instability; examining the significance of feeling safe for resilience of adolescents in sub-Saharan Africa; and as an informative measure for a model of human-animal interactions.[62,63,64,65] In addition, researchers have validated an Italian version of the scale in a nonclinical sample and the scale was found to have a three-factor structure with good convergent, divergent, and test–retest validity and robust psychometric properties.[66]

As previously explored (in Chapters 3 and 5), in healthcare environments, where stress and trauma are often prevalent, PVT highlights the importance of fostering psychological safety to support the well-being of both patients and healthcare professionals. By ensuring a sense of safety, healthcare professionals are better able to regulate their emotions, connect with others, and perform effectively in high-pressure situations, ultimately enhancing overall care and recovery. As such, we recently conducted a study that validated the NPSS as a reliable and multidimensional tool for assessing psychological safety in health and social care settings. The study highlights the importance of psychological safety for health and social care workers and provides a valuable measure to support interventions aimed at fostering safer and more supportive work environments.[67]

Most traditional psychometric measures focus on pathology rather than prevention and positive adaptation. The NPSS aims to facilitate psychological safety development and can be used to mitigate risk factors and promote protective factors helping prevent mental health difficulties.

The NPSS can be employed in a wide range of settings, such as psychological therapy/counseling, and it is free for therapeutic and research purposes. For example, it could track change in your client's feelings of psychological safety within the therapy setting, across the course of therapy, or in a particular situation (such as when attending the hospital for an appointment). It could be used to evidence and support improvements in care toward psychologically informed healthcare. It could be implemented to establish feelings of psychological safety for healthcare professionals and trainees to support practice and learning. A copy of the scale and handbook can be found in the Appendix.

Gendlin's Focusing and Felt Sense

What is split off, not felt, remains the same. When it is felt, it changes. Most people don't know this! They think that by not permitting the feeling of their negative ways they make themselves good. On the contrary, that keeps these negatives static, the same from year to year. A few moments of feeling it in your body allows it to change. If there is in you something bad or sick or unsound, let it inwardly be and breathe. That's the only way it can evolve and change into the form it needs.

—Dr. Eugene Gendlin

Developed in the 1960s by the American philosopher and student of Carl Rogers, Dr. Eugene Gendlin, *experiential focusing* is an embodiment practice.

This process of inner enquiry, self-understanding, and change could be useful in therapy to improve body awareness and self-compassion for your client.

Focusing is a mind–body process that involves getting in touch with the *felt sense*. The "felt sense" is Gendlin's term for a holistic sense, experienced via the body, that encompasses and describes the wholeness of how you are in general. Gendlin discovered that when someone pays attention to this felt sense of something, and stays with that experience, allowing it to be there fully, it changes, and the way the person is holding the issue or problem changes too. Focusing is a six-step process that helps us find our implicit embodied knowing about an issue in our life. Turning attention inward and listening with compassion allows a felt sense, a whole sense of the situation, to form. As such, focusing is a way of listening deeply to this experiential sense of who we are and how we are.

Focusing: Six Steps

1. Clearing a space: get out of your head and into your peaceful, inner body knowing
2. Identify a felt sense: a bodily knowing
3. Find a handle: words or an image that capture the bodily knowing
4. Resonate: check if those words fit with that bodily knowing
5. Inquire: Ask the bodily felt sense an open-ended question
6. Receive the experience

—adapted from Gendlin, *Focusing*[68]

Gabor Mate's Seven A's of Healing

Emotional competence is what we need to develop if we are to protect ourselves from the hidden stresses that create a risk to health, and it is what we need to regain if we are to heal.

Gabor Mate[69]

In his book, *When the Body Says No: The Cost of Hidden Stress*, Gabor Maté, a Hungarian-born Canadian physician, describes that to rid the body of stress and associated inflammation we must turn our attention toward our mental and emotional health too.[70] He notes that three factors that lead to stress universally include uncertainty, lack of information, and loss of control, all of which can be an ongoing part of life with an LTC. Maté describes seven steps toward mental and physical healing. While of course, it is important to recognize that there will likely be ongoing health difficulties, it can be helpful to consider this framework from the perspective of clients who are experiencing chronic health problems to help them manage their condition and optimize their health:

Gabor Mate's Seven Steps Applied to LTCs

Acceptance: This involves meeting ourselves where we are, fully accepting ourselves, and recognizing we are worthy of compassion. For example, "Today I am in pain, tired, and anxious but I am still a person worthy of compassion." Or "My body is doing its best for me, and I will listen to it, look after myself, and try to meet my needs for rest, recovery, and self-care."

Awareness: Being aware of what our bodies tell us is important for healing. When we are aware of these feelings, we can make informed choices about how to respond. This can be difficult for people who have coped with distressing feelings through avoidance. Sensitively working toward improved awareness is important. For example, "Today I am tired, I need to listen to my body and rest." Or "My symptoms seem to have worsened, I need to see my doctor."

Anger: Harboring anger and resentment can cause more harm than good. Anger is a normal response to injustice, yet often it is considered a negative emotion (especially for women) and we learn to suppress it. Yet, this can breed hostility and aggression and can leak out in angry and misdirected outbursts or become self-directed, leading to self-criticism, shame, and low mood. It can also lead to stress in the body or turned inward to depression. Being able to experience, express, and consider anger in a productive and healthy way is crucial to healing. For example, "It is unfair that I must face another medical procedure, it is okay for me to feel angry about this. I can work through this feeling and then let it go." Or "It is not fair that my employer is not supporting me in the workplace, I need to speak to human resources and my union representative to ensure I get the support that I am entitled to."

Autonomy: Developing personal boundaries and knowing yourself honestly will help self-management of any chronic health issues. For example, "I understand my personal limits, and I have the right to communicate them to my partner and explain that I need time by myself to rest."

Attachment: Being connected to others is a lifeline to healing. This involves allowing ourselves to become vulnerable in safe relationships. For example, "I am feeling anxious about going for another hospital appointment, I am going to ask my close friend to take me. I will be less anxious if they drive and then I will not need to worry about finding a space to park my car. They will also help to distract me in the waiting area, remember what the doctor says during my appointment, and we can do something nice afterward if we feel up to it."

Assertion: Recognizing that each of us has a right to be here, to think and feel, to love and be loved. For example, "Even though I can't work, I have as much right to be part of society as anyone else." Or "Just because I was born with a heart condition, does not mean I am not entitled to a happy life."

Affirmation: Maté describes two types of affirmation. Affirming our creative selves (e.g., through art, music, writing) and by connecting to something bigger, a higher purpose or power. For example, "I will take some art materials into hospital with me so that I can draw, I find this helps me to stay calm." Or "I will create a sense of purpose from my experiences by campaigning for improved care for children with the same condition."

Attending the hospital chapel helped me cope with my most recent stay in hospital, which lasted 338 days, with me waiting for, and having, a heart transplant. Whilst I don't consider myself particularly religious, I do acknowledge a spiritual side to my character. As such the chapel provided a safe haven to go to, which I used particularly when I was struggling psychologically. I recall after about 6 months of waiting, my own health was in decline, a transplant patient friend was struggling medically to a significant extent post-transplant, and it was my wedding anniversary. To face all these factors simultaneously was difficult and I remember thinking at the time that I was broken. The chapel gave me a quiet space (there was usually nobody else in there) to have a cry, gather my thoughts and ultimately, tell myself that I'm in the right place and that it was time to "go again." This meant to come to an acceptance of the reality of my situation and to recognize that all the resources of the hospital were endeavoring to support me here.

—Richard, 60 years old, congenital heart condition, heart transplant recipient, United Kingdom

Emotional Regulation

Healthy *emotional regulation* can help to alleviate and prevent mental health problems and promote healing from medical trauma for people with an LTC. Emotional regulation is the ability to effectively monitor, evaluate, and change our emotions, which is fundamental to everyday functioning. This includes having an awareness of and being able to notice and label emotions, being able to tolerate unpleasant feelings, recognize patterns, and manage feelings in a healthy way. Emotional regulation is not something we are born with; rather it is a set of skills that we can build on to improve our health and well-being.[71]

By working with your client to help them accept a normal emotional response to difficult life experiences, termed "*radical acceptance*,"[72] they will be better able to validate their feelings, learn to manage them, and problem-solve what they need to do to feel better. This is particularly important for clients that have learned to suppress their feelings or have felt dismissed and invalidated during healthcare encounters.

Rather than suppressing or resisting feelings, research has shown that exploring and labeling emotions helps to make them less distressing. It is important for clients to learn how to recognize their emotions and label them because they carry important messages about their needs. Working with clients and helping them listen to their bodies and what messages their feelings are telling them will help them respond to situations in a thoughtful and empathetic way. An emotion wheel, or wheel of emotions, a visual tool to help individuals identify and verbalize their emotions, may be useful. The following sentence can help client's better link feelings, triggers, and needs.

- I feel ... because ... and I need ....

For example:

- I feel *scared* because *I am going back to the hospital for a check-up*, and I need *to take someone supportive with me.*
- I feel *sad* because *I need to have more treatment*, and I need to *take time to work through this.*
- I feel *confused* because *I do not understand what is happening to me*, and I need *to speak to my healthcare team.*
- I feel *stressed* because *I cannot keep on top of everything*, and I need *to ask others for help.*

Empowering your clients with psychoeducation, for example by helping them to *map their nervous system*, collaboratively exploring their triggers, *glimmers* (what helps them to feel grounded, safe, and connected[73]) and resource regulation can help. Be mindful to consider any limitations and symptoms of their health condition. Remind your client that, when needed, it is okay to live one day, hour, or moment at a time and that resilience allows vulnerability.

Working with your client to develop soothing techniques that draw on the senses can also help them feel psychologically safer. This could include holding in mind comforting images, looking at photographs from a happy and relaxing time, thinking about someone who offered them unconditional love and acceptance, going for a walk-in nature, watching something comforting on the TV, feeling something soothing such as a cozy or weighted blanket or comfortable clothing or holding a grounding object such as a pebble or patting a pet. Smells can also be soothing, such as using a relaxing moisturizer, candle, essential oils, the smell of nature, or baking. Comforting sounds may also help, such as bird song, relaxing music, or their own favorites. You could work with your client to create a soothing box where they can keep all the things that help them feel safer, that they can turn to when they are feeling overwhelmed. They may find it helpful to create a bag of soothing items like this to take with them during a hospital stay.

Cognitive Defusion

Cognitive defusion techniques work by helping people become more psychologically flexible in their thinking, especially when their thoughts get in the way of functioning or living by their values.[74] They enable individuals to detach from their thoughts rather than treat them as fact. Cognitive defusion is associated with improved emotional regulation, reduced impulsivity and self-criticism and includes the following techniques.

> **Cognitive Defusion Techniques**
>
> *Naming Your Thoughts:* This technique is the practice of naming and labeling thoughts, for example, if your client has a self-critical thought they can note, "I notice that I'm having a critical thought." This allows them to acknowledge it without giving it any power or influence. This technique involves noticing the distressing thought when it comes to mind, labeling it, and allowing it to come and go without trying to make anything happen.
> *Thought Bubbles:* The thought bubbles technique takes naming the thoughts a step further, whereby your client imagines that they are putting the distressing thought inside a thought bubble and then allowing it to drift away.
> *Mindful Observation:* Mindful observation is a technique for your client to connect with the present moment and experience it with full awareness. This practice can help them to build their capacity for awareness and grounding in the here

> and now. It may help them to choose something to focus on from their five senses, such as their breath, music, a color, or smell. Ask them to focus their attention on the chosen object, notice any details or sensory information about it, and observe without judgment, noticing any thoughts, images, or body sensations that come up. If their mind wanders, ask them to simply notice that and gently bring their attention back.
>
> *Singing Your Thoughts:* Singing their thoughts can be a creative and fun way for your client to defuse distressing thoughts and it can help them to externalize their thoughts.
>
> *Metaphor Creation:* One of the most common metaphors for thought defusion is clouds in the sky. Ask your client to imagine that their thoughts are clouds in the sky, to notice them without judgment, and then allow them to softly and gently float away and out of their awareness. They may prefer to create their own thought defusion metaphor.
>
> *Word Repetition:* The next time your client has a distressing thought, get them to say it aloud or repeat it in their head over and over quickly. This can take the thought out of context and help to reduce its impact.
>
> *Observing Self:* Get your client to imagine stepping back and observing their thoughts from the perspective of an impartial third party. This can help them to detach and gain distance from the thought.

Enhancing Self-Compassion

Neff and Germer describe self-compassion as having three parts, namely self-kindness, common humanity, and mindfulness.[75] Self-kindness means not being harsh or judgmental of ourselves, accepting that we cannot be perfect, and offering ourselves the understanding that we often do loved ones. Common humanity involves the recognition that all human beings are flawed and a work in progress. It involves looking at the broader context with compassion and recognizing that our experiences are not unique, and the human condition is universal. By doing so we can reach out to others for support during hardship rather than feeling ashamed, hiding ourselves away and becoming isolated in our suffering. Mindfulness refers to being aware of the present moment in an open and balanced manner.

Respecting and working with our body is the basis for *self-compassion*.[76] However, as discussed, this can be challenging when you have a long-term health condition and uncomfortable symptoms because living with a chronic health condition can negatively affect self-concept and trust in one's body. When your body is the source of your distress it is common to go into battle with it to cope, for example, by fighting fatigue and pain by pushing through and not listening to the body. Over time, this can worsen symptoms leading to a boom-and-bust cycle, self-criticism, and low mood. Further, self-care may seem pointless if you feel like your body has let you down, which may lead to poor diet, inactivity, and risk taking.

It can be useful to take a *cognitive-behavioral approach* (CBT) to challenging any underlying unhelpful thoughts, unfounded beliefs, and internalized stigma that clients may have developed about themselves, other people, and the world, and unhelpful rules and strategies that they have developed to compensate for them, that in turn maintain their distress.[77] While perfectly understandable considering their experiences, some of these beliefs can be unhelpful and negative, for example, "*I am unlovable,*" "*I am defective,*" or "*I am a failure.*"

To compensate for these unhelpful beliefs, you may find that your client has formed *rules* such as "*I won't reveal my true self or I will be rejected,*" "*I can't make any mistakes, or I will get caught out,*" or "*I can't exert myself, or I will get very unwell.*" While these rules may have helped them out at one time, it is likely that they are outdated, keep the original negative belief in place, and hold them back in life. Further, they may contribute to unhelpful "compensatory" behaviors, such as perfectionism, disordered eating, risk-taking, appeasement, or social withdrawal, that support a vicious cycle of distress.

Working collaboratively with your clients to help them recognize any unhelpful core beliefs and rules, allows them to start to challenge them using cognitive strategies such as cognitive diffusion, restructuring, Socratic questioning, and guided discovery. Of course, it is important to note that sometimes these unhelpful beliefs and rules are grounded in painful childhood experiences and taking time to process any underlying trauma, pain, or grief is important.

Often, clients learn to cope with distressing feelings such as anxiety with *reassurance seeking* and *checking behaviors*. This may include seeking reassurance from doctors, searching for answers online, or engaging in checking behaviors such as repeatedly examining a lump or checking their heart rate. While this provides a temporary quick fix, it reinforces a vicious cycle of anxiety and/or low mood. Over time, these quick fix behaviors can undermine their confidence, support the cycle, make their distress worse in the longer term, and get in the way of day-to-day functioning. It can be useful to tackle these safety behaviors with clients by developing an "exposure hierarchy" at the same time as developing healthy coping strategies such as breathing techniques, coping statements, and relaxation exercises. It may also be useful to work with your client to empower them to discuss any underlying anxieties they have about their health with their healthcare providers and to establish red flag symptoms. This will put them in a more informed position to so they can distinguish between benign symptoms and ones that do require medical follow-up because such anxieties or earlier negative health experiences may understandably underlie any checking and reassurance-seeking behaviors.

Using a cognitive behavioral approach, it can also help to work with clients to recognize their triggers. A trigger is a situation that may provoke a distressing memory, or uncomfortable feelings and unhelpful behaviors. Once these situations are identified, it will be easier for your client to take steps to prepare themselves to manage the feelings they evoke. Thought diaries can help to establish patterns of triggers, thoughts, distressing feelings, physical symptoms, and behaviors.

Working with your client to increase activity levels, using activity scheduling, can help to improve low mood especially if they have withdrawn from the things they previously enjoyed. To support a sense of well-being it is important to achieve a balance between pleasurable activities and ones that provide a sense of accomplishment (e.g., pleasure and mastery).

A compassion-focused therapy approach can also be useful.[78] As described in Chapter 1, traumatic experiences can lead to an overdeveloped "threat system" and underdeveloped "soothing system." Working therapeutically with clients to help them develop their "soothing system" through co-regulation, developing self-compassion, emotional regulation, and challenging any overreliance on the "drive system" can be beneficial. To this end, a loving kindness meditation is included in the Appendix.

Further, *coming out* as disabled or being more open with others about their health condition and expressing *disability pride* can offer protection against psychological effects of stigma.[79]

Helping Your Client to Work with Their Body

- ✓ Validate any additional (hidden) barriers, challenges, and injustices
- ✓ Promote self-care and pacing
- ✓ Avoid "compare and despair" with healthy peers

> ✓ Promote assertive communication about any challenges
> ✓ Acknowledge strengths, resilience, and determination
> ✓ Challenge negative self-talk, beliefs, and unhelpful coping strategies (reassurance seeking, safety/checking behaviors, alcohol/drug misuse)
> ✓ Encourage them to find supportive and positive people (beware toxic positivity)
> ✓ Encourage them to focus on what they can do

Recognizing Grief, Loss, and Anger

Living with an LTC can also mean facing significant losses.[80] Some of these losses may be hard for clients to recognize because they involve the loss of something they never knew, such as a "normal" childhood, activities others can take for granted, social inclusion, and missed opportunities and life choices. For some there may be loss associated with being unable to have children or as big a family as they had hoped. There can be a decline in health status or not having energy or stamina to do some of the activities they previously enjoyed. There can be anticipation of a decline in health and loss of what they expected life to look like, facing another surgery, being at risk of a sudden traumatic medical event or reduced life expectancy. Your client may report feeling sad, without understanding why, when they are grieving about their situation.

Other people can complicate these feelings of grief. For example, by assuming that because your client has lived with an LTC for many years they should be able to cope with it or by underestimating the daily impact. This can make it harder for them to recognize, acknowledge, and understand your client's feelings of grief. It can also be complicated by feelings of "survivor's guilt" or messaging they have received about being brave, strong, and inspiring.

Working with clients to help them link their experiences with their feelings can help emotional processing and healing. In time, it is important to work with your client on rebuilding and find new meaning to life.

Denial is a common defense mechanism when experiencing a loss. Denial offers protection from the reality of a situation. In the short term it can help people with a health condition process, integrate, and adjust. While this is normal, it becomes problematic when it is prolonged. Over time it can affect the way your client takes care of themselves or prevent them from seeking help. Prolonged denial is associated with depression and anxiety and may impede an individual's ability to adhere to doctor's recommendations, develop healthy life choices, and recognize that they need more support.[81]

Anger is also a normal response to adversity, stigma, and injustice. We feel angry when something is unfair, which can motivate us to address any injustice; this is known as "righteous anger." There are many understandable reasons why people may feel angry, such as in response to the unfairness of living with an LTC or if they face discrimination. Helping clients to recognize this feeling, identifying the reasons for it and finding healthy ways to express it are important.

Story Writing

Seriously ill people are wounded not just in body but in voice. They need to become storytellers in order to recover the voices that illness and its treatment often takes away.

—Arthur Frank[82]

Encouraging your clients to write about their health story can help them to make sense of it, has been shown to be therapeutic, and offers an opportunity to gain new insights into their experiences. Studies reveal that when people write about the most stressful events in their lives, they experience better health evaluations related to their illness.[83] Writing about their experiences can be understandably emotional, so it is important to encourage them to pace themselves. Remind them that they may feel a range of emotions and it is important for them to take care of themselves. If they feel overwhelmed, then it is time to step away and do something soothing or distracting for a while. They may prefer to share their experiences in another creative way such as through art, music, dance, or acting.

Therapeutic Letter Writing

Some clients report difficult encounters with healthcare professionals, colleagues, loved ones, or friends where they did not have the opportunity to safely express their feelings, or they were silenced or invalidated when they tried. Writing a letter (one that they will not actually send) can be a powerful means to help them process this encounter and an opportunity to make sense of their feelings.

> **Instructions for Therapeutic Letter Writing**
>
> - Find a safe time and space where you will not be interrupted.
> - Get a pen and paper or a computer and write a letter to the person or people who triggered your feelings (e.g., a workplace or childhood bully, medical professional who would not listen, a critical parent, or even the universe for the cards you have been dealt).
> - Be as expressive as you can, do not worry about making sense, jumping about through different timelines, spelling, or grammar. The purpose is to find your voice, tell your side of the story, and express your feelings.
> - Write down how you felt (at the time and now) and the impact this event(s) has had on you.
> - This can be a very emotive task so you may want to do it in short chunks (5–10 mins), putting the letter away and coming back to it when you feel ready.
> - You may also find that as you process one thing other events come to mind that you want to add because often difficult emotions are layered.
> - As you are processing your feelings you may feel more emotional, and dream and think about the event(s) more than usual. This is okay, it means you are processing what has happened. Be self-compassionate and look after yourself.
> - When you feel the letter is finished, add a final paragraph saying that you will no longer be consumed by what happened, that you are moving forward positively and taking control of your life on your terms. It does not matter if you do not feel like this yet, this is your first step toward liberating yourself from these past hurts.
> - If there is someone in your life that you can trust, such as a partner, parent, or therapist, you may want to share the letter with them. Having someone bear witness to your story can be therapeutic, however, this step is not necessary for positive change.
> - You may instead choose to do something symbolic, such as burning the letter, to mark moving forward and letting go.

Reintegration and Connection

Bonding with a cohort of other patients who were waiting for similar procedures at the same time on the ward helped us cope. We were able to share experiences, talk about how we were (or weren't) coping psychologically and form a bond via group meals, movie nights and just chatting in the day room. The provision of the day room

and lovely courtyard garden attached to our ward proved vital in this regard and actually only became available after I entered the ward, as it had been seconded to Staff only use during and post COVID.
—Richard, 60 years old, congenital heart condition, heart transplant recipient, United Kingdom

Social support is one of the most protective factors for our mental health, yet as described in Chapter 1, this can be challenging when you have a serious health condition because often your peers are not going through the same challenges and because of enacted, anticipated, and internalized stigma. Establishing community and finding connection with others who "get it" through peer support and mentorship (boundaried) can be powerful for people with an LTC. However, this can be difficult if they meet someone with the same condition who is not doing as well (e.g., has faced a significant decline in their health) or who is keeping a lot better (e.g., has been able to have children or work full-time, when your client has not). Preparing your client for these different scenarios and working through any issues that arise is important. Some nonprofit organizations offer peer mentorship programs where mentors have gone through rigorous selection and training.

It can be helpful to work with your clients to explore their social network. We all have different needs including emotional, practical, intellectual, and fun that cannot be met by just one person. As such, it is healthy to have a network of different people[84] with realistic expectations about what each relationship can offer.

A common barrier to accessing support for people with an LTC can be unhelpful, or toxic, positivity. This is when someone minimizes or denies their experiences with overly optimistic "feel good" quotes or statements such "But you look so well," "You are lucky to be alive," or "I get tired or feel pain too, you've just got to keep on fighting." These types of comments can shut down the opportunity for your client to open up about how they are really feeling or to explore the challenges that they face. This can leave them feeling invalidated, silenced, frustrated, and alone in their experience. Comments that superficially seem complimentary, such as "You are always so brave," "God gives his toughest battles to his strongest soldiers," or "Look on the bright side," can also prevent them from opening up about any difficulties because they may worry that if they do share distress, it will be interpreted as meaning that they are no longer coping well, are being overly negative, or becoming a burden. Comparisons with other people who seemingly have it worse or sayings such as "Everything happens for a reason" or "Happiness is a choice" can be equally frustrating. At times, healthcare providers can also seem dismissive of illness experiences with comments like "Other patients don't experience that symptom" or "You shouldn't be feeling that" or "Don't worry this won't hurt." This may prevent your client from sharing genuine anxieties and asking important questions for fear of being labeled a "difficult" or "anxious" patient. Overt microaggressions like "It can't be that bad because you were able to (work/shop/go out)," "You just use your illness when it suits you" or "You are attention seeking" can add to this toll. Over time your client may understandably build up resentment, which can lead them to withdrawing from relationships, passive aggressive behavior, or even angry outbursts.

If this is a pattern that your client has noticed in relationships, then working with them to kindly but firmly address this behavior in others by explaining how these comments make them feel and what they need to feel better supported can help. Some people genuinely do not know what to say to offer support and struggle with being empathic, especially if they have always enjoyed good health. Often, they fall back on these trite phrases or idioms without understanding the impact they have. Or they might even regret what they have said afterward. Sometimes we expect loved ones to be mind readers and then feel let down when they cannot figure out what is wrong with us, yet we have not even properly tried to explain it to them. In this case, it can be helpful for your client to inform family, friends, and colleagues a bit more about their condition and how it affects them, which can help their relationships deepen. If there are people in your client's life who continue to make them feel like this, even after they have tried to address this issue, then it may be time to set some firm boundaries around contact and to look for support elsewhere.

Helping your client to understand the importance of social support, (boundaried) peer support, and psychological support can help them to manage health difficulties (see Figure 7.1). Using psychoeducation about assertive communication skills for dealing with loved ones and healthcare providers and for handling toxic positivity may also be indicated.

My boyfriend was my most important support during my third operation. It was important to me that he saw me immediately after the operation. During the bowel resection, the exchange with other patients helped me a lot. They coached me through the treatment. It was helpful that the person next to me had the same operation. We were very supportive of each other during the days in hospital afterwards. Talking to someone who has experienced something similar has helped me the most in processing my story.

—Lou, 48, bowel endometriosis, Germany

212   Beyond the Medical Gaze

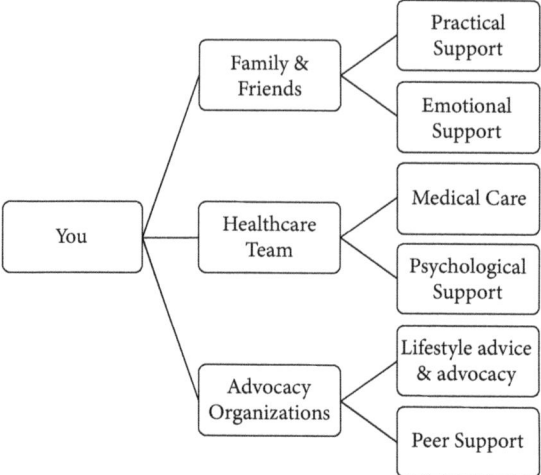

Figure 7.1 Therapists can help their clients map their social network using the above diagram to establish any gaps in meeting their needs.

Assertive Communication for Someone with an LTC Might Include:

- Explaining to others that they cannot commit to an event because they are unsure how they will feel.
- Let others know that they will need to take rest breaks.
- Explaining to others that they may not be able to take part in certain events or will only be able to take part for a shorter period (e.g., "*I can come along for the meal but can't stay on for drinks afterwards*").
- Letting others know how their health affects them and asking others for their understanding.
- Asking family and friends to be considerate and let them know if they are unwell before meeting up because catching, even a common cold, can significantly affect their health.
- Assertively correcting others if they make wrong assumptions or say things that are unhelpful, negative, or discriminatory.
- Asking for a meeting with their manager to discuss how their condition affects them and negotiating reasonable adjustments to make their workload manageable.

Learning from Practice: Developing an ACHD Support Group

By Meredith Kalbacker, LCSW
Mount Sinai Fuster Heart Hospital's Adult Congenital Heart Disease Center, New York

Patients living with adult congenital heart disease (ACHD) face unique medical challenges that contribute to emotional, behavioral, and social difficulties. As the advanced social work practitioner within Mount Sinai Fuster Heart Hospital's Adult Congenital Heart Disease Center led by Dr. Ali N. Zaidi in New York City, I witnessed firsthand this patient population experience psychosocial difficulties related to living with ACHD.

In the outpatient clinic, I continued to meet patient after patient experiencing symptoms of health anxiety, depression, and post-traumatic stress disorder. I found myself in a unique situation where I was meeting numerous patients a week who reflected on themes of isolation and difficulties of relating to their heart-healthy peers and thought, *"if we could just knock down these clinic walls and connect this patient to the patient in the room next door, they could know that they are by no means alone."* I became eager to find ways to connect these patients in the hope that it could improve their emotional, behavioral, social, and in turn health outcomes.

In January 2023, I began to research information on ACHD support groups and found that there was limited research data on this specific form of group. Kovac et al.'s 2018 "Randomized Controlled Pilot Trial of a Psychosocial Intervention for Adults with Congenital Heart Disease"[85] was the first trial of a group psychosocial intervention targeting this patient population. The trial indicated there were several barriers to ACHD support group participation, including scheduling and transportation. I also began to reach out to social workers at other ACHD centers in and outside of the United States to learn if they were providing support groups and to gather any feedback on how to run a successful group.

As I began to consider the structure of this group, I came across the book Healing Hearts and Minds: A Holistic Approach to Coping Well with Congenital Heart Disease, written by Tracy Livecchi and Liza Morton.[86] This book provides evidenced-based and digestible coping and self-care strategies for adults living with CHD. In addition to providing psychoeducation around CHD, the book weaves powerful personal stories into the narrative from patients living with CHD. After reading the book, I reached out to the authors to see if they would be open to the initiation of an ACHD Support Group in the format of a book club starting with their book Healing Hearts and Minds. Livecchi and Morton supported the book club concept and provided thoughtful feedback on the support group's format and progressive development.

Continued

Continued

Before initiating the group, I conducted a needs-assessment to understand what kind of support our ACHD center's patients were looking for and to understand any potential barriers to attendance. Based on the assessment results, the support group was offered virtually biweekly. Group members were encouraged to read one chapter of the book Healing Hearts and Minds between each group session. Mount Sinai Hospital's Social Work Department provided funding for book copies lent to any group member who was not able to access the book independently. During each group session, members reviewed and reflected on the key themes from the most recently read chapter and I provided psychoeducation as needed around mental health concepts. While the majority of the group sessions were held online, by attendee request the group came together in-person twice over the course of the year for a picnic.

Some of the barriers of the group included that for members to attend the group, they needed to be cognitively able to read and to speak in the English language. Group members needed to have some form of access to the internet and the ability to navigate Zoom. Within any support group, the facilitator is not able to completely control the ways individuals may communicate and interact with one another on or offline outside of the support group. Future support groups must establish clear and safe guidelines and ground rules around appropriate communication inside and outside of the organized ACHD support group. Future ACHD support groups should find ways to support patients who do not speak English and who are not able to navigate online communication formats.

From my perspective as the ACHD social worker, the impact the ACHD support group appeared to have on patients was seen via patients' expressions of feelings of **comfort**, and **an increased sense of connection** being able to communicate with and relate to other individuals with CHD. Many group members had never met another patient with CHD and appreciated the opportunity to share stories from their pediatric hospital visits, reflect on limitations they may have faced, discuss scars they may have, and show excitement over shared medical providers.

Group members showed signs of **newfound confidence** in finding themselves in the position to provide support to other members and feel like "experts" on the topic of life with a chronic, ever-present health condition. For example, patients found themselves offering encouragement before another group member's upcoming heart surgery or sharing strategies about ways to manage an anxiety-inducing upcoming major life event. Many of these patients had been used to being dependent on others due to their CHD, so to flip the script and be able to be "experts" on something based on their own lived experience appeared to be empowering and confidence building. It was wonderful to metaphorically "break down" the walls between the patient clinic rooms and see how patients with CHD could collectively and naturally support one another's psychosocial needs and in doing so support their own.

Empowering Self-Management

Understandably, clients with a serious medical condition may be more dependent on parents, loved ones, and medical care providers. This can undermine autonomy, particularly for those with a health condition from childhood. Studies have found that parental attitudes and overprotectiveness can also influence the ability of children with an LTC to launch into adulthood,[87] adding a barrier to independence. Sensitively working with your client toward developing their independence, as much as possible, will empower them to take charge of their life. It is important to recognize that taking charge of their life will mean different things for different individuals depending on their symptoms, life circumstances, relationships, employment status, and finances.

Conversely, for some people, they may find it challenging to accept being more dependent on others and the task of therapy may involve helping them communicate their needs and accept more help. Relationships are reciprocal so sensitively establishing how they contribute to relationships will help to build a sense of autonomy and confidence.

Helping Your Client Prepare for Medical Experiences

Studies have shown that being psychologically prepared for medical care is beneficial to physical, psychological, and emotional health. It is important to recognize and validate that healthcare appointments can trigger memories from past medical experiences or fears about the future for clients. Having to return to where they have previously experienced difficult news, painful interventions, and feeling unwell can be particularly challenging. They may be asked to strip off clothing for medical examinations or procedures which can leave them feeling even more vulnerable, exposed, cold, and in the "patient role."[88] Working with your clients on empowering them to develop a positive working relationship with their medical team can help. It may also be helpful to advocate for them, about their emotional and psychological well-being, with their healthcare providers.

As previously discussed, social support is one of the most protective factors for our mental health and well-being. During medical experiences, the soothing presence of a loved one has health benefits across the lifespan;[89] therefore encouraging your client to take a loved one with them to appointments may help. Although it is equally as important to bear in mind some clients may prefer to attend on their own.

Clients may have mixed feelings about appointments and hospital stays. If they spent a lot of time in hospital as children, it could feel like a "second home." They may have strong relationships with their care team and positive memories of times with people who did their best to take care of them at their most vulnerable. At times, they may even feel "safer" and in the best hands in the hospital if they are unwell or for rest if they have been battling debilitating symptoms. They may feel relieved and hopeful that something is going to be done to make them feel better. Some individuals report that after a long hospital stay, it can be hard to go home after living in the "safety bubble" of the hospital with their care team on hand.

At the same time, medical procedures can be painful and frightening. They can be overwhelming, can cause feelings of helplessness, and may give a sense of life threat. It can be frightening to experience physical symptoms, especially when they may indicate a worsening of their condition or that further medical explorations or interventions may be needed. Clients may also experience a range of feelings when dealing with new symptoms, hospitalizations, or finding out that they need to have surgery. These feelings may include, but not be limited to sadness, fear, anger, frustration, or anxiety.

Working with your client to develop skills to help them during stressful medical experiences can help. For example, meditation practice in the medical setting has a compelling evidence base as an adjunctive therapy for supporting health and well-being for many health conditions.[90] Clients may also benefit from relaxation exercises, breathing grounding, distraction, and somatic techniques which can be found in the Appendix as handouts.

An Invincible Summer: Spirituality, Finding Meaning and Post-Traumatic Growth

I was a minister's daughter, and religion was a significant part of my formative years, providing a sense of community and support for me and my family, particularly when times were challenging. I had a constant stream of visitors during hospital stays and knew my community kept me in their prayers when

I underwent serious cardiac surgeries. As I child I found it comforting and containing to believe in a higher benevolent power and that, despite what I was going through, there was a sense of purpose beyond my understanding. My father retired due to ill health when I was 13 years old, which meant that we had to move from our manse to a completely different area. Moving away from our home and social support network and having to make new friends at a new school was particularly challenging at a time when my health became even more challenging. While I have questioned organized religion since then, I have kept a sense of spirituality that helps me at times of adversity.

Studies have found that religiousness and positive religious coping styles are predictors of well-being, for example, post cardiac surgery.[91] Religiosity has been linked with greater use of adaptive emotion regulation strategies (e.g., cognitive reappraisal and acceptance) and less use of strategies that are linked to less adaptive outcomes (e.g., rumination).[92] However, negative religious coping such as religious discontent and making punitive religious reappraisals, such as feeling abandoned or punished by God, are associated with worse overall mental health, depressive symptoms, and lower life satisfaction for women with breast cancer.[93]

As such, it is important for therapists to be culturally sensitive to their client's religious and spiritual beliefs, since these may shape how they understand and cope with their illness, treatment, their relationships, and community.

As I entered the process of going for my recent operation (a heart transplant), I understood that it would not be without risk and potentially life changing. (The mortality risk of the operation was described as 20% in the consent form.) Therefore, for me, it was vital to understand why I was doing this, to make sense of it. . . . I was influenced by the writing of Viktor Frankl, the psychologist who endured terrible suffering in the second world war. He said "This is the core of the human spirit. . . . If we can find something to live for—if we can find some meaning to put at the center of our lives—even the worst kind of suffering becomes bearable." I also made the link between Frankl and the philosopher Nietzsche, who said: "He who has a why to live can bear almost any how." This is the line I reflected most on. In my personal situation, and with the support of 2 separate NHS therapists, I was able to articulate what was important to me, and what would motivate me to get up each day and keep going, in face of the challenges of this particular process. In my case, what I re-discovered in myself was a burning desire and overwhelming curiosity to see how my children's lives would pan out in the future. More specifically to that, I had this hope and dream of becoming a

> *grandad to their, hopefully in the future, children ... at times when I was down, these thoughts would re-emerge and give me spirit to carry on and face the challenge.*
> —Richard, 60 years old, congenital heart condition, heart transplant recipient, United Kingdom

It is possible for people living with an LTC to live a full, meaningful, and purposeful life, given the right support and their place as full members of society. It can also be helpful for people to create meaning from challenging experiences. Sensitively exploring the silver linings, while avoiding assumptions or clichés, with your client can help. Appreciating the strengths they have developed because of adversity is important. Living with a serious LTC can provide clarity and focus that some people only find near the end of their life. For many, it becomes easier to keep perspective on what and who matters, feel gratitude for the small stuff, and to make the most of life. When you have had to manage chronic symptoms, you also learn how to efficiently use your energy and time. When you must overcome major health crises daily inconveniences are comparatively welcome. Living with an LTC can hone determination, grit, and humor through necessity; you do not realize how strong you are until there is no other choice. Being humbled by times of dependency on others develops deep empathy and compassion.[94] Taking time to focus on such personal strengths, how they have helped your client cope with their experiences and been honed and strengthened by what they have come through can help.

Such positive change following adversity is known as *post-traumatic growth*, which encompasses five broad areas including increased personal strength, changed priorities, more meaningful relationships, changed philosophies, and spiritual development.[95] One study found that 90% of trauma survivors reported experiencing at least one aspect of post-traumatic growth after a stressful encounter.[96]

> *In the depth of winter, I finally learned that within me there lay an invincible summer.*
> —Albert Camus[97]

We can proactively develop post-traumatic growth. Several factors are known to provide a pathway to healing and personal growth following adversity, including having the opportunity to share our story, to feel heard and understood by others and ourselves. This is one of the main reasons that therapy can be helpful. Social support and nourishing relationships also protect us from mental health problems and having strong role models can inspire us. Feeling empowered to manage our health condition and being able to manage and regulate our emotions is also associated with post traumatic growth. Additionally, a growing body of evidence has shown the benefits of gratitude on our physical health and well-being through gratitude interventions such as keeping a gratitude journal. Post-traumatic growth can be helped by:[98]

- Social support
- Sense of control
- Help seeking
- Find personal meaning and goals
- Building resilience and coping skills
- Emotional release and regulation
- Psychological support

Finding Meaning, Purpose, and Hope

It helps me to find meaning in what I have been through; volunteering for patient organizations, dedicating research, and working with patients in similar situations—being part of creating the support system I was missing as a child.
   —**Lene, 27 years-old, congenital heart condition, clinical psychologist, Norway**

When you are living with an LTC, you can start to lose your sense of self beyond the symptoms, investigations, and treatments. Particularly, if you have had to give up earlier parts of your life, goals, and ambitions. Health changes can mean your client's life goals may shift and change for many reasons. While it is natural for your client to feel sad if they must let go of some of their goals, it is important for them to replace or change their plans. We are meaning-seeking animals, and we all need a sense of purpose and hope in life. It is important for your client to have realistic and value-driven goals to motivate them across different areas of their lives; this is called "committed action" in ACT.[99] This may include relationship goals, career and educational goals, and goals involving their hobbies and interests and personal growth. Usually, goals are underpinned by our values and what is important to us. It can be helpful to take some time with your client to consider their values and what matters to them across different areas of their life such as:

- Relationships (e.g., spending time with my family is important to me)
- Leisure and fun (e.g., learning how to paint is important to me)
- Work and education (e.g., being able to work part-time matters to me)
- Personal growth (e.g., taking time to practice meditation matters to me)

They can then explore and set realistic goals for each area. It may help them to break their goals down into more achievable steps.

> **Exercise: Goal Setting**
>
> SMART criteria can help with goal setting, this involved the following steps:[100]
>
> **Specific**—select a specific goal you want to work on (e.g., to learn to play the guitar).
> **Measurable**—make sure progress is measurable (e.g., achieve Grade 1).
> **Assignable**—state who will do it (e.g., you).
> **Realistic**—make sure your goal is doable, given available resources (e.g., you have access to a guitar and someone to teach you).
> **Time-related**—state a deadline for achieving your goal (e.g., start lessons by the end of this month).

Savoring

Savoring can be a helpful technique to help clients focus on positive experiences. This can involve savoring the past, present, or future. When using these techniques be sensitive to the client's health circumstances and be careful to validate challenges.

> *Savoring the past*: Ask your client to spend a few minutes thinking about a happy, joyful, or pleasant event that happened to them in the last week or month. Ask them to recall the people, smells, sounds, physical sensations, and sights that they experienced. Ask them to try to recreate the positive emotions that they felt around the time of the event. As they are savoring, invite them to let their thoughts wander to anything else about the joyful experience that makes them feel good. Then, ask them to mentally hold on to whatever feels good, take a deep breath, and pay attention to how these emotions feel in their body.
>
> *Savor the present*: Encourage your client to pay attention when they experience something positive. Whenever they notice themselves feeling good, mentally hold on by thinking about the positive emotions and what caused them.
>
> *Savor the future*: Encourage your client to strive for (achievable) goals and think about positive experiences to come.

Case Studies for Therapists

Case Study 1

You receive a new referral for a client. During the introductory session, the 27-year-old teacher describes her experiences which are contributing to her increasing anxiety and low mood. Around a year ago she collapsed at work, and she was taken by ambulance to hospital. She thought she was going to die. She later found out she had a problem with the electrical rhythm of her heart, and she was rushed to theater and fitted with an implantable cardioverter defibrillator (ICD). She was medically approved to return to work after 6 weeks of recovery. She cut her hours down to part-time and asked for "reasonable adjustments" to her workload. She finds it hard to distinguish between anxiety and an abnormal heart rhythm and she constantly checks her heart rate on her fitness watch. She is terrified her ICD is going to shock her. When she expressed her concerns to her consultant, he told her this was extremely unlikely and that it was time for her to get on with her life. Yet, she heard from other patients when she was in the hospital about someone experiencing their ICD shocking them in a false alarm. She also has nightmares and flashbacks about being in an ambulance and being rushed to the theater.

She reports that colleagues are treating her differently. She overheard one of them complaining about her "using her condition" to dump work onto them and her line manager has started to put pressure on her to resume her normal duties and return to work full-time. Since going part-time, she has been struggling financially too.

She lives with her husband, but is worried about intimacy with him. They were planning to start a family, but she is now scared that she won't be able to carry a pregnancy or that she might pass on her condition. She feels ashamed of her scar, which she hides, and she no longer feels able to wear lots of her clothes. Her family make jokes about her being a "bionic woman" and while she laughs along, she feels irritated. Everyone keeps telling her how brave she is and how lucky she is to be alive, so she does not want to complain and has become increasingly withdrawn. No-one else she knows has been through this and she feels very alone.

Case Study 2

Martin has been self-referred to your care. He was diagnosed with multiple sclerosis 2 years ago. He is a 45-year-old, self-employed builder and divorced father of 2 teenage boys. He sought medical advice because his hands kept going numb and he was struggling to keep up at work. He was shocked by the diagnosis and feels like he has been unable to take it in. At the time, he put it to the back of his mind and stopped going to any medical appointments. However, his symptoms recently got a lot worse. He feels tired all the time, cannot think straight, and has noticed that his speech is sometimes slurred. He has been feeling incredibly low. He has been unable to work for 6 months, has been struggling financially and is getting increasingly into debt. His partner of 4 years left him 1 year after his diagnosis, and he does not see the point in dating again. He used to go to sports games with his friends. However, he has gradually withdrawn from them. He no longer finds any pleasure in meeting up with them, does not have the energy to keep putting on a brave face, and worries that they may notice his speech slurring. The last time this happened they made a joke about it assuming he was drunk. He laughed along but felt angry and embarrassed. The only things keeping him going are his two sons and elderly mother. However, he has been unable to keep up with childcare payments to his ex-wife for his children and he worries a lot about what the future holds. He does not want to be a burden to his family and has recently experienced suicidal thoughts.

Case Study 3

Susan was diagnosed with breast cancer last year. She has undergone a mastectomy and radiotherapy, and is now having chemotherapy. She is 35 years old and had a 6-month-old baby when she was diagnosed. She is angry because she consulted her doctor about a lump in her breast a month after her baby was born and at the time her doctor dismissed it as being normal. It was only when she went back to them and insisted on further investigation that a diagnosis was made. Her partner has been supportive, but she has felt unattractive since the mastectomy and losing her hair, so she pushes him away. Despite being told that she is responding well to treatment, she is terrified that the cancer may be terminal and that she will not live to see her daughter grow up. After each chemotherapy session she feels exhausted for days and guilty about the impact this has on her as a mum and wife. She feels that she is missing precious time with her young baby, due to being unwell, and worries about the impact this may have had on her little girl. She struggles with going to hospital for treatment because it brings back lots of difficult memories. She cannot sleep the night before appointments, and she becomes very anxious leading up to them. Some of her friends have distanced themselves from her since her diagnosis and she has not felt well enough to go to mother and baby classes to meet new mums. She is feeling down and worried about the future.

Case Study 4

Matthew is a 21-year-old man referred by his cardiology team. He needs open heart surgery but is refusing treatment. He has a serious congenital cardiac condition. He underwent open heart surgery when he was a toddler and again when he was 8 years old. Since then he has attended a routine annual check-up with his cardiac team. He moved to adult care providers when he was 18 years old, and he was missing from care for a year during his late teens. He started re-attending appointments when he became symptomatic. He says that he cannot face going back to hospital for open heart surgery. Growing up everyone used to call him a "heart warrior" and tell him how brave he was. He feels like he is letting everyone down. Since being told that he needs further surgery he has been having terrible nightmares about being in hospital as a child, waking up in a cold sweat. He has also been experiencing flashbacks. He finds it difficult to recall exactly what happened to him, but the smell of disinfectant and loud noises triggers the flashbacks. He can vaguely recall being in a lot of pain, being held down to have a chest drain removed and the smell of blood. He describes feeling anxious all of the time, low and helpless. He also feels angry that this is happening to him when no one else his age must go through this. He says that nobody understands what he is going through and there is no point even trying to explain his feelings to his parents, girlfriend, or friends. He has dropped out of college, has been drinking heavily, and driving recklessly. He says that there is no point looking after himself because he will die young anyway.

Reflective Questions for Each Case Study

- What do you notice about your inner/private responses (physical sensations, emotions, thoughts, action urges) when reading about and imagining the client?
- How would you work with this client, considering their health condition?
- What do you consider important in relation to:

  ° Your relationship with them
  ° Developing a psychological formulation
  ° The focus of therapy
  ° Collaboratively developing goals
  ° Avoiding ableism or discrimination within the therapeutic encounter?

- If this client were to leave the session feeling like they could trust you and feel psychologically safe with you, what do you think would have been some ingredients of the therapeutic session?

Final Reflective Exercise: Psychologically Informed Healthcare

At the start of this book, you were invited to reflect on your practice, the organizational context you work in, and your training experience. It may be helpful to revisit these reflections and see if the answers to the reflective questions have changed.

- What is your current understanding about the psychological and emotional impact of living with a serious health condition?
- How has this been affected by your personal experience, or that of your loved ones?
- What is your current understanding about the potential psychological and emotional impact of working in a healthcare profession?
- Were these issues adequately covered in your training program?
- Do you think they are adequately addressed in healthcare policy and practice?
- What organizational and structural facilitators and barriers are there to acknowledging and meeting the emotional and psychological needs of people who are experiencing health difficulties and healthcare staff, in healthcare settings?
- How can we work to improve this individually, organizationally, and systemically?
- What does practicing psychologically informed healthcare mean to you?
- How do your reflections compare to those you made at the beginning of this book?
- How do you plan to take this forward: in your day-to-day work, over the medium and longer term?

APPENDICES: FURTHER RESOURCES AND HANDOUTS

Appendix 1: Grounding and Mindfulness Exercises
Appendix 2: Sleep Hygiene Tips
Appendix 3: Dealing with Emotions
Appendix 4: Somatic Exercises
Appendix 5: Loving Kindness Meditation
Appendix 6: Nurturing Self-Compassion
Appendix 7: Self-Compassionate Letter Writing
Appendix 8: Self-Soothing Touch
Appendix 9: Shaking it off
Appendix 10: SOBER: Stress Interruption Technique
Appendix 11: Patient Prompt Sheet
Appendix 12: Managing Anxiety About Seeing the Doctor
Appendix 13: Pacing, Planning, and Prioritizing
Appendix 14: Building Resilience
Appendix 15: European Association for Children in Hospital (EACH) Charter
Appendix 16: ISupport Rights-Based Standards for Children Having a Health Care Procedure (Test, Treatment, Examination, or Intervention)
Appendix 17: Neuroception of Psychological Safety Scale—Generic Version (NPSS-G)
Appendix 18: Neuroception of Psychological Safety Scale (NPSS): Manual and Scoring Guide

APPENDIX 1

Grounding and Mindfulness Exercises

Grounding exercises are a way to bring yourself back to the present moment when you become overwhelmed by distressing feelings. They are especially useful for people experiencing intense emotions or recovering from traumatic experiences. Grounding exercises can help if you are feeling very anxious. They are also useful if you are feeling angry, upset, or frightened or when you experience a flashback, nightmare, intrusive memory, or ruminating thoughts. Grounding can be used anywhere at any time, and no one else needs to know you are doing it. Please note that these suggested interventions are recommended to be conducted under a therapist's guidance, since mindfulness meditation practices can exacerbate past trauma.

5,4,3,2,1 Method: Describe (aloud if possible) five things you can see, four things you touch, three things you can hear, two things you can smell, and one thing you can taste.

Grounding Object: A grounding object is a comforting item that carries a positive meaning for you that you can use to distract yourself if you feel overwhelmed by focusing on the color and textures of the object. It should be small enough to carry with you, such as a pebble, a soft piece of cloth, or a necklace.

Grounding Phrase: You can also produce a phrase to remind you that you are living in the present moment. This might be something like *I have survived the past and I am safe now* or *This too will pass*. It is important to produce a phrase that is meaningful for you. It can be useful to write it down and keep it somewhere so you can look at it when you feel overwhelmed.

Grounding Activities: Other ways to ground yourself in the present include running cool water over your hands and noticing how it feels, reaching out and touching objects around you, noticing your body and how it feels sitting or standing. You can also make use of aromatherapy by using essential oils or a diffuser and think about your own strategies to ground yourself in the present moment.

Mindfulness Breathing Exercise: Make sure you are sitting or lying comfortably and bring your attention to your breath by placing one hand on your stomach. Imagine there is a balloon in your stomach that inflates each time you breathe in. Notice the sensations in your body as you breathe in and out. Thoughts will come to your mind, and that is okay. Try to just notice them without judgment and pull your attention back to your breath. Repeat this process breathing in and out. You can build up the time you spend on this exercise.

Box Breathing: Inhale deeply for four counts, then exhale for four counts, and repeat the cycle for four minutes several times a day.

Mindfulness Activity: Choose a normal daily activity, this might be making a cup of tea, eating an apple, going for a walk, or lying in your bed drifting off to sleep. The next time you do this try to keep yourself in the present moment. Pay close attention to what you are doing, what do you smell? See? Hear? Taste? What do you feel? Again, thoughts will enter your mind but just notice them nonjudgmentally, let them go, and shift your attention back to what you are doing. Stay in the present moment and fully experience it, just being in the here and now.

Meditation: Meditation is a simple practice available to everyone; if practiced regularly, it can help us to develop the ability to become calmer and more mindful in our day-to-day life. Regular meditation practice can have mental and physical health benefits. There are many types of meditation techniques, which are influenced by a variety of traditions, cultures, religions, and spiritual beliefs. You may wish to begin with practice for 5 minutes or so and then build up the time slowly. The goal is not to empty your mind completely, but rather to release any crowded thoughts you may have that may be causing stress. As with any type of activity, be sure to speak with your healthcare provider about the possible risks and benefits in relation to your health situation. Examples of ways some people meditate:

- Daily walks in nature
- Daily prayer
- Reading poetry or scripture and reflecting
- Guided meditation in a class or on an app
- Yoga
- Qi gong
- Tai chi
- Deep, calm breathing

Distraction: Distraction helps by taking our attention away from our distressing feelings, for example, when you are sitting in a doctor's waiting area or when you feel overwhelmed with worrying thoughts. Distraction can help to reduce anxiety levels and distress, for example, during conscious medical procedures. By distracting yourself you can keep distress levels in check and help to prevent a panic attack or cycle of anxiety (for example, health anxiety or obsessive thoughts). Different things work for different people, please find some suggestions to try below.

Distraction Techniques

- Doing a puzzle (e.g., crossword, word search, sudoku)
- Coloring or practicing a form of art
- Call or message someone for a chat
- Read a magazine
- Watch TV
- Listen to music
- Go for a walk
- Spending time with your pet
- Counting backward from 50 to 0, 100 to 0
- Saying the alphabet backward

APPENDIX 2
Sleep Hygiene Tips

- Try to go to bed the same time each night and get up at the same time each morning
- Make sure your bedroom is dark enough; install block out blinds, if needed
- Keep the bedroom quiet when sleeping
- Use your bed only for sleep and for sex
- Try to eat your last big meal at least 3 hours before bedtime
- Keep an eye on alcohol consumption, as it can disrupt your natural sleep cycle
- Avoid caffeine (including hidden caffeine, e.g., in soft drinks) and sugar in the evenings
- Create a relaxing routine each night and repeat (cup of decaf tea, bath, reading, stretching)
- Get regular physical activity each day
- Get regular exposure to outdoor light
- Try guided meditation or other relaxation exercises before going to sleep

Sleep tips, what to avoid:

- Caffeine in the late afternoon and evening
- Daytime naps
- Excessive television, internet use, or mobile phone scrolling at night
- Stimulating activity just before bed (scary movie, emotional discussion)
- The use of alcohol or nonprescription drugs to get to sleep
- Eating a big meal right before you sleep
- Taking another person's sleeping pills

APPENDIX 3

Dealing with Emotions

Emotional Release: Emotional release is finding a healthy way to express how you are feeling. This might be writing it down, punching a pillow, or "getting it off your chest" by talking to a trusted friend. Other strategies include exercise such as going for a fast walk, playing a musical instrument, or using art as a way of expressing yourself. Finding healthy ways to communicate how you are feeling, such as speaking assertively to others or having a good cry can also help to release your emotions. Crying releases the stress hormone cortisol, and it may activate our parasympathetic nervous system, which helps our body to rest and feel calmer.

Live One Day at a Time: If you are having a lot of anxiety and worry about the worst scenario, try to stay in the moment and not think more than one day or even one hour at a time. Sometimes thinking too far into the future can increase difficult feelings.

Worry Time: Some people who experience a lot of worrying thoughts, especially about their health, find it helps to set aside a certain time or times each day, for about 10–15 minutes, to simply "worry." During this time, it can be helpful to keep a journal to jot down whatever concerns you. It can help to separate the worries into two columns: what you can control and what you cannot control.

Positive Affirmations, Coping Statements, and Self-Compassion: Self-compassion is linked to good mental health. Positive coping statements can help us get through distressing emotions. Some statements that may help are listed below. It could be helpful to add some of your own—try asking yourself what you would like someone to say to you when you feel distressed and write down the answer. If that is too difficult, ask yourself what you would say to a friend or child in a similar situation. Here are some examples of the affirmations that you can draw on the next time you feel this way.

- This will pass
- Feelings are normal and temporary
- My feelings are valid
- I got through this before
- This feels bad, but it is a normal human response and it will pass
- Everything is temporary
- I am allowed to feel upset
- I am a good and worthwhile person
- My life has meaning and purpose
- I can deal with this
- I am good enough
- This is tough, what do I need to do to cope or feel better?
- I am worthy
- I am more than my accomplishments or failures
- It is okay to cry
- Everyone makes mistakes
- Even although I am feeling this, I accept myself

It can be hard to remember these statements when you are feeling overwhelmed. It might help to write some of these statements on a card and keep it somewhere safe, such as your wallet or phone, to look at the next time you are feeling distressed. You might also want to hang some inspirational affirmations around your home as reminders.

APPENDIX 4

Somatic Exercises

Please note that these suggested interventions are recommended to be entertained under a therapist's guidance, since somatic practices can exacerbate past trauma.

Clearing a Space:[1]

- Lie down, or sit in a way that is comfortable for you, and loosen any clothing that is too tight.
- Pay attention to your breathing (try the breathing exercise described previously for a few minutes).
- Ask yourself, "What's between me and feeling perfectly all right?"
- Spend a moment with this issue, noticing how you carry it in your body for a few seconds.
- Think about how this issue physically manifests as a tension in your body.
- Ask yourself, "What is the 'feel' of this thing?"
- Do not try to go into the issue or try to solve the problem, just notice how it feels in your body.
- Try to find some words or an image for the feeling or the "quality" for example, "scared, frustrating, annoying."'
- Imagine wrapping this issue; the physical tension, and the feelings it brings up like a parcel and set it outside of yourself for a moment.
- You may experience a "sigh" of relief as you imagine lifting it and setting it outside.
- See if you can set it outside for a while.
- You can come back and solve it later, but for now see if your body can be free of it for a moment.
- Repeat this process for any other items that you are carrying.
- Continue in this way until all the issues have been named and set outside yourself.
- Enjoy the experience of the "cleared space" in your body.
- You may want to create a word or an image for this good feeling state, so that you can come back here whenever you want.

The Diver's Response: When mammals hit the cold water, it automatically triggers a physiological relaxation response. It is especially effective and useful when in an extreme emotional state. Before you try this make sure to get the okay from your medical team, as this simple technique will bring down your adrenaline, calm your breathing, and slow your heart rate. One way to start this is by taking a cold shower and making sure to get the cold water on your face. A quicker way to get this response is to grab something cold like a soft drink can or a cold wet cloth and place it on or over your face.

Sighing: We naturally sigh or yawn a few times each hour. Sighing can help to rest the autonomic nervous system. You can induce the exaggerated inhale and exhale of a sigh or yawn.

Prolonged Exhale: Taking a long out-breath helps to create calm in your vagus nerve. Breathe in through your nose and do a prolonged exhalation through your mouth.

Stretching: Stretching is an underrated stress reliever. You may have noticed stretching and yawning is something pets use a lot to relieve stress. It automatically releases muscle tension and can help with body aches. There is no prescribed routine or time requirement and there are many different stretches you can find online, depending on the body parts that need attention.

Hum, Sing, or Gargle: The muscles on the back of the throat activate the vagus nerve as they move, and you can stimulate them by humming, sighing, or gargling.

Massage: Massaging can stimulate the vagus nerve, for example going for a facial massage, reflexology foot massage. Lightly massaging your face can help.

Acupuncture: Some research suggests that traditional acupuncture points may stimulate the vagus nerve.

Safe place—Guided Visualization: Guided visualization can reduce levels of anxiety, for example, before surgery. It can help to create a safe place in your mind. This can be based on a genuine experience, or it can be imagined. It is a place where you feel happy and secure. For example, it might be lying on a beach or in front of a cozy fire. Use all your senses to make this as real as possible. Think about the colors, skin sensations, what you can touch, what you can smell, what you can hear. For example, imagine a gentle breeze, the feeling of the sun on your skin, the sound of the waves lapping. You may find it helpful to take some time to describe it in as much detail as possible, drawing on all your senses, your safe place. Sometimes writing a description of your safe place helps in this process. There are lots of free ways to access guided visualization exercises online or on meditation applications.

Resourcing the Vagal Brake:

- ✓ Emotional release (e.g., screaming into a pillow, writing, music)
- ✓ Connecting with a trusted other
- ✓ Grounding exercises
- ✓ Yoga
- ✓ Mindfulness-based movement
- ✓ Meditation practice
- ✓ Being in nature
- ✓ Breath work and sighing
- ✓ Savoring
- ✓ Body scanning
- ✓ Self-regulation (e.g., hug self), hum, sing, or laugh
- ✓ Play, dance, and creativity
- ✓ Snuggle a pet
- ✓ Autonomic touchstones
- ✓ A cold shower or splash face with cold water
- ✓ Music helps us feel embodied and helps to regulate the nervous system

Overcoming Feeling Numb: Gently squeeze your forearms with opposite hands. Also increase your awareness by noticing the environment through the five senses. What do you see, hear, smell? If you can, try touching or tasting something mindfully.

APPENDIX 5

Loving Kindness Meditation

Loving kindness meditation can be traced to early Buddhism, and it can be practiced for increased compassion toward self, toward another individual, and/or toward the greater community in general. It is a meditation which can invoke feelings of compassion, self-love, kindness, empathy, and warmth. It can help you make peace with your body.

Please note that it is recommended to be conducted under a therapist's guidance, since mindfulness meditation practices can exacerbate past trauma.

Create a quiet, private space for yourself. Adjust the temperature and lighting and cut out any distractions. Get comfortable and take some deep, controlled breaths. For the first session, set a timer for 2 minutes (or the amount of time that feels right for you). This will help you to remain focused on your breathing and your intention of increased self-love and compassion. You can, of course, increase the time and build on it if you decide to practice this each day.

Imagine someone in your life (past or present) who was kind to you and cared for you unconditionally in a healthy, positive way. This could be a family member, friend, kind empathetic stranger, or beloved pet. Try to visualize that person or pet; breathe in that love and those feelings of empathy, kindness, and acceptance. If you have difficulty identifying someone, then imagine how you would like to be treated, or how you would offer love and kindness to someone in need, and turn that feeling onto yourself.

Repeat the following statements with the intention of increasing those positive, loving feelings within yourself and toward yourself. Continue to breathe deeply and smoothly as you continue to visualize yourself wrapped in the warmth of love and acceptance.

> May I be safe and protected.
> May I experience peace and calm.
> May I be content and happy.
> May I be filled with strength and well-being.

Now say or wish the same thoughts to someone else. Someone whom you love deeply. It could be a child, a spouse, a parent. Or, if no one comes to mind, you may direct it to someone you have never met or to an imaginary person but again, say or think:

> May you be safe and protected.
> May you experience peace and calm.
> May you be content and happy.
> May you be filled with strength and well-being.

Repeat three times, first by imagining someone in your community who you know is struggling; second, by wishing well to a difficult person in your life; and finally, by sending this message out to all the people of the world.[2]

APPENDIX 6

Nurturing Self-Compassion

We can work on nurturing self-compassion and kindness. When you are feeling distress try the following technique. It may help to place your hands over your heart[3]

- ***Awareness.*** Pay attention to the fact that you are experiencing some sort of suffering (e.g., emotional pain, mental pain, physical pain).
- ***Normalizing.*** Recognize that suffering is universal, it is not your fault or failing, you are not to blame, and you are not alone.
- ***Kindness.*** Meet this suffering with feelings of kindness, care, warmth, and concern toward yourself.
- ***Alleviation.*** Focus your energy on how to alleviate the suffering. This may include comfort and caring actions, providing a helpful perspective, or finding the strength and courage to take other necessary actions to address the problem being faced.

APPENDIX 7

Self-Compassionate Letter Writing

Self-Compassionate Letter Writing: Writing a compassionate letter to yourself has been found to increase happiness and feelings of self-compassion and reduce symptoms of depression.[4] If you want to try, use these follow steps:

- Choose a time when you are unlikely to be disturbed and have peace and calm.
- Identify something that makes you feel ashamed, insecure, or unhappy about yourself. Acknowledge how it makes you feel as honestly as you can.
- Write a letter to yourself expressing compassion, understanding, and acceptance of this part of yourself. It might help to recall someone who loves and accepts you unconditionally or what you might say to someone else you love unconditionally such as a child.
- In a compassionate way consider the wider context such as your upbringing, challenges you have faced, and other contributing factors.
- Draw from your wisdom to give yourself understanding and advice on how to cope, focusing on constructive changes you can make to manage this perceived flaw. Avoid judging yourself.
- You may want to keep the letter to read the next time you become overwhelmed with self-criticism.[5]

APPENDIX 8

Self-Soothing Touch

Self-soothing touch is an alternative to touch from others as a means of stress relief which has been found to reduce cortisol responses to psychosocial stress.[6] Self-soothing touch is an expression of self-compassion that can create physical and emotional soothing and calmness. Be gentle with yourself. If you find yourself experiencing distress or feeling uncomfortable you can take a few moments to take a break and let everything settle. Please note that these suggested interventions are recommended to be entertained under a therapist's guidance, since self-soothing practices can exacerbate past trauma.

Self soothing touch includes:

- Putting one hand on your cheek
- Cradling your face in your hands
- Putting a hand over your heart
- Cupping your hands together
- Rubbing your feet together

Self-soothing hug

- Find a comfortable and quiet space to sit in a chair or lie down on the floor.
- Place one hand below the opposite armpit and place the other hand on top of the opposite arm, between the elbow and the shoulder, hugging yourself.
- Draw your attention to the sensation of being held.
- You might want to imagine you are hugging yourself.
- Pay attention to the physical sensations in your body around the areas you are touching.
- Explore the sensations on the hand under the armpit, like temperature and pressure.
- Explore the sensations on the skin and muscles of the arm being hugged by the other hand.
- Explore the sensations of feeling your arms across the chest.
- Connect to the emotional experience this creates within you—maybe you feel safe and held.
- Keep exploring your physical and emotional experience, connecting to the pleasant sensations that arise.

APPENDIX 9

Shaking It Off

This technique can help you self-soothe calm your nervous system. Animals often shake themselves to release the excess energy produced from the stress response calmness. This technique allows your body to connect with the trembling sensation produced by a stressful event and enables your system to settle. Be gentle with yourself. If you find yourself experiencing distress or feeling uncomfortable while doing this exercise, you can always stop for a while and let everything settle.

- Find a space where you feel comfortable and safe for shaking.
- You can do this by either lying on the floor or standing up.
- Let the energy move through your body as you shake your legs and feet.
- Shake the energy off by shaking your arms and hands.
- It might be helpful to imagine that you are shaking off the sand from your body after going to the beach.
- Explore any other movements that might feel good for your body.
- Come back to a resting position, sitting, or lying down.
- Use the relaxing breathing technique to bring balance.

APPENDIX 10

SOBER: Stress Interruption Technique

The SOBER practice prompts you to become more mindful to promote self-awareness and emotional regulation. It consists of applying the following five steps for stress interruption[7]:

- Stop what you are doing. Take a moment, interrupting your usual reaction to stress.
- Observe what is happening in your body and mind. Imagine you are standing back from the situation, observing how you think and feel.
- Breathe. Settle your attention on your breath, noticing the movements of your body.
- Expand awareness to your whole body and surroundings. Attend to the rest of your body, your experience, and what is happening around you.
- Respond with awareness. Having taken a moment, choose how you wish to respond.

APPENDIX 11

Patient Prompt Sheet

When you are feeling unwell or anxious it can be hard to remember all of the things that you would like to speak to your healthcare providers about. This sheet is designed to help you prepare in advance of your appointment and to remember any important information. You can use it to write down any questions you have. You can then take it with you to your appointment as a prompt. During and after your visit you can also use it to make any notes or reminders about what has been discussed.

My Questions Before My Appointment

Questions about my health condition(s):
e.g., What should I expect in terms of symptoms?

Questions about my treatment:
e.g., What treatment options do I have? or When and how will I get my test results back?

Questions about my medication:
e.g., What side effects might there be?

Other things that are important to me *(this may include any difficult healthcare experiences you have experienced in the past that you feel it is important for your healthcare providers to know about)*:
e.g., I prefer to have my partner with me during my appointments.

Other questions, concerns or worries I have:
e.g., When will my next appointment be and what should I do if things get worse in the meantime? Are there any condition-specific patient support organizations that I can contact? Is there a specialist nurse I can contact?

After My Appointment

Notes about my visit:
e.g. The doctor that I saw was called Dr Smith and she was a Consultant Cardiologist. She is referring me for breathing tests. I should get an appointment within four months for this.

Things I need to remember:
e.g. My new medication is… and I have to take it once each morning.

APPENDIX 12

Managing Anxiety About Seeing the Doctor

It is completely understandable that visiting the doctor can bring on anxiety. This is especially true for those who have a chronic or serious illness or who have had difficult medical experiences in the past. This anxiety can get in the way of scheduling preventative care visits or may lead to delaying important follow-up appointments. However, avoidance of medical follow-up and care can negatively affect health outcomes. These tips may help you during doctor's appointments.

Social support: Social support is one of the most protective factors for our mental health and well-being. During medical experiences, the soothing presence of a loved one has health benefits. Research studies have shown that compassion can help us to feel safer and more resilient. As such, it can help to ask a caring family member or friend to go with you to hospital appointments. They can also help you to remember any new care instructions or recommendations; it can also give them a better understanding about what is going on medically for you.

Acknowledge your feelings and practice self-compassion: Go easy on yourself and look after yourself as much as possible. Medical appointments can be difficult, and it is understandable if you feel anxious, angry, or a bit down. This does not mean that you are not coping, it just means you are having a normal response to a challenging situation. Plan something pleasant to do before and/or after your appointment, reach out to loved ones to talk through your experience, or do something that helps you feel safer. Learning and practicing relaxation techniques such as grounding, deep breathing and relaxation exercises, meditation, and mindfulness can help you leading up to and after your appointment.

Assertive communication: Communicating assertively will better enable you to make the most of your appointment with your doctor. Many people report feeling disempowered during medical consultations and it is common to revert to the "patient role" at this time. If this is the case, it can be useful to write down any questions you have in advance and take this list with you to make sure each one is answered. If possible, you may find it useful to ask your doctor, by contacting their medical secretary, what you can expect during your appointment in advance. You can also let your doctor or someone on his/her team know how difficult appointments are for you. If your doctor's "bedside manner" is contributing to your feelings, you might want to consult with a different doctor to see if their style helps to increase your sense of safety and trust. It may also help to take someone with you to provide a backup "memory" or to advocate for you.

If you have met difficult medical experiences in the past that make your care more challenging or evoke strong feelings, then you can let your doctor know this. You can ask them to write this in your medical notes so that added time and care can be taken for any procedures that you find particularly difficult. For example, if you have a needle phobia you can ask to be referred to a therapist for treatment. Following this you can ask for added time, support, and, if it helps, to lie down before the blood is taken and added recovery time afterward.

Prepare for your appointment: Plan your appointment in advance to minimize stress on the day. This will help you to ensure that there is enough time in your day, and that you have planned for travel time, parking, check-in time, and where you need to go. Depending on your condition and financial situation you may be entitled to transport or assistance to and from your appointment.

Patiently waiting: Unfortunately, medical appointments are often delayed, so it can be useful to bring along something to distract you while waiting to be seen. Different things work for different people, depending on your interests, however, knitting, journaling, reading, a fidget toy or playing a word game on your phone can help. You could also listen to relaxing music or relaxation exercises on your phone. If you find that you have been waiting for a long time, let the people at reception know, in case you have been missed. You can also ask them how much longer you are likely to wait.

Self-care: Visiting your doctor is an important part of self-care. Staying on top of your recommended appointments is one of the ways you can maximize your overall health, contributing to a better quality of life. Often people will report feeling a sense of relief after their appointment is over and sometimes recount that the anticipation leading up to the day was more difficult than the appointment itself.

APPENDIX 13

Pacing, Planning, and Prioritizing

The three P's, pacing, planning, and prioritizing, are useful for self-management of chronic symptoms such as fatigue or pain. It is common for people with chronic symptoms to overdo it on good days or push themselves through tiredness or pain and suffer for it after; this cycle is known as "boom and bust." However, to gain control of chronic symptoms and function optimally it is important to listen to your body and recognize your limits.

It can help you to think of yourself as a container that has most of your energy at the start of each day (or whenever the best time of day is for you). Try and not use your energy up too fast, leaving you depleted by the end of the day. Using your energy wisely throughout the day will help you sustain it and make the most out of your it. Ideally you will pace yourself so that you have a little left by the end of your day. Occasionally you might need to borrow energy from the next day, for example to attend a special event such as a wedding. If this is the case, and you come home depleted then you can plan a "rest day" afterward to compensate.

Some people with chronic symptoms find it useful to split the day up into three parts (morning, afternoon, and evening), and make commitments in only two of the parts, allowing themselves to rest and recover for the other third. It is also okay to prioritize what matters to you rather than using your energy on things that are less important to you. It can be hard to say no, but it is important to assertively communicate what it means for you to pace yourself and manage your symptoms with others.

You may also find it useful to use labor-saving devices, take frequent microbreaks, and, if needed, use disability access. Working part-time or flexibly can also make a big difference.

APPENDIX 14

Building Resilience

In addition to any physical symptoms, people living with a chronic health condition often need to manage the impact of their health condition on their relationships, finances, and life choices. Understandably, this can take an emotional and psychological toll and increase vulnerability to more serious mental health difficulties, such as anxiety and depression. As such, it is important to take steps to support overall well-being. Resilience enables us to successfully adapt to life's challenges and overcome hardship, trauma, or stress. Personal resilience is not fixed; it can be preserved, honed, and strengthened by ensuring quality social support, by developing healthy coping strategies and by creating meaning and purpose in life. Paying attention to the following areas can help to maintain and enhance resilience for people living with a long-term condition.

Nourish self-care and self-compassion: Make sure you are practicing self-care by eating well, taking exercise (as much as possible), and connecting with nature. Many of us are in "chronic sleep debt," but sleep is essential to well-being and recovery, so try to get enough rest. When you are struggling with chronic symptoms, such as pain or fatigue, it can feel like you are in a battle with your body. You may become self-critical if you are not functioning as well as you want to and you might push yourself too hard and end up in a "boom and bust" cycle. This can affect your mood and self-esteem. Accepting your medical condition and learning to pace yourself and work with your body are essential to managing your condition. Combating self-critical thoughts and developing self-compassion are key to supporting resilience. It can also help to limit exposure to stressful news and "compare and despair" social media content.

Allow yourself to grieve and process difficult feelings: Grief is a normal and understandable response to loss. For people with a health condition, losses may include deteriorating health, missed education and employment opportunities, an inability to take part in some activities, or being unable to have children. It is important to recognize your grief and allow yourself to work through it. It is understandable if you feel sad, anxious, angry, or down at times. This does not mean that you are not resilient, it just means you are having a normal response to a challenging situation. Resilience also means allowing yourself to be vulnerable, expressing difficult feelings, and seeking help when you need it.

Seek pleasure and purpose: If you can no longer take part in activities that used to bring you joy or are unable to work toward goals that you once had, make sure that you proactively find replacement activities and set yourself new meaningful goals. We need to experience a balance of rewarding and enjoyable experiences to support our health and reduce stress, and we thrive when we have purpose and meaning in life.

Build a supportive network: Social support is one of the most protective factors for our mental health and resilience. Since no one person can meet all our needs, it is important to set up a network of people in our lives. Surround yourself with supportive and positive people, setting boundaries with people who bring you down. Some friends may offer practical support, others a shoulder to cry on, while others may bring fun. Sometimes we expect loved ones to be mind-readers and feel let down if they cannot figure out what is wrong with us, creating tensions. It can be helpful to share with loved ones more about your condition, how it affects you, and how they can support you, while ensuring you are giving back, as much as possible.

Self-management: You are an essential partner in your healthcare team, and building a trusting relationship with them is vital. Learn as much as you can about your condition to become a "patient expert," or get someone who can advocate for you. It is common to revert to the "patient role" during encounters with doctors, yet communicating assertively with medical professionals is key to managing a long-term condition. Before appointments, it can be useful to write down any questions you have in advance. It may also help to take someone supportive with you.

Evaluate your coping strategies: Sometimes our go-to coping strategies are no longer serving us well, or better options have become available to us. Common unhelpful coping strategies include the misuse of substances or alcohol, overspending, and isolating yourself from friends and family. More helpful strategies include talking to a trusted friend, physical exercise, distraction, mindfulness, meditation, reading, movies and TV series, spending time outdoors, connecting with others with the same health condition, or finding a creative outlet that brings you joy. If you are struggling, you could attend therapy to help you process your feelings and manage your condition.

Focus on what you can control: Depending on your medical condition, there may be things in life that you cannot do. This can be understandably frustrating, and for many people it can be difficult to accept. This does not mean that you cannot live a full, meaningful life. It can help you to consider what you can control and what you cannot control. There may be feelings of loss connected to things that are out of your control. However, when you process these feelings, it will be easier to refocus on the aspects of your life that you can control.

Nurture and build on your resilience: In addition to the challenges, many people who face adversity also report unexpected benefits of living with a long-term condition. This positive adaptation, called post-traumatic growth, can include increased personal strength and resilience.

APPENDIX 15

European Association for Children in Hospital (EACH) Charter

The 10 principles of the EACH Charter[8] relate to the rights of the child as stipulated in the UNCRC. While the EACH charter has been widely accepted, implementation of each statement is still a goal for many.

> **Article 1**: Children shall be admitted to hospital only if the care they require cannot be equally well provided at home or on a day basis.
> **Article 2**: Children in hospital shall have the right to have their parents or parent substitute with them at all times.
> **Article 3 (1)**: Accommodation should be offered to all parents and they should be helped and encouraged to stay.
> **Article 3 (2)**: Parents should not need to incur additional costs or suffer loss of income.
> **Article 3 (3)**: In order to share in the care of their child, parents should be kept informed about ward routine and their active participation encouraged.
> **Article 4 (1)**: Children and parents have the right to be informed in a manner appropriate to their age and understanding.
> **Article 4 (2)**: Steps should be taken to mitigate physical and emotional stress.
> **Article 5 (1)**: Children and parents have the right to informed participation in all decisions involving their healthcare.
> **Article 5 (2)**: Every child shall be protected from unnecessary medical treatment and investigation.
> **Article 6 (1)**: Children shall be cared for together with children who have the same developmental needs and shall not be admitted to adult wards.
> **Article 6 (2)**: There should be no age restrictions for visitors to children in hospital.
> **Article 7**: Children shall have full opportunity for play, recreation and education suited to their age and condition and shall be in an environment designed, furnished, staffed, and equipped to meet their needs.
> **Article 8**: Children shall be cared for by staff whose training and skills enable them to respond to the physical, emotional, and developmental needs of children and families.
> **Article 9**: Continuity of care should be ensured by the team caring for children.
> **Article 10**: Children shall be treated with tact and understanding and their privacy shall be respected at all times.

APPENDIX 16

ISupport Rights Based Standards for Children Having a Health Care Procedure (Test, Treatment, Examination, or Intervention)

- The standards[9] have been developed by an expert international collaborative group through extensive consultation with children, parents, and professionals.
- The standards are framed by a commitment to prioritize the rights of a child (United Nations Convention on the Rights of the Child, 1989) and ensure that their short- and long-term physical, emotional and psychological well-being are of central importance in any practice and decision-making related to health care procedures.
- These international standards recognize that all children have rights that should be respected regardless of their age, disability, race, religion or belief, sex, sexual orientation, ethnicity, language, ability, or any other status.
- These standards aim to provide broad principles for practice to support all children aged from 0 to 18 years undergoing a health care procedure. These standards should be applied in practice to recognize and respect each individual child's needs, competence, ability, preferences and experience.

The intention of these standards and how they should be applied in practice are outlined below.

These standards intend to:

- Propose an approach to minimize any anxiety, distress and harm experienced by children when undergoing health care procedures;
- Propose an approach to establish trust with children undergoing health care procedures;
- Contribute to describing good procedural practice with children;
- Define and promote supportive holding as an approach to prioritize children's rights and well-being;
- Challenge the use of restraining holds for health care procedures, whether intended or labeled as such, by raising awareness that whilst restraining holds occur in procedural practice and may be necessary to provide lifesaving care for children or prevent significant harm, holding a child against their will can be harmful and should be minimized, openly acknowledged and documented;
- Support health professionals and other health care workers (hereafter referred to as professionals) in advocating for children's rights and positive procedural experiences;
- Be of value internationally and across different clinical settings;
- Support "open and transparent" reflection and learning between professionals, children, and parents/carers;
- Act as broad principles which will need consideration and adaptation within different local regulations, laws, and resources; and
- Act as broad principles, to be considered alongside professional judgment.

The standards do not intend to:
- Endorse the use of restraining holds with children; rather they call for an honest and transparent acknowledgment and documentation of when such holds are used within a health care procedure;
- Override or replace country or discipline specific laws, regulations, frameworks, policies, standard operating procedures, or guidance; and
- Provide specific guidance on the use of pharmacological interventions for procedures, for example procedural sedation and/or analgesia

Standards for Children Having a Health Care Test, Treatment, Examination, or Intervention – Healthcare Professional's Version

To achieve good practice for children undergoing health care procedures, professionals should recognize that:

1. **A child has rights to be cared for by professionals who have the appropriate knowledge and skills to support their physical, emotional and psychological well-being and rights before, during and after their procedure.**
   a) A child is cared for by a professional who has the appropriate knowledge and skills and who is competent to conduct the procedure.
   b) A child is cared for by a professional who has access to appropriate equipment and resources (e.g., staff, environment) to conduct the procedure.
   c) A child is cared for by a professional who has confirmed the clinical need for the procedure.
   d) A child is cared for by a professional who has the appropriate knowledge and skills to assess a child's individual needs, competence, abilities, preferences, and experiences.
   e) A child is cared for by a professional who demonstrates respect for children's rights and who can work in a child-centered manner to support and advocate for these rights.
   f) A child is cared for by a professional who has the appropriate knowledge and skills to promote procedural comfort and to reduce the potential for traumatic procedural experiences.
   g) A child is cared for by a professional who can work in partnership with a child and their parents/carers and who can utilize the skills and knowledge of the wider multidisciplinary team (if available).

2. **A child has rights to be communicated with in a way which supports them to express (verbally or behaviorally) their views and feelings and for these views and feelings to be listened to, taken seriously and acted upon.**
   a) A child is communicated with directly in an open, honest, supportive and caring way to appropriately acknowledge their feelings and in a way a child can understand and that is consistent with their individual needs, competence, abilities, preferences, and experiences at the time of the procedure.
   b) A child is provided with the time and environment to develop trust and rapport with those present at their procedure.
   c) A child is provided with the time and environment to feel able to communicate and freely express their views and feelings before, during and after their procedure.
   d) A child is encouraged and supported to express their views and feelings freely without pressure, coercion or manipulation.
   e) A child is encouraged and supported to recognize and communicate their rights.
   f) A child's parents/carers are supported to recognize and communicate their child's views, choices and rights.

3. **A child has rights to be supported to make procedural choices and decisions and for these choices to be acted upon to help them gain some control over their procedure.**
    a) A child is assumed to have the ability to be involved in choices about their procedure even when they are not able to make bigger decisions on their own.
    b) A child is provided with sufficient information, including alternate options and the potential outcomes of those options, in ways that enable them to form their own views and be involved in decisions about their procedure.
    c) A child is actively encouraged from the earliest opportunity and throughout the procedure to share their views, feelings, procedural preferences and choices. This may include analgesia, methods of distraction, relaxation techniques, positioning, who supports them for their procedure and sources of comfort.
    d) A child is supported through their choices and decisions to have optimal control during their procedure.
    e) A child and their parents/carers are provided with the opportunity to discuss previous procedural experiences to inform procedural choices and decisions.
    f) A child's parents/carers are supported by a professional who works with them to consider their child's views, preferences and choices for pharmacological and non-pharmacological interventions.
    g) A child's views and expressions of refusal must be listened to, considered, taken seriously and given due weight.

4. **A child has rights to be provided with meaningful, individualized and easy to understand information to help them prepare and develop skills to help them cope with their procedure.**
    a) A child is provided with tailored, easy to understand, meaningful, honest and appropriately timed information to help them prepare for a procedure, understand what is happening and have the opportunity to ask questions to check their understanding.
    b) A child shall receive specific, honest and clear information at key points before, during and after their procedure.
    c) A child's questions and expressions of concern should be responded to in a calm and honest manner in accordance to their individual needs, competence, abilities, preferences and experiences.
    d) A child's parents/carers are provided with tailored, appropriately timed, easy to understand, meaningful and honest information to ensure they are aware and prepared for their child's procedure and have been able to ask questions to understand what is happening and their role in supporting their child before, during and after a procedure.

5. **A child has the right for their short- and long-term best interests and well-being to be a priority in all procedural decisions.**
    a) A child's best interests must be prioritized in all decisions and actions before, during and after a procedure. A child's interests should be prioritized over those of their parents/carers, professionals and the institution.
    b) A child's short- and long-term best interests are openly considered and collectively discussed by health professionals, parents/carers and the child (where appropriate) in the preparation phase prior to the procedure.
    c) A child is protected from harm; any potential or actual harm to a child caused by unnecessary procedures or overriding their expressions of dissent should be carefully considered and mitigated wherever possible.
    d) A child is supported to feel calm, secure and settled during a procedure.
    e) A child who becomes upset or resistant before or during a procedure is helped as quickly as possible, if it does not cause harm, to take a supported break. Professionals should reconsider the procedural plan.

f) A child and their parents/carers are supported after a procedure to talk through and reflect on positive or any challenging aspects.

g) A child's health records will include clear documentation of what worked well during a procedure and what procedural support or techniques would help for future procedures.

6. **A child has the right to be positioned for a procedure in a supportive hold (if needed) and should not be held against their will.**

    a) A supportive hold involves supporting a child to feel calm, secure, and settled during a procedure. In a supportive hold a child agrees to the procedure and positioning and/or does not express signs of refusal.

    b) Supportive holding is a way of providing comfort to the child and helping them to maintain a good position for the procedure.

    c) A child is only held using a supportive hold for their procedure.

    d) A child is encouraged to express their views and choices about who will supportively hold them for their procedure.

    e) A restraining hold is any action to prevent a child moving freely against their choice or will while expressing signs of refusal.

    f) Regardless of who holds a child, if it is against their will (expressed verbally and/or behaviorally) the hold is a restraining hold. A restraining hold should be recognized as such and not labeled as a clinical, supportive or comfort hold.

    g) A child is not held against their will (restrained) at any point in a procedure unless the procedure is lifesaving or where there is a likelihood of significant harm if the procedure is not carried out.

    h) Any child who has been subjected to a restraining hold during a procedure must receive appropriate support from a professional to help them understand their experience and re-build trust.

    i) A child's health records will include clear documentation if they have been held without their agreement (restraining hold), regardless of who held the child. This would include the rationale for using a restraining hold, who made the decision that a restraining hold was necessary, the restraining hold/technique(s) used, and the outcome for the child.

Standards for Children Having a Health Care Test, Treatment, Examination, or Intervention – Child's Version

- These standards show health professionals* the best way to prepare and support me if I need a health care test, treatment, examination or intervention (procedure).
- The statements are based on my rights as a child** to make sure my well-being is the most important thing when making choices and decisions about my procedure.
- The statements and my rights apply no matter who I am, how old I am, where I live, if I have a disability, what I think, who I identify as, what my religion is or how I communicate.

When communicating with me you will...

- Communicate with me directly in a caring, clear and supportive way.
- Communicate with me in a way I can understand.

---

* A health professional is anyone providing health care to me.

** These Rights-based standards for children undergoing clinical procedures are framed by the United Nations Convention for the Rights of the Child which are a list of rights which apply to every child under the age of 18 years old, no matter where they live in the world.

- Check my understanding of what has been communicated.
- Ask me and my parents/carers how I want to share my ideas.
- Let me have time to share my ideas.

When making choices and decisions with me you will...

- Help me be involved in choices about my procedure even when I am not able to make big decisions on my own.
- Offer me choices and options to help me manage my procedure. These options might include things to distract me, things to help me relax, who stays with me, pain medicine and the best position for me to be in for my procedure.
- Support me to share my ideas and choices, before, during and after my procedure.
- Talk with me about what is best for me before my procedure starts.
- Pay attention to my views and choices, and if I say or show I mean "no" you will take this seriously.
- Act on my choices and decisions whenever possible.

When sharing information with me and helping me prepare you will...

- Give me information that is honest and easy to understand.
- Help me understand what is happening and give me time to ask questions if I want.
- Give my parents/carers information to make sure they understand what is happening and have the chance to ask questions.

When acting in a way where my well-being comes first you will...

- Think about what is best for me in all decisions and actions before, during and after my procedure.
- Make sure that what is best for me comes first before what is best for my parents/carers, the health professionals and the hospital or clinic.
- Help me to feel calm and listened to during my procedure.
- Support me to take a break if I become upset or show I mean "stop" or "no" to help everyone rethink how to help me have my procedure.
- Consider how it will make me feel if you do not listen when I say or show I mean "stop" or "no."
- Support me after my procedure to help me understand my experience.
- Write down in my health records what helped me and what did not help me to make it better next time.

If you are holding me to help me keep still you will...

- Only hold me in a supportive hold which helps me feel calm, safe and settled.
- Ask me how I would like to be held and who I would like to hold me.
- Explain to me why I am being held.
- Stop holding me if I say or show that I want you to.
- Not hold me against my wishes or expect my parent/carer to hold me against my wishes to get a procedure done, unless the health professional in charge decides it is lifesaving or I will be really harmed if it is not completed.
- If I have been held for a procedure against my wishes you should explain why and discuss with me what follow-up support I would like.
- If I have been held for a procedure you will write down notes about this in my health records.

For further materials including a prep sheet, cartoons and case studies please visit the ISupport website at: isupportchildrensrights.com.

APPENDIX 17
Neuroception of Psychological Safety Scale—Generic Version (NPSS-G)

Please rate how well the following statements describe your feelings <u>over the past week</u>.
Strongly Disagree (score = 1), *Disagree* (score = 2), *Neither Agree or Disagree* (score = 3), *Agree* (score = 4), *Strongly Agree* (score = 5).

1	I felt valued	1	2	3	4	5
2	I felt comfortable expressing myself	1	2	3	4	5
3	I felt accepted by others	1	2	3	4	5
4	I felt understood	1	2	3	4	5
5	I felt like others got me	1	2	3	4	5
6	I felt respected	1	2	3	4	5
7	There was someone who made me feel safe	1	2	3	4	5
8	There was someone that I could trust	1	2	3	4	5
9	I felt comforted by others	1	2	3	4	5
10	I felt heard by others	1	2	3	4	5
11	I felt like people would try their best to help me	1	2	3	4	5
12	I felt cared for	1	2	3	4	5
13	I felt wanted	1	2	3	4	5
14	I didn't feel judged by others	1	2	3	4	5
15	I felt able to empathize with other people	1	2	3	4	5
16	I felt able to comfort another person if needed	1	2	3	4	5
17	I felt compassion for others	1	2	3	4	5
18	I wanted to help others relax	1	2	3	4	5
19	I felt like I could comfort a loved one	1	2	3	4	5
20	I felt so connected to others I wanted to help them	1	2	3	4	5
21	I felt caring	1	2	3	4	5
22	My heart rate felt steady	1	2	3	4	5
23	Breathing felt effortless	1	2	3	4	5
24	My voice felt normal	1	2	3	4	5
25	My body felt relaxed	1	2	3	4	5
26	My stomach felt settled	1	2	3	4	5
27	My breathing was steady	1	2	3	4	5
28	I felt able to stay still	1	2	3	4	5
29	My face felt relaxed	1	2	3	4	5

APPENDIX 18

Neuroception of Psychological Safety Scale (NPSS): Manual and Scoring Guide

NPSS Development and psychometric properties described in:

Morton, L., Cogan, N., Kolacz, J., Calderwood, C., Nikolič, M., Bacon, T., Pathe, E., Williams, D., Porges, S. (2022) A new measure of feeling safe: Developing psychometric properties of the neuroception of psychological safety scale (NPSS). Psychological Trauma; Theory, Research, Practice and Policy.

This measure is free to use for research and educational purposes.

1. **Interpretation Guidelines**
   1. **General**
      This scale provides a standardized measure of psychological safety informed by The Polyvagal Theory. Higher scores indicate stronger feelings of psychological safety.
   2. **The importance of context**
      It is important to note that feelings of safety are likely to differ depending on context (for example, being at work versus being at home).

      Please note that the general form can be modified depending on the context of the research question. If a specific context is needed, we recommend editing the instructions of the text with the following addition:

      Please rate how well the following statements describe your feelings during (specify a particular situation, timeframe, or experience). For example: "Your experiences at work over the past week," "Your recent hospital stay," or "Your time spent on social media over the past week." All such modifications should be explicitly described in publications, presentations, and other dissemination of research.

2. **NPSS Scoring**
   1. **Response Conversion to Numbers**
      For each item, assign values to the responses according to the numbering below:

Response	Value
Strongly Disagree	1
Disagree	2
Neither Agree nor Disagree	3
Agree	4
Strongly Agree	5

   2. **Score Calculation**
      Total score and subscale values can then be calculated by sum or mean of the items. Subscale groupings are below.
   3. **Missing Values**
      Participants should be allowed to skip items that they cannot accurately report. It is preferable to have missing values for scoring than unreliable responses.

Calculation of mean scores will be more robust to missing item values than sum scores, which affect the range of possible values. When missing values are present in the data, imputation may be used if needed. Scores for participants with high levels of missing item data should be interpreted with caution.

NPSS Subscale Overview:

Domain	Subscale	Description	Item Count
Social	Social Engagement Subscale	Higher scores on this subscale reflect the evaluation of the environment as non-threatening and safe for social engagement. These scores reflect feelings of being accepted, understood, cared for, being able to express oneself without being judged, and having someone to trust.	14
Compassion	Compassion Subscale	Higher scores on this subscale reflect the ability to be compassionate and feeling connected, empathetic, caring, and wanting to help others.	7
Bodily	Bodily Sensations Subscale	Higher scores reflect internal sensations of the body in a state of calm capturing the feeling of relaxation in the face and the body, steady heartbeat, and breath, and settled stomach.	8

NPSS Item Subscale Scoring: Overview

Subscale	Item	Item Number
Social Engagement	I felt valued	1
	I felt comfortable expressing myself	2
No items: 14	I felt accepted by others	3
Max Sub Score = 70	I felt understood	4
	I felt like others got me	5
	I felt respected	6
	There was someone who made me feel safe	7
	There was someone that I could trust	8
	I felt comforted by others	9
	I felt heard by others	10
	I felt like people would try their best to help me	11
	I felt cared for	12
	I felt wanted	13
	I didn't feel judged by others	14

Subscale	Item	Item Number
Compassion	I felt able to empathize with other people	15
No items = 7	I felt able to comfort another person if needed	16
	I felt compassion for others	17
Max Sub-Score	I wanted to help others relax	18
=35	I felt like I could comfort a loved one	19
	I felt so connected to others I wanted to help them	20
	I felt caring	21
Body Sensations	My heart rate felt steady	22
	Breathing felt effortless	23
No Items =8	My voice felt normal	24
Max sub-score = 40	My body felt relaxed	25
	My stomach felt settled	26
	My breathing was steady	27
	I felt able to stay still	28
	My face felt relaxed	29

Afterword

As a girl, when I was struggling with my health condition, my dad suggested writing down how I was feeling. So I did; in personal diaries, essays and poems. While this provided an outlet for my feelings I didn't have the words or insights to fully articulate my experiences. It has taken decades for me to make sense of the complex social, emotional, and psychological terrain associated with living with a serious lifelong health condition. Learning, research, and personal therapy have helped me find the words which I have shared in this book. I hope they are helpful to others, in the way I needed back then.

As someone who has depended on healthcare lifelong, I passionately believe that *psychologically informed healthcare* should be a top priority for anyone who is involved in modern healthcare policy, practice, or education. It is my hope that one day soon, we will look back and wonder why there was ever a time when psychological and emotional health was not supported in this way.

Psychologically informed healthcare is a framework, and of course there have always been many aspects of healthcare compatible with this thinking. My hope is this book will help to elevate and standardize psychologically informed healthcare across all settings, to ease conversations, and to promote creative solutions to make life easier for those of us living with a long-term health condition, for our loved ones, and for those involved in our care. Of course, this is an ongoing and changing landscape as our understanding about the mind–body link improves and we continue to work together to improve well-being.

Notes

1. Preface

1. Dasmahapatra, H. K., Jamieson, M. P., & Brewster, G. M. (1986). Permanent cardiac pacemaker in infants and children. *Thoracic Cardiovascular Surgery 34*: 230–235
2. Reid, J. M., Coleman, E. N., & Doig, W. (1982). Complete congenital heart block: Report of 35 cases. *British Heart Journal, 48*, 236–239
3. Morton, L. (2018). Born with a heart condition: The clinical implications of the polyvagal theory. In S. Porges & D. Dana (Eds.), *Clinical application of the polyvagal theory*. Norton Professional Books.
4. Foucault, M. (1963). *The birth of the clinic: An archaeology of medical perception*. Routledge.

2. Positionality Statement

1. Braun, V., & Clarke, V. (2024). Reporting guidelines for qualitative research: A values-based approach. *Qualitative Research in Psychology, 22*(2), 399–438. https://doi.org/10.1080/14780887.2024.2382244

3. Quotes

1. Bevan, A. (1952). *In place of fear* (p. 100). London Heinemann.
2. Chisholm, B. (1954). *Outline for a study group on world health and the survival of the human race: Material drawn from articles and speeches by Brock Chisholm*. World Health Organization.

4. Chapter 1

1. Woolf, V. (1930). *On being ill*. The Hogarth Press.
2. *TIME* magazine. (2015). *What happened when a baby girl got a heart transplant from a baboon*, October 26, 2015.
3. Gatzoulis, M. A., Swan, L., Therrien, J., & Pantley, G. A. (2010). *Adult congenital heart disease: A practical guide* (2nd ed.). Blackwell.
4. Hacker, K. (2024). The burden of chronic disease. *Mayo Clinic Proceedings: Innovations, Qual & Outcomes, 8*(1), 112–119. https://doi.org/:10.1016/j.mayocpiqo.2023.08.005. PMID: 38304166; PMCID: PMC10830426.
5. Bogart, K. R., Lund, E. M., & Rottenstein, A. (2018). Disability pride protects self-esteem through the rejection identification model. *Rehabilitation Psychology, 63*(1), 155–159. https://doi.org/10.1037/rep0000166
6. Morton, L., Cogan, N., Kolacz, J., et al. (2022). A new measure of feeling safe: Developing psychometric properties of the Neuroception of Psychological Safety Scale (NPSS). *Psychological Trauma: Theory, Research, Practice, and Policy, 16*(4), 701–708. https://doi.org/10.1037/tra0001374

7. Nightingale, F. (1858). *Notes on nursing: What it is, and what it is not*. Appleton and Company.
8. World Health Organization. (1948). *Summary reports on proceedings minutes and final acts of the International Health Conference held in New York from 19 June to 22 July 1946*. https://apps.who.int/iris/handle/10665/85573
9. Hickman, B., Pourkazemi, F., Pebdani, R. N., Hiller, C. E., & Fong Yan, A. (2022). Dance for chronic pain conditions: A systematic review. *Pain Medicine*, 23(12), 2022–2041. https://doi.org/10.1093/pm/pnac092. PMID: 35736401; PMCID: PMC9714531.
10. Marin, C. E., Kfouri, P. P., Callegaro, D., et al. (2021). Patients and neurologists have different perceptions of multiple sclerosis symptoms, care, and challenges. *Mult Scler Relat Disord*, 102806.
11. Mula, M., & Sander, J. W. (2016). Psychosocial aspects of epilepsy: A wider approach. *BJPsych Open*, 2(4), 270–274. https://doi.org/10.1192/bjpo.bp.115.002345
12. Davis, H. E., McCorkell, L., Vogel, J. M., et al. (2023). Long COVID: Major findings, mechanisms, and recommendations. *Nat Rev Microbiol*, 21, 133–146. https://doi.org/10.1038/s41579-022-00846-2
13. Thomas, C., Faghy, M. A., Owen, R., et al. (2023). Lived experience of patients with Long COVID: A qualitative study in the UK. *BMJ Open*, 13, e068481. https://doi.org/10.1136/bmjopen-2022-068481
14. Kalra, S., Jena, B. N., & Yeravdekar, R. (2018). Emotional and psychological needs of people with diabetes. *Indian J Endocrinol Metab*, 22(5), 696–704. https://doi.org/10.4103/ijem.IJEM_579_17. PMID: 30294583; PMCID: PMC6166557.
15. Jordan, N., & D'Cruz, D. (2016). Current and emerging treatment options in the management of lupus. *Immunotargets Ther*, 5, 9–20. https://doi.org/10.2147/ITT.S40675. PMID: 27529058; PMCID: PMC4970629.
16. Stavropoulou, A., Vlamakis, D., Kaba, E., et al. (2021). "Living with a stoma": Exploring the lived experience of patients with permanent colostomy. *Int J Environ Res Public Health*, 18(16), 8512. https://doi.org/10.3390/ijerph18168512. PMID: 34444262; PMCID: PMC8393572.
17. Lévesque, V., Laplante, L., Shohoudi, A., et al. (2020). Implantable cardioverter-defibrillators and patient-reported outcomes in adults with congenital heart disease: An international study, *Heart Rhythm*, 17(5, Part A), 768–776. https://doi.org/10.1016/j.hrthm.2019.11.026.
18. Holland, E., Matthews, K., Macdonald, S., et al. (2024). The impact of living with multiple long-term conditions (multimorbidity). on everyday life: A qualitative evidence synthesis. *BMC Public Health* 24, 3446. https://doi.org/10.1186/s12889-024-20763-8
19. Holland, E., Matthews, K., Macdonald, S. et al. (2024). The impact of living with multiple long-term conditions (multimorbidity). on everyday life: A qualitative evidence synthesis. *BMC Public Health* 24, 3446. https://doi.org/10.1186/s12889-024-20763-8
20. National Institute for Health and Care Research. (n.d.). *Improving how we work with patients, carers and the public. NIHR strategic commitments for public partnerships 2025–2030*. https://www.nihr.ac.uk/about-us/what-we-do/Improving-how-we-work-with-patients-carers-and-the-public.htm. Accessed March 2024.
21. Holland, E., Matthews, K., Macdonald, S. et al. (2024). The impact of living with multiple long-term conditions (multimorbidity). on everyday life: A qualitative evidence synthesis. *BMC Public Health* 24, 3446. https://doi.org/10.1186/s12889-024-20763-8
22. Agarwal, S., Birk, J. L., Abukhadra, S. L., et al. (2022). Psychological distress after sudden cardiac arrest and its impact on recovery. *Curr Cardiol Rep*, 24(10), 1351–1360. https://doi.org/10.1007/s11886-022-01747-9. Epub 2022 Aug 3. PMID: 35921024; PMCID: PMC9561080.

23. Guggenbühl-Craig, A. (1998). *Power in the helping profession.* Spring.
24. Hinz, A., Herzberg, P. Y., Lordick, F., et al. (2019). Age and gender differences in anxiety and depression in cancer patients compared with the general population. *Eur J Cancer Care* (Engl), *28*(5), e13129. https://doi.org/10.1111/ecc.13129
25. Bremner, J. D. (2006). Traumatic stress: Effects on the brain. *Dialogues Clin Neurosci, 8*(4), 445–461. https://doi.org/10.31887/DCNS.2006.8.4/jbremner. PMID: 17290802; PMCID: PMC3181836.
26. Clark, C. R., McFarlane, A. C., Morris, P., et al. (2003). Cerebral function in posttraumatic stress disorder during verbal working memory updating: A positron emission tomography study. *Biol Psychiatry, 53*(6), 474–481. https://doi.org/10.1016/s0006-3223(02)01505-6. PMID: 12644352.
27. Spinazzola, J., van der Kolk, B., & Ford, J. D. (2018). When nowhere is safe: Interpersonal trauma and attachment adversity as antecedents of posttraumatic stress disorder and developmental trauma disorder. *Journal of Traumatic Stress, 31*(5), 631–642. https://doi.org/10.1002/jts.22320. PMID: 30338544; PMCID: PMC6221128.
28. Rauch, S. L., van der Kolk, B. A., Fisler, R. E., et al. (1996). A symptom provocation study of posttraumatic stress disorder using positron emission tomography and script-driven imagery. *Arch Gen Psychiatry, 53*(5), 380–387. https://doi.org/10.1001/archpsyc.1996.01830050014003. PMID: 8624181.
29. Porges, S. W. (2022). Polyvagal theory: A science of safety. *Front Integr Neurosci, 16*, 871227. https://doi.org/10.3389/fnint.2022.871227. PMID: 35645742; PMCID: PMC9131189.
30. Porges, S. W. (2022). Polyvagal theory: A science of safety. *Front Integr Neurosci, 16*, 871227. https://doi.org/10.3389/fnint.2022.871227. PMID: 35645742; PMCID: PMC9131189.
31. Porges, S. W. (2022). Polyvagal theory: A science of safety. *Front Integr Neurosci, 16*, 871227. https://doi.org/10.3389/fnint.2022.871227. PMID: 35645742; PMCID: PMC9131189.
32. Schwarz, A. (2020). *A practical guide to complex PTSD: Compassionate strategies for childhood trauma.* Rockridge Press.
33. Schwartz, A. (2016). *The complex PTSD workbook: A mind–body approach to regaining emotional control and becoming whole.* Althea Press.
34. Nuredini, G., Saunders, A., Rajkumar, C., & Okorie, M. (2020). Current status of white coat hypertension: Where are we? *Ther Adv Cardiovasc Dis.* 14, 1753944720931637. https://doi.org/10.1177/1753944720931637. PMID: 32580646; PMCID: PMC7318827.
35. Hannibal, K. E., & Bishop, M. D. (2014). Chronic stress, cortisol dysfunction, and pain: A psychoneuroendocrine rationale for stress management in pain rehabilitation. *Phys Ther, 94*(12), 1816–1825. https://doi.org/10.2522/ptj.20130597. Epub 2014 Jul 17. PMID: 25035267; PMCID: PMC4263906.
36. van der Kolk, B. A. (2014). *The body keeps the score: Brain, mind, and body in the healing of trauma.* Viking.-
37. Gajwani, R., & Minnis, H. (2023). Double jeopardy: Implications of neurodevelopmental conditions and adverse childhood experiences for child health. *Eur Child Adolesc Psychiatry, 32*, 1–4. https://doi.org/10.1007/s00787-022-02081-9
38. Morton, L. (2020). Using psychologically informed care to improve mental health and wellbeing for people living with a heart condition from birth: A statement paper. *Journal of Health Psychology, 25*(2), 197–206. https://doi.org/10.1177/1359105319826354
39. Dale, L. P., Cuffe, S. P., Kolacz, J., et al. (2022). Increased autonomic reactivity and mental health difficulties in COVID-19 survivors: Implications for medical providers. *Front Psychiatry, 13*, 830926. https://doi.org/10.3389/fpsyt.2022.830926

40. Surwit, R. S., Schneider, M. S., & Feinglos, M. N. (1992). Stress and diabetes mellitus. *Diabetes Care, 15*, 1413–1422.
41. Habek, M. (2019). Immune and autonomic nervous system interactions in multiple sclerosis: Clinical implications. *Clin Auton Res, 29*, 267–275. https://doi.org/10.1007/s10286-019-00605-z
42. Capone, C., Buyon, J. P., Friedman, D. M., & Frishman, W. H. (2012). Cardiac manifestations of neonatal lupus: A review of autoantibody-associated congenital heart block and its impact in an adult population. *Cardiol Rev, 20*(2), 72–76. https://doi.org/10.1097/CRD.0b013e31823c808b. PMID: 22183063; PMCID: PMC3275696.
43. Horsch, A., Garthus-Niegel, S., Ayers, S., Chandra, P., Hartmann, K., Vaisbuch, E., & Lalor, J. (2024). Childbirth-related posttraumatic stress disorder: Definition, risk factors, pathophysiology, diagnosis, prevention, and treatment. *Am J Obstet Gynecol, 230*(3S), S1116–S1127. https://doi.org/10.1016/j.ajog.2023.09.089. Epub 2024 Jan 9. PMID: 38233316.
44. Horsch, A., Garthus-Niegel, S., Ayers, S., Chandra, P., Hartmann, K., Vaisbuch, E., & Lalor, J. (2024). Childbirth-related posttraumatic stress disorder: definition, risk factors, pathophysiology, diagnosis, prevention, and treatment. *Am J Obstet Gynecol, 230*(3S), S1116–S1127. https://doi.org/10.1016/j.ajog.2023.09.089. Epub 2024 Jan 9. PMID: 38233316.
45. Heyne, C. S., Kazmierczak, M., Souday, R., et al. (2022). Prevalence and risk factors of birth-related posttraumatic stress among parents: A comparative systematic review and meta-analysis. *Clin Psychol Rev, 94*, 102157. https://doi.org/10.1016/j.cpr.2022.102157.
46. Neaton, K., Voldanova, L., Kiely, T., & Nagle, C. (2024). Non-pharmacological treatments for shivering post neuraxial anaesthesia for caesarean section: A scoping review. *Contemp Nurse, 60*(1), 42–53. https://doi.org/10.1080/10376178.2024.2310256.
47. Mothers and Babies: Reducing Risk through Audits and Confidential Enquiries across the UK (MBRRACE-UK). *Maternal mortality UK 2020–22*. January 2024.
48. Howell, E. A. (2018). Reducing Disparities in Severe Maternal Morbidity and Mortality. *Clin Obstet Gynecol, 61*(2), 387–399. https://doi.org/10.1097/GRF.0000000000000349.
49. Mothers and Babies: Reducing Risk through Audits and Confidential Enquiries across the UK (MBRRACE-UK). *Maternal mortality UK 2020–22*. January 2024.
50. Nowak, A. L., Anderson, C. M., Mackos, A. R., Neiman, E., & Gillespie, S. L. (2020). Stress during pregnancy and epigenetic modifications to offspring DNA: A systematic review of associations and implications for preterm birth. *J Perinat Neonatal Nur, 34*(2), 134–145. https://doi.org/10.1097/JPN.0000000000000471. PMID: 32332443; PMCID: PMC7185032.
51. Alhusen, J. L., Ray, E., Sharps, P., & Bullock, L. (2015). Intimate partner violence during pregnancy: Maternal and neonatal outcomes. *J Womens Health* (Larchmt), 24(1), 100–106. https://doi.org/10.1089/jwh.2014.4872. Epub 2014 Sep 29.
52. Smith, L. K., Dickens, J., Bender Atik, R., Bevan, C., Fisher, J., & Hinton, L. (2020). Parents' experiences of care following the loss of a baby at the margins between miscarriage, stillbirth and neonatal death: A UK qualitative study. *BJOG, 127*(7), 868–874. https://doi.org/10.1111/1471-0528.16113. Epub 2020 Feb 21. PMID: 31976622; PMCID: PMC7383869.
53. Smith, L. K., Dickens, J., Bender Atik, R., Bevan, C., Fisher, J., & Hinton, L. (2020). Parents' experiences of care following the loss of a baby at the margins between miscarriage, stillbirth and neonatal death: a UK qualitative study. *BJOG, 127*(7), 868–874. https://doi.org/10.1111/1471-0528.16113. Epub 2020 Feb 21. PMID: 31976622; PMCID: PMC7383869.

54. Sanders, M. R., & Thompson, G. S. (2021). *Polyvagal theory and the developing child: Systems of care for strengthening kids, families, and communities.* W. W. Norton.
55. Bowlby, J. (1988). *A secure base: Parent–child attachment and healthy human development.* Tavistock professional book. Routledge.
56. Bowlby, J. (1951). *Maternal care and mental health.* World Health Organization.
57. Bowlby, J. (1969). *Attachment and loss.* Basic Books.
58. Siegel, D. J. (2012). *The developing mind: How relationships and the brain interact to shape who we are* (2nd ed.). The Guilford Press.
59. Narvaez, D. (2018). Basic needs and fulfilling human potential. In D. Narvaez (Ed.), *Basic needs, wellbeing and morality*, 51–89. Palgrave Pivot. https://doi.org/10.1007/978-3-319-97734-8_5
60. Narvaez, D. (2018). Basic needs and fulfilling human potential. In D. Narvaez (Ed.), *Basic needs, wellbeing and morality*, 51–89. Palgrave Pivot. https://doi.org/10.1007/978-3-319-97734-8_5
61. Christian-Brandt, A. S., Santacrose, D. E., Farnsworth, H. R., & MacDougall, K. A. (2019). When treatment is traumatic: An empirical review of interventions for pediatric medical traumatic stress. *Am J Community Psychol, 64*(3–4), 389–404. https://doi.org/10.1002/ajcp.12392. Epub 2019 Oct 16. PMID: 31617588.
62. Gilbert, P. (2014). The origins and nature of compassion focused therapy. *British Journal of Clinical Psychology, 53*(1), 6–41.
63. Helfricht, S., Latel, B., & Fisher, J. E. (2008). Surgery related post traumatic stress disorder in parents of children undergoing cardiopulmonary bypass surgery: A prospective cohort study. *Pediatric Critical Care Medicine, 9*(2), 217–223.
64. Kazak, A., Alderfer, M., Rourke, M. T., Simms, S., Streisand, R., & Grossman, J. R. (2004). Posttraumatic stress disorder (PTSD) and posttraumatic stress symptoms (PTSS) in families of adolescent childhood cancer survivors. *Journal of Pediatric Psychology, 29*(3), 211–219. https://doi.org/10.1093/jpepsy/jsh022
65. Robertson, J. (1970). *Young children in hospital* (2nd ed.). Tavistock Publications.
66. Bliss for babies born premature or sick (2023). *Locked out: The impact of COVID-19 on neonatal care.*
67. Anand, K. J., & Hickey, P. R. (1987). Pain and its effects in the human neonate and fetus. *New England Journal of Medicine, 317*, 1321–1329.
68. Porter, F. L., Porges, S. W., & Marshall, R. E. (1988). Newborn pain cries and vagal tone: Parallel changes in response to circumcision. *Child Development, 59*(2), 495–505. https://doi.org/10.2307/1130327
69. Anand, K. J., & Hickey, P. R. (1987). Pain and its effects in the human neonate and fetus. *New England Journal of Medicine, 317*, 1321–1329.
70. Campbell-Yeo, M., Eriksson, M., & Benoit, B. (2022). Assessment and management of pain in preterm infants: A practice update. *Children (Basel), 9*(2), 244. https://doi.org/10.3390/children9020244. PMID: 35204964; PMCID: PMC8869922.
71. Cruz, M. D., Fernandes, A. M., & Oliveira, C. R. (2016). Epidemiology of painful procedures performed in neonates: A systematic review of observational studies. *Eur J Pain, 20*(4), 489–498. https://doi.org/10.1002/ejp.757
72. Campbell-Yeo, M., Eriksson, M., & Benoit, B. (2022). Assessment and management of pain in preterm infants: A practice update. *Children (Basel), 9*(2), 244. https://doi.org/10.3390/children9020244. PMID: 35204964; PMCID: PMC8869922.
73. Wilson, W. M., Smith-Parrish, M., Marino, B. S., & Kovacs, A. H. (2015). Neurodevelopmental and psychosocial outcomes across the congenital heart disease lifespan. *Progress in Paediatric Cardiology, 39*, 113–118.

74. Morton, L. (2020). Using psychologically informed care to improve mental health and wellbeing for people living with a heart condition from birth: A statement paper. *Journal of Health Psychology, 25*(2), 197–206. https://doi.org/10.1177/1359105319826354
75. Corrigan, P. W., Rafacz, J., & Rüsch, N. (2011). Examining a progressive model of self-stigma and its impact on people with serious mental illness. *Psychiatry Research, 189*(3), 339–343. PMC3185170; PMID:21715017
76. Earnshaw, V. A., & Quinn, D. M. (2012). The impact of stigma in healthcare on people living with chronic illnesses. *J Health Psychol, 17*(2), 157–168. https://doi.org/10.1177/1359105311414952. Epub 2011 Jul 28. PMID: 21799078; PMCID: PMC8919040.
77. Benfer, N., Howell, M. K., Lucksted, A., Romero, E. G., & Drapalski, A. L. (2023). Self-stigma and PTSD: Conceptualization and implications for research and treatment. *Psychiatric Services, 74*(10), 1081–1083, appi.ps.20220397. https://doi.org/10.1176/appi.ps.20220397
78. Quenneville, A. F., Badoud, D., Nicastro, R., et al. (2020). Internalized stigmatization in borderline personality disorder and attention deficit hyperactivity disorder in comparison to bipolar disorder. *J Affect Disord, 262*, 317–322.
79. Mahajan, A. P., Sayles, J. N., Patel, V. A., et al. (2008). Stigma in the HIV/AIDS epidemic: A review of the literature and recommendations for the way forward. *AIDS, 22*(Suppl 2), S67–79. https://doi.org/10.1097/01.aids.0000327438.13291.62. PMID: 18641472; PMCID: PMC2835402.
80. Sayles, J. N., Ryan, G. W., Silver, J. S., Sarkisian, C. A., & Cunningham, W. E. (2007). Experiences of social stigma and implications for healthcare among a diverse population of HIV positive adults. *Journal of Urban Health, 84*(6), 814–828.
81. Quinn, D. M., & Chaudoir, S. R. (2009). Living with a concealable stigmatized identity: The impact of anticipated stigma, centrality, salience, and cultural stigma on psychological distress and health. *Journal of Personality and Social Psychology, 97*(4), 634–651.
82. Morton, L. (2020). Using psychologically informed care to improve mental health and wellbeing for people living with a heart condition from birth: A statement paper, *Journal of Health Psychology, 25*(2), 197–206.
83. Swan, L., Windram, J., Burchill, L., et al. (2023). Sexual health and well-being in adults with congenital heart disease: An international society of adult congenital heart disease statement. *Journal American College of Cardiology: Advances, 2*(10), Article 100716. https://doi.org/10.1016/j.jacadv.2023.100716
84. McGrath, M., Low, M. A., Power, E., McCluskey, A., & Lever, S. (2021). Addressing sexuality among people living with chronic disease and disability: A systematic mixed methods review of knowledge, attitudes, and practices of health care professionals. *Arch Phys Med Rehabil, 102*(5), 999–1010. https://doi.org/10.1016/j.apmr.2020.09.379.
85. Swan, L., Windram, J., Burchill, L., et al. (2023). Sexual health and well-being in adults with congenital heart disease: A international society of adult congenital heart disease statement. *Journal American College of Cardiology: Advances, 2*(10), Article 100716. https://doi.org/10.1016/j.jacadv.2023.100716
86. Bogart, K. R., & Dunn, D. S. (2019). Ableism special issue introduction. *Journal of Social Issues, 75*, 650–664. https://doi.org/10.1111/josi.12354
87. Morton, L., Calderwood, C., Cogan, N., Murphy, C., Nix, E., & Kolacz, J. (2021). An exploration of psychological trauma and positive adaptation in adults with congenital heart disease during the COVID-19 pandemic. *Journal of Patient Experience, 9*(1), 82–94.
88. Livecchi, T., & Morton, L. (2023). *Healing hearts and minds: A holistic approach to coping well with congenital heart disease.* Oxford University Press.

89. Namkung, E. H., & Carr, D. (2020). The psychological consequences of disability over the life course: Assessing the mediating role of perceived interpersonal discrimination. *Journal of Health and Social Behavior, 61*(2), 190–207. https://doi.org/10.1177/0022146520921371
90. Gong, C. L., Zhao, H., Wei, Y., et al. (2020). Lifetime burden of adult congenital heart disease in the usa using a microsimulation model. *Pediatr Cardiol, 41*(7), 1515–1525. https://doi.org/10.1007/s00246-020-02409-9
91. Birkeland Nielsen, M., Shahid Emberland, J., & Knardahl, S. (2017). Workplace bullying as a predictor of disability retirement: A prospective registry study of norwegian employees. *J Occup Environ Med, 59*(7), 609–614. https://doi.org/10.1097/JOM.0000000000001026
92. Hackett, R. A., Steptoe, A., Lang, R. P., & Jackson, S. E. (2020). Disability discrimination and well-being in the United Kingdom: A prospective cohort study. *BMJ Open, 10*(3), e035714. https://doi.org/10.1136/bmjopen-2019-035714. PMID: 32169928; PMCID: PMC7069317.
93. Gong, C. L., Zhao, H., Wei, Y., et al. (2020). Lifetime burden of adult congenital heart disease in the usa using a microsimulation model. *Pediatr Cardiol, 41*(7), 1515–1525. https://doi.org/10.1007/s00246-020-02409-9
94. Eisenberger, N. I. (2012). The neural bases of social pain: Evidence for shared representations with physical pain. *Psychosom Med, 74*(2), 126–135. https://doi.org/10.1097/PSY.0b013e3182464dd1.
95. Gilbert, P. (2014). The origins and nature of compassion focused therapy. *British Journal of Clinical Psychology, 53*(1), 6–41.
96. Alves, T., van Munster, M. A., Alves, I. dos S., & Souza, J. V. de. (2022). The "normal" physical education classes: The ableism facing the inclusion of disabled students. *Disability and Society, 39*(2), 469–484. https://doi.org/10.1080/09687599.2022.2071679
97. Ives, Clayton, B., Brittain, I., & Mackintosh, C. (2021). "I'll always find a perfectly justified reason for not doing it": Challenges for disability sport and physical activity in the United Kingdom. *Sport in Society, 24*(4), 588–606. https://doi.org/10.1080/17430437.2019.1703683
98. Giese, M., & Ruin, S. (2018). Forgotten bodies: An examination of physical education from the perspective of ableism. *Sport in Society, 21*(1), 152–165. https://doi.org/10.1080/17430437.2016.1225857
99. Smith, B., Mallick, K., Monforte, J., & Foster, C. (2021). Disability, the communication of physical activity and sedentary behaviour, and ableism: A call for inclusive messages. *British Journal of Sports Medicine, 55*(20), 1121–1122. https://doi.org/10.1136/bjsports-2020-103780
100. Fennell, M. J. (1997). Low self-esteem: A cognitive perspective. *Behavioural and Cognitive Psychotherapy, 25*, 1–26.
101. Rimes, K. A., Smith, P., & Bridge, L. (2023). Low self-esteem: A refined cognitive behavioural model. *Behavioural and Cognitive Psychotherapy, 51*(6), 579–594. https://doi.org/10.1017/S1352465823000048
102. Hatzenbuehler, M. L. (2009). How does sexual minority stigma "get under the skin"? A psychological mediation framework. *Psychol Bull, 135*(5), 707–730. https://doi.org/10.1037/a0016441. PMID: 19702379; PMCID: PMC2789474.
103. Gilbert, P. (2009). *The compassionate mind.* Robinson.
104. Gilbert, P. (2014). The origins and nature of compassion focused therapy. *British Journal of Clinical Psychology, 53*(1), 6–41.
105. Gilbert, P. (2009). *The compassionate mind.* Robinson.

106. Freedman, V. A., Carr, D., Cornman, J. C., & Lucas, R. (2017). Aging, mobility impairments and subjective wellbeing. *Disability and Health Journal, 10*(4), 525–531.
107. Brown, R. L., & Barrett, A. E. (2011). Visual impairment and quality of life among older adults: An examination of explanations for the relationship. *J Gerontol B Psychol Sci Soc Sci, 66*(3), 364–373. https://doi.org/10.1093/geronb/gbr015.
108. Yang, Y. (2006). How does functional disability affect depressive symptoms in late life? The role of perceived social support and psychological resources. *Journal of Health and Social Behavior, 47*(4), 355–372. https://doi.org/10.1177/002214650 604700404
109. Anie, K. A., Egunjobi, F. E., & Akinyanju, O. O. (2010). Psychosocial impact of sickle cell disorder: Perspectives from a Nigerian setting. *Global Health, 6*(2). https://doi.org/10.1186/1744-8603-6-2.
110. Hinz, A., Herzberg, P. Y., Lordick, F., et al. (2019). Age and gender differences in anxiety and depression in cancer patients compared with the general population. *Eur J Cancer Care* (Engl), *28*(5), e13129. https://doi.org/10.1111/ecc.13129. Epub 2019 Jul 9. PMID: 31290218.
111. Meentken, M. G., van Beynum, I. M., Legerstee, J. S., Helbing, W. A., & Utens, E. M. (2017). Medically related post-traumatic stress in children and adolescents with congenital heart defects. *Front Pediatr, 5*, 20. https://doi.org/10.3389/fped.2017.00020. PMID: 28243582; PMCID: PMC5303720.
112. Naser, A. Y., Hameed, A. N., Mustafa, N., Alwafi, H., Dahmash, E. Z., Alyami, H. S., & Khalil H. (2021). Depression and anxiety in patients with cancer: A cross-sectional study. *Front Psychol, 12*, 585534. https://doi.org/10.3389/fpsyg.2021.585534. PMID: 33935849; PMCID: PMC8081978.
113. Sloan, M., et al. (2023). Prevalence and identification of neuropsychiatric symptoms in systemic autoimmune rheumatic diseases: An international mixed methods study. *Rheumatology, 63*(5), 1259–1272. https://doi.org/10.1093/rhe/kead369
114. Ziarko, M., Siemiątkowska, K., Sieński, M., Samborski, W., Samborska, J., & Mojs, E. (2019). Mental health and rheumatoid arthritis: Toward understanding the emotional status of people with chronic disease. *Biomed Res Int, 2019*, 1473925. https://doi.org/10.1155/2019/1473925. PMID: 30886858; PMCID: PMC6388315.

5. Chapter 2

1. Damasio, A. R. (1994). *Descartes' error: Emotion, reason, and the human brain*. G. P. Putnam.
2. Foucault, M. (1963). *The birth of the clinic: An archaeology of medical perception*. Routledge.
3. Endometriosis UK. (n.d.) *Endometriosis UK diagnosis survey 2023 report March*. endometriosis-uk.org
4. Morton, L. (2020). Using psychologically informed care to improve mental health and wellbeing for people living with a heart condition from birth: A statement paper. *Journal of Health Psychology, 25*(2), 197–206. https://doi.org/10.1177/1359105319826354
5. Appignanesi, L. (2008). *Mad, bad and sad: A history of women and the mind doctors from 1800 to the present*. Virago Pres.
6. Knaak, S., Mantler, E., & Szeto, A. (2017). Mental illness-related stigma in healthcare: Barriers to access and care and evidence-based solutions. *Health Manage Forum, 30*(2), 111–116. https://doi.org/10.1177/0840470416679413. Epub 2017 Feb 16. PMID: 28929889; PMCID: PMC5347358.

7. Gruber, J., Lordan, G., Pilling, S., Propper, C., & Saunders, R. (2022). The impact of mental health support for the chronically ill on hospital utilisation: Evidence from the UK. *Social Science and Medicine, 294*, 114675. https://doi.org/10.1016/j.socscimed.2021.114675.
8. Van Lieshout R. J., & Macqueen G. (2008). Psychological factors in asthma. *Allergy Asthma Clin Immunol, 4*(1), 12–28. https://doi.org/10.1186/1710-1492-4-1-12. Epub 2008 Mar 15. PMID: 20525122; PMCID: PMC2869336.
9. DiMatteo, M. R., Lepper, H. S., & Croghan, T. W. (2000). Depression is a risk factor for noncompliance with medical treatment: Meta-analysis of the effects of anxiety and depression on patient adherence. *Arch Intern Med, 160*(14), 2101–2107. https://doi.org/10.1001/archinte.160.14.2101. PMID: 10904452.
10. Khan, M., Monaghan, M., Klein, N., Ruiz, G., & John, A. S. (2015). Associations among depression symptoms with alcohol and smoking tobacco use in adult patients with congenital heart disease. *Congenital Heart Dis, 10*, E243–E249.
11. Barnett, K., Mercer, S. W., Norbury, M., Watt, G., Wyke, S., & Guthrie, B. (2012). Epidemiology of multimorbidity and implications for health care, research, and medical education: a cross-sectional study. *Lancet, 380*(9836), 37–43. https://doi.org/10.1016/S0140-6736(12)60240-2. Epub 2012 May 10. PMID: 22579043.
12. Morton, L. (2020). Using psychologically informed care to improve mental health and wellbeing for people living with a heart condition from birth: A statement paper. *Journal of Health Psychology, 25*(2), 197–206. https://doi.org/10.1177/1359105319826354
13. Morton. L. (2021). Waiting patiently [blog]. *British Medical Journal.*
14. McCarthy. K., McGee, H. M., & O'Boyle, C. A. Outpatient clinic waiting times and non-attendance as indicators of quality. *Psychol Health Med*, 2000; 5, 287–293. https://doi.org/10.1080/713690194
15. Morton. L. (2021). Waiting patiently [blog]. *British Medical Journal.*
16. Cogan, N., Morton, L., Georgiadis, E., Butler, S. H., Fleck, V. J., & Johnstone, J. (2024). Exploring the perspectives of healthcare professionals concerning the use and utility of the hospital gown to develop theoretically informed behaviour change interventions. *Public Health Open Access, 8*(1), 000265.
17. Morton, L., Cogan, N., Kornfält, S., Porter, Z., & Georgiadis, E. (2020). Baring all: The impact of the hospital gown on patient wellbeing. *British Journal of Health Psychology, 25*(3), 452–473.
18. Morton, L., Cogan, N., Kornfält, S., Porter, Z., & Georgiadis, E. (2020). Baring all: The impact of the hospital gown on patient wellbeing. *British Journal of Health Psychology, 25*(3), 452–473.
19. Album, D., Johannessen, L. E. F., Rasmussen, E. B. (2017). Stability and change in disease prestige: A comparative analysis of three surveys spanning a quarter of a century. *Social Science & Medicine, 180*, 45–51.
20. Livecchi, T., & Morton, L. (2023). *Healing hearts and minds: A holistic approach to coping well with congenital heart disease.* Oxford University Press.
21. Crenshaw, K. W., Gotanda, N., Peller, G., & Thomas, K. (1995). *Critical race theory: The key writings that formed the movement* (p. 101). Faculty Books.
22. Holland, E., Matthews, K., Macdonald, S., et al. (2024). The impact of living with multiple long-term conditions (multimorbidity) on everyday life: A qualitative evidence synthesis. *BMC Public Health, 24*, 3446. https://doi.org/10.1186/s12889-024-20763-8
23. Fricker, M. (2007). *Epistemic injustice: Power and the ethics of knowing.* Oxford University Press.
24. Rosen, L. T. (2021). Mapping out epistemic justice in the clinical space: Using narrative techniques to affirm patients as knowers. *Philosophy, Ethics, and Humanities in Medicine, 16* (1), 1–6.

25. Heggen, K. M., & Berg, H. (2021). Epistemic injustice in the age of evidence-based practice: The case of fibromyalgia. *Humanit Soc Sci Commun, 8*, 235. https://doi.org/10.1057/s41599-021-00918-3
26. Rose, R. (2012). *Life story therapy with traumatized children: A model for practice*. Jessica Kingsley.
27. Booth, R. (2022). Helping us heal: How creative life story work supports individuals and organisations to recover from trauma. *Journal of Social Work Practice, 36*(1), 119–127. https://doi.org/10.1080/02650533.2021.2025349
28. Morton, L. (2023). The injustice of losing my childhood medical history. The Alliance, 21st Feb, 2024, https://www.alliance-scotland.org.uk/blog/opinion/the-injustice-of-losing-my-childhood-medical-history/
29. Ashdown, L., & Jones. L. (2024). The time for patient partnership in medical education has arrived: Critical reflection through autoethnography from a physician turned patient. *Med Teach, 46*(10), 1322–1327. https://doi.org/10.1080/0142159X.2024.2308065.
30. Lown, B. A., Rosen, J., & Marttila, J. (2011). An agenda for improving compassionate care: A survey shows about half of patients say such care is missing. *Health Aff* (Millwood), *30*(9), 1772–1778. https://doi.org/10.1377/hlthaff.2011.0539. PMID: 21900669.
31. Chaney, S. (2021). Before compassion: Sympathy, tact and the history of the ideal nurse. *Medical Humanities, 47*, 475–484.
32. Francis, R. (2013). *Report of the Mid Staffordshire NHS Foundation Trust Public Enquiry*. The Stationery Office.
33. Morse, D. S., Edwardsen E. A., & Gordon, H. S. (2008). Missed opportunities for interval empathy in lung cancer communication. *Arch Intern Med, 168*(17), 1853–1858. https://doi.org/10.1001/archinte.168.17.1853. PMID: 18809811; PMCID: PMC2678758.
34. Morton, L., Cogan, N., Kornfält, S., Porter, Z., & Georgiadis, E. (2020). Baring all: The impact of the hospital gown on patient wellbeing. *British Journal of Health Psychology, 25*(3), 452–473.
35. Tai-Seale, M., Olson, C. W., Li, J., et al. (2017). Electronic health record logs indicate that physicians split time evenly between seeing patients and desktop medicine. *Health Aff* (Millwood), *36*(4), 655–662. https://doi.org/10.1377/hlthaff.2016.0811.
36. Trzeciak, S., & Mazzarelli, A. (2019). *Compassionomics: The revolutionary scientific evidence that caring makes a difference*. Studer Group.
37. Kennedy, M., Bray, L., Saron, H., & Brady, L. M. (2024). Scoping communication training in undergraduate children's nursing programmes: A mixed method study examining delivery methods and content. *Nurse Education in Practice, 79*, 104056. https://doi.org/10.1016/j.nepr.2024.104056.
38. Mehta, K. K., Salam, S., Hake, A., et al. (2024). Cultivating compassion in medicine: A toolkit for medical students to improve self-kindness and enhance clinical care. *BMC Med Educ, 24*, 291. https://doi.org/10.1186/s12909-024-05270-z
39. Chaney, S. (2021). Before compassion: Sympathy, tact and the history of the ideal nurse. *Medical Humanities, 47*, 475–484.
40. Li, W. W., Heward, C., Merrick, A., Astridge, B., & Leow, T. (2024). Prevalence of experiencing public humiliation and its effects on victims' mental health: A systematic review and meta-analysis. *Journal of Pacific Rim Psychology, 18*. https://doi.org/10.1177/18344909241252325
41. Li, W. W., Heward, C., Merrick, A., Astridge, B., & Leow, T. (2024). Prevalence of experiencing public humiliation and its effects on victims' mental health: A systematic review and meta-analysis. *Journal of Pacific Rim Psychology, 18*. https://doi.org/10.1177/18344909241252325

42. Wigg, L., Li, W. W., & Leow, T. A (2024). Systematic review and meta-analysis on teaching by humiliation in medical training: Its frequency and impact on the mental health outcomes of medical trainees. *Med Sci Educ*, 35, 569–585. https://doi.org/10.1007/s40670-024-02213-7
43. Cheng, M. Y., Neves, S. L., Rainwater, J., et al. (2020). Exploration of mistreatment and burnout among resident physicians: A cross-specialty observational study. *Med Sci Educ*, 30, 315–321. https://doi.org/10.1007/s40670-019-00905-z
44. Li, W. W., Heward, C., Merrick, A., Astridge, B., & Leow, T. (2024). Prevalence of experiencing public humiliation and its effects on victims' mental health: A systematic review and meta-analysis. *Journal of Pacific Rim Psychology*, 18. https://doi.org/10.1177/18344909241252325
45. Doherty, M., McCowan, S., & Shaw, S. C. (2023). Autistic SPACE: A novel framework for meeting the needs of autistic people in healthcare settings. *Br J Hosp Med (Lond)*, 84(4), 1–9. https://doi.org/10.12968/hmed.2023.0006.
46. Nightingale, F. (1858). *Notes on nursing: What it is, and what it is not*. Appleton and Company.
47. Burger, P., Van den Ende, E. S., Lukman, W., et al. (2022). Sleep in hospitalized pediatric and adult patients: A systematic review and meta-analysis, *Sleep Medicine*, 4, 100059. https://doi.org/10.1016/j.sleepx.2022.100059.
48. Jagriti, P., Manish, T., Rajni, P., & Divya, S. (2022). Noise pollution in intensive care unit: A hidden enemy affecting the physical and mental health of patients and caregivers. *Noise and Health*, 24(114), 130–136. https://doi.org/10.4103/nah.nah_79_21
49. Berglund, B., Lindvall, T., & Schwela, D. H., & World Health Organization Occupational and Environmental Health Team. (1999). *Guidelines for community noise*. World Health Organization. https://iris.who.int/handle/10665/66217
50. Tronstad, O., Patterson, S., Zangerl, B., et al. (2024). The introduction of a sound reduction bundle in the intensive care unit and its impact on sound levels and patients. *Aust Crit Care*, 37(5), 716–726. https://doi.org/10.1016/j.aucc.2024.02.011. Epub 2024 Apr 11. PMID: 38604917.
51. Jagriti, P., Manish, T., Rajni, P., & Divya, S. (2022). Noise pollution in intensive care unit: A hidden enemy affecting the physical and mental health of patients and caregivers. *Noise and Health*, 24(114), 130–136. https://doi.org/10.4103/nah.nah_79_21
52. Morton, L. (2020). Using psychologically informed care to improve mental health and wellbeing for people living with a heart condition from birth: A statement paper. *Journal of Health Psychology*, 25(2), 197–206. https://doi.org/10.1177/1359105319826354
53. Roseman, A. S., Morton, L., & Kovacs, A. H. (2020). Health anxiety among adults with congenital heart disease. *Current Opinion in Cardiology*, 36, 98–104.
54. World Health Organization. (2013). *Health 2020: A European policy framework and strategy for the 21st century*. Regional office for Europe.

6. Chapter 3

1. Engel, G. L. (1977). The need for a new medical model: A challenge for biomedicine. *Science*, 196(4286), 129–136. https://doi.org/10.1126/science.847460. PMID: 847460.
2. Engel G. L. The need for a new medical model: A challenge for biomedicine. *Psychodyn Psychiatry*, 40(3), 377–396. https://doi.org/10.1521/pdps.2012.40.3.377. PMID: 23002701.
3. Chris J., Main, Steven Z. George. Psychologically Informed Practice for Management of Low Back Pain: Future Directions in Practice and Research. *Physical Therapy*, 91(5), 820–824, https://doi.org/10.2522/ptj.20110060

4. van der Kolk, B. A. (2014). *The body keeps the score: Brain, mind, and body in the healing of trauma*. Viking.
5. Gilbert, P. (2014). The origins and nature of compassion focused therapy. *British Journal of Clinical Psychology, 53*(1), 6–41.
6. Hupcey, J. E. (2020). Feeling safe: The psychosocial needs of ICU patients. *J Nurs Scholarsh, 32*(4), 361–367. https://doi.org/10.1111/j.1547-5069.2000.00361.x. PMID: 11140200.
7. Porges, S. W. (2022). Polyvagal theory: A science of safety. *Front Integr Neurosci, 16*, 871227. https://doi.org/10.3389/fnint.2022.871227. PMID: 35645742; PMCID: PMC9131189.
8. Porges, S. W. (2022). Polyvagal theory: A science of safety. *Front Integr Neurosci, 16*, 871227. https://doi.org/10.3389/fnint.2022.871227. PMID: 35645742; PMCID: PMC9131189.
9. Porges, S. W. (2022). Polyvagal theory: A science of safety. *Front Integr Neurosci, 16*, 871227. https://doi.org/10.3389/fnint.2022.871227. PMID: 35645742; PMCID: PMC9131189.
10. Carter, C. S. (2022). Sex, love and oxytocin: Two metaphors and a molecule. *Neurosci Biobehav Rev, 143*,104948. https://doi.org/10.1016/j.neubiorev.2022.104948. Epub 2022 Nov 5. PMID: 36347382; PMCID: PMC9759207.
11. Müller, J., et al. (2018). Number of thoracotomies predicts impairment in lung function and exercise capacity in patients with congenital heart disease. *Journal of Cardiology, 71*(1), 88–92.
12. Rogers, C. R. (1959). A theory of therapy, personality, and interpersonal relationships, as developed in the client-centered framework. *Psychology: A Study of a Science, 3*, 184–256.
13. Wong, A. M. F. (2020). *The art and science of compassion, a primer: Reflections of a physician-chaplain*. Oxford University Press.
14. Neff, K. D., & Germer, C. (2017). Self-Compassion and Psychological Wellbeing. In J. Doty (Ed.). *Oxford Handbook of Compassion Science*, Chap. 27. Oxford University Press.
15. Jacob, J. G., Romate., J, Allen, J. G., & Rajkumar, E (2024). Compassionate communication: A scoping review. *Frontiers in Communication, 8*. https://www.frontiersin.org/journals/communication/articles/10.3389/fcomm.2023.1294586
16. Lown, B. A., Rosen, J., & Marttila, J. (2011). An agenda for improving compassionate care: A survey shows about half of patients say such care is missing. *Health Aff* (Millwood), *30*(9), 1772–1778. https://doi.org/10.1377/hlthaff.2011.0539. PMID: 21900669.
17. Tehranineshat, B., Rakhshan, M., Torabizadeh, C., & Fararouei, M. (2019). Compassionate care in healthcare systems: A systematic review. *Journal of the National Medical Association, 111*(5), 546–554. https://doi.org/10.1016/j.jnma.2019.04.002
18. Field, T. M., Diego, M., & Hernandez-Reif, M (2010). Preterm infant massage therapy research: A review. *Infant Behavioral Development, 33*(2), 115–124.
19. Mollon, D. (2014). Feeling safe during an inpatient hospitalization: A concept analysis. *J Adv Nurs, 70*(8), 1727–1737. https://doi.org/10.1111/jan.12348. Epub 2014 Jan 2. PMID: 24383463.
20. Holt-Lunstad, J., Birmingham, W. A., & Light, K. C. (2008). Influence of a "warm touch" support enhancement intervention among married couples on ambulatory blood pressure, oxytocin, alpha amylase, and cortisol. *Psychosom Med, 70*(9), 976–985. https://doi.org/10.1097/PSY.0b013e318187aef7.
21. Egbert, L. D., Battit, G. E., Welch, C. E., & Bartlett, M. K. (1964). Reduction of postoperative pain by encouragement and instruction of patients: A study of doctor–patient rapport. *N Engl J Med., 270*, 825–827.

22. Kim, S. S., Kaplowitz, S., & Johnston, M. V. (2004). The effects of physician empathy on patient satisfaction and compliance. *Eval Health Prof*, *27*(3), 237–251. https://doi.org/10.1177/0163278704267037. PMID: 15312283.
23. Porges, S. W. (2021). *Polyvagal safety: Attachment, communication, self-regulation*. Norton Press.
24. National Institutes of Health. (2014). *The science of compassion: Future directions in end-of-life and palliative care*.
25. Mehta, K. K., Salam, S., Hake, A., et al. (2024). Cultivating compassion in medicine: A toolkit for medical students to improve self-kindness and enhance clinical care. *BMC Med Educ*, *24*, 291. https://doi.org/10.1186/s12909-024-05270-z
26. Bagacean, C., Cousin, I., Ubertini, A. H., et al. (2020). Simulated patient and role play methodologies for communication skills and empathy training of undergraduate medical students. *BMC Med Educ*, *20*(1), 491. https://doi.org/10.1186/s12909-020-02401-0. PMID: 33276777; PMCID: PMC7716460.
27. Neff, K. D., & Germer, C. (2017). Self-compassion and psychological wellbeing. In J. Doty (Ed.), *Oxford handbook of compassion science*, 478–492. Oxford University Press.
28. Dyer, E., Swartzlander, B. J., & Gugliucci, M. R. (2018). Using virtual reality in medical education to teach empathy. *J Med Libr Assoc*, *106*(4), 498–500. https://doi.org/10.5195/jmla.2018.518. Epub 2018 Oct 1. PMID: 30271295; PMCID: PMC6148621.
29. Porges, S. W. (2021). *Polyvagal safety: Attachment, communication, self-regulation*. Norton Press, N. Y.
30. Roche, H., Morton, L., & Cogan, N. (2025). Barriers and facilitators to psychological safety during medical procedures among individuals diagnosed with chronic illnesses in childhood. *MDPI*. https://doi.org/10.20944/preprints202503.0513.v1
31. Cogan, N., Campbell, J., Morton, L., Young, D., & Porges, S. (2024). Validation of the Neuroception of Psychological Safety Scale (NPSS). Among Health and Social Care Workers in the UK. *International Journal of Environmental Research and Public Health*, *21*(12), 1551. https://doi.org/10.3390/ijerph21121551
32. Porges, S. W. (2021). *Polyvagal safety: Attachment, communication, self-regulation*. Norton Press, N. Y.
33. Morton, L. (2015). The heart of medicine: Growing up with pioneering treatment. *British Medical Journal*, *351*, h3881. https://doi.org/10.1136/bmj.h3881
34. Hauser, D. J., & Schwarz, N. (2015) The War on Prevention: Bellicose Cancer Metaphors Hurt (Some) Prevention Intentions. *Personality and Social Psychology Bulletin*, *41*(1), 66–77. https://doi.org/10.1177/0146167214557006
35. Hayes, S. C., Levin, M. E., Plumb-Vilardaga, J., Villatte, J. L., & Pistorello, J. (2013). Acceptance and commitment therapy and contextual behavioral science: Examining the progress of a distinctive model of behavioral and cognitive therapy. *Behav Ther*, *44*(2), 180–198. https://doi.org/10.1016/j.beth.2009.08.002. Epub 2011 Jun 1. PMID: 23611068; PMCID: PMC3635495.
36. Bradshaw, J., Siddiqui, N., Greenfield, D., Sharma, A. Kindness, Listening, and Connection: Patient and Clinician Key Requirements for Emotional Support in Chronic and Complex Care. *J Patient Exp*, 9:23743735221092627. doi: 10.1177/23743735221092627.
37. Chute, A., Johnson, S., & Pawliuk, B. (2023). *Professional communication skills for health studies*. MacEwan Open Books. https://doi.org/10.31542/b.gm.3. Used under a CC BY-NC-SA 4.0 licence.
38. Chute, A., Johnson, S., & Pawliuk, B. (2023). *Professional communication skills for health studies*. MacEwan Open Books. https://doi.org/10.31542/b.gm.3. Used under a CC BY-NC-SA 4.0 licence.

39. Barney, C., & Shea, S. C. (2007). The art of effectively teaching clinical interviewing skills using role-playing: A primer. *Psychiatric Clinics of North America, 30*, 31–50. https://doi.org/10.1016/j.psc.2007.03.001
40. Osborn, D., & Costas, L. (2013). Role-playing in counselor student development. *Journal of Creativity in Mental Health, 8*(1), 92–103. https://doi.org/10.1080/15401383.2013.763689
41. Monden, K. R., Gentry, L., & Cox, T. R. (2016). Delivering bad news to patients. *Proc (Bayl Univ Med Cent), 29*(1), 101–102. https://doi.org/10.1080/08998280.2016.11929380. PMID: 26722188; PMCID: PMC4677873.
42. Baile, W. F., Buckman, R., Lenzi, R., Glober, G., Beale, E. A., & Kudelka, A. P. (2000). SPIKES-A six-step protocol for delivering bad news: Application to the patient with cancer. *Oncologist, 5*(4), 302–311. https://doi.org/10.1634/theoncologist.5-4-302. PMID: 10964998.
43. Ptacek, J. T., Ptacek, J. J., & Ellison, N. M. (2001). "I'm sorry to tell you . . .": Physicians' reports of breaking bad news. *J Behav Med, 24*(2), 205–217. https://doi.org/10.1023/a:1010766732373. PMID: 11392920.
44. Thestrup, J., Sørensen, J. L., Esbjørn, B. H., et al. (2025). Paediatric patient perceptions of healthcare professionals: Contributions to a communication curriculum. *Eur J Pediatr, 184*, 75. https://doi.org/10.1007/s00431-024-05911-x
45. Krauss, B. A., Leroy, P. L., & Krauss, B. S. (2024). Establishing trust with children. *Eur J Pediatr, 183*(10), 4185–4193. https://doi.org/10.1007/s00431-024-05704-2. Epub ahead of print. PMID: 39136756.
46. Krauss, B. A., Leroy, P. L., & Krauss, B. S. (2024). Establishing trust with children. *Eur J Pediatr*. https://doi.org/10.1007/s00431-024-05704-2. Epub ahead of print. PMID: 39136756.
47. Chapman, L., Wicks, G., & Friend, A. (2022). Adolescents in hospital, which wards are they admitted to and is this appropriate? *BMJ Paediatrics Open, 6*. https://doi.org/10.1136/bmjpo-2022-RCPCH.1
48. Thestrup, J., Sørensen, J. L., Esbjørn, B. H., et al. (2025). Paediatric patient perceptions of healthcare professionals: Contributions to a communication curriculum. *Eur J Pediatr, 184*, 75. https://doi.org/10.1007/s00431-024-05911-x
49. South Wales and South West Congenital Heart Disease Network Newsletter. (2025). January 2025, p. 8. https://www.swswchd.co.uk/image/blog/0.%20New%20Year%202025%20SWSW%20CHD%20Network%20Newsletter%20Final%20as%20at%20%2014-01-2025%20v1.0.pdf
50. NICE. (2016). NICE guideline, Babies, children and young people's experience of healthcare, Published: 25 August 2021.
51. Thestrup, J., Sørensen, J. L., Esbjørn, B. H., et al. (2025). Paediatric patient perceptions of healthcare professionals: Contributions to a communication curriculum. *Eur J Pediatr, 184*, 75, https://doi.org/10.1007/s00431-024-05911-x
52. National Institute on Ageing. *Talking with your older patients*. https://www.nia.nih.gov/health/health-care-professionals-information/talking-your-older-patients
53. Montgomery, E. (2013). Feeling safe: A metasynthesis of the maternity care needs of women who were sexually abused in childhood. *Birth, 40*(2), 88–95. https://doi.org/10.1111/birt.12043. PMID: 24635462.
54. Loomis, B., Epstein, K., Dauria, E. F., & Dolce, L. (2019). Implementing a trauma-informed public health system in San Francisco, California. *Health Education and Behavior, 46*(2), 251–259. https://doi.org/10.1177/1090198118806942
55. Fennell, M. J. (1997). Low self-esteem: A cognitive perspective. *Behavioural and Cognitive Psychotherapy, 25*, 1–26.

56. Tyrer, P., Cooper, S., Crawford, M., et al. (2011). Prevalence of health anxiety problems in medical clinics. *Journal of Psychosomatic Research*, 71(6), 392–394. https://doi.org/10.1016/j.jpsychores.2011.07.004
57. Roseman, A. S., Morton, L., & Kovacs, A. H. (2020). Health anxiety among adults with congenital heart disease. *Current Opinion in Cardiology*, 36, 98–104.
58. American Psychiatric Association. (2013). *Desk reference to the diagnostic criteria from DSM-5 (R)*. American Psychiatric Association Publishing.
59. Myers, C. (1915). A contribution to the study of shell shock: Being an account of three cases of loss of memory, vision, smell, and taste, admitted into the Duchess of Westminster's war hospital, Le Touquet. *The Lancet*, 185(4772), 316–320.
60. Morton, L. (2020). Using psychologically informed care to improve mental health and wellbeing for people living with a heart condition from birth: A statement paper. *Journal of Health Psychology*, 25(2), 197–206. https://doi.org/10.1177/1359105319826354
61. Seng, J. S., Graham-Bermann, S. A., Clark, M. K., McCarthy, A. M., & Ronis, D. L. (2005). Posttraumatic stress disorder and physical comorbidity among female children and adolescents: Results from service-use data. *Pediatrics*, 116(6), e767–76. https://doi.org/10.1542/peds.2005-0608. PMID: 16322133.
62. Parker, A. M., Sricharoenchai, T., Raparla, S., Schneck, K. W., Bienvenu, O. J., & Needham, D. M. (2015). Posttraumatic stress disorder in critical illness survivors: A metaanalysis. *Crit Care Med*, 43(5), 1121–1129. https://doi.org/10.1097/CCM.0000000000000882. PMID: 25654178.
63. Vilchinsky, N., Ginzburg, K., Fait, K., & Foa, E. B. (2017). Cardiac-disease-induced PTSD (CDI-PTSD): A systematic review. *Clin Psychol Rev*, 55, 92–106. https://doi.org/10.1016/j.cpr.2017.04.009. Epub 2017 Apr 25. PMID: 28575815.
64. Abbey, G., Thompson, S. B., Hickish, T., & Heathcote, D. (2015). A meta-analysis of prevalence rates and moderating factors for cancer-related post-traumatic stress disorder. *Psychooncology*, 24(4), 371–381. https://doi.org/10.1002/pon.3654. Epub 2014 Aug 22. PMID: 25146298; PMCID: PMC4409098.
65. Vermetten, E., & Bremner, J. D. (2003). Olfaction as a traumatic reminder in posttraumatic stress disorder: case reports and review. *J Clin Psychiatry*, 64(2), 202–207. https://doi.org/10.4088/jcp.v64n0214. PMID: 12633130.
66. Abu, H. H., Tohid, H., Mohd, A. R., Long, B.M. B., Muthupalaniappen, L., Omar, K., et al. (2013) Factors influencing insulin acceptance among type 2 diabetes mellitus patients in a primary care clinic: A qualitative exploration. *BMC Fam Pract*. 2013;14:164.
67. Foa, E. B. (2010). Cognitive behavioral therapy of obsessive-compulsive disorder. *Dialogues Clin Neurosci*, 12(2), 199–207. https://doi.org/10.31887/DCNS.2010.12.2/efoa. PMID: 20623924; PMCID: PMC3181959.
68. Aguglia, A., Signorelli, M. S., Albert, U., et al. (2018). The impact of general medical conditions in obsessive-compulsive disorder. *Psychiatry Investig*, 15, 246–253. https://doi.org/10.30773/pi.2017.06.17.2
69. Meier, S. M., Mattheisen, M., Mors, O., et al (2016). Mortality among persons with obsessive-compulsive disorder in Denmark. *JAMA Psychiatry*, 73, 268–274. https://doi.org/10.1001/jamapsychiatry.2015.310
70. Papola, D., Ostuzzi, G., Tedeschi, F., et al. (2023). CBT treatment delivery formats for panic disorder: A systematic review and network meta-analysis of randomised controlled trials. *Psychol Med*, 53(3), 614–624. https://doi.org/10.1017/S0033291722003683. Epub 2022 Dec 9. PMID: 37132646; PMCID: PMC9975966.
71. Cackovic, C., Nazir, S., & Marwaha, R. (2025). *Panic disorder*. StatPearls Publishing. Available from https://www.ncbi.nlm.nih.gov/books/NBK430973/

72. Health Quality Ontario. (2017). Psychotherapy for major depressive disorder and generalized anxiety disorder: A health technology assessment. Ont Health Technol Assess Ser, 17(15), 1–167. PMID: 29213344; PMCID: PMC5709536.
73. Sareen, J., Cox, B. J., Clara, I., & Asmundson, G. J. (2005). The relationship between anxiety disorders and physical disorders in the U. S. National Comorbidity Survey. *Depress Anxiety*, 21(4), 193–202. https://doi.org/10.1002/da.20072. PMID: 16075453.
74. Hinz, A., Herzberg, P. Y., Lordick, F., et al. (2019). Age and gender differences in anxiety and depression in cancer patients compared with the general population. *Eur J Cancer Care (Engl)*, 28(5), e13129. https://doi.org/10.1111/ecc.13129. Epub 2019 Jul 9. PMID: 31290218.
75. Naser, A. Y., Hameed, A. N., Mustafa, N., Alwafi, H., Dahmash, E. Z., Alyami, H. S., & Khalil, H. (2021). Depression and anxiety in patients with cancer: A cross-sectional study. *Front Psychol*, 12, 585534. https://doi.org/10.3389/fpsyg.2021.585534. PMID: 33935849; PMCID: PMC8081978.
76. DiMatteo, M. R., Lepper, H. S., & Croghan, T. W. (2000). Depression is a risk factor for noncompliance with medical treatment: Meta-analysis of the effects of anxiety and depression on patient adherence. *Arch Intern Med*, 160(14), 2101–2107. https://doi.org/10.1001/archinte.160.14.2101. PMID: 10904452.
77. BPS. (2017). *Position statement: Understanding and preventing suicide: A psychological perspective*.
78. Hersche, R., Roser, K., Weise, A., Michel, G., & Barbero, M. (2022). Fatigue self-management education in persons with disease-related fatigue: A comprehensive review of the effectiveness on fatigue and quality of life, *Patient Education and Counseling*, 105(6), 1362–1378. https://doi.org/10.1016/j.pec.2021.09.016
79. NICE. (2016). NICE guideline, Babies, children and young people's experience of healthcare, Published: 25 August 2021.
80. Steffens, N. M., Tucholka, J. L., Nabozny, M. J., Schmick, A. E., Brasel, K. J., & Schwarze, M. L. (2016). Engaging patients, health care professionals, and community members to improve preoperative decision making for older adults facing high-risk surgery. *JAMA Surg*, 151(10), 938–945. https://doi.org/10.1001/jamasurg.2016.1308. PMID: 27368074; PMCID: PMC5071104.

7. Chapter 4

1. Nightingale, F. (1858). *Notes on nursing: What it is, and what it is not*. Appleton and Company.
2. The Guardian. (2024, January 3). https://www.theguardian.com/uk-news/2024/jan/03/childrens-ideas-help-transform-glasgow-hospital-unit-murals
3. Burger, P., Van den Ende, E. S., Lukman, W., et al. (2022). Sleep in hospitalized pediatric and adult patients: A systematic review and meta-analysis. *Sleep Medicine*, 4, 100059. https://doi.org/10.1016/j.sleepx.2022.100059
4. Tronstad, O., Patterson, S., Zangerl, B., et al. (2024). The introduction of a sound reduction bundle in the intensive care unit and its impact on sound levels and patients. *Aust Crit Care*, 37(5), 716–726. https://doi.org/10.1016/j.aucc.2024.02.011. Epub 2024 Apr 11. PMID: 38604917.
5. Jagriti, P., Manish, T., Rajni, P., & Divya, S. (2022). Noise pollution in intensive care unit: A hidden enemy affecting the physical and mental health of patients and caregivers. *Noise and Health*, 24(114), 130–136. https://doi.org/10.4103/nah.nah_79_21
6. Jagriti, P., Manish, T., Rajni, P., & Divya, S. (2022). Noise pollution in intensive care unit: A hidden enemy affecting the physical and mental health of patients and caregivers. *Noise and Health*, 24(114), 130–136. https://doi.org/10.4103/nah.nah_79_21

7. Jongerden, I. P., Slooter, A. J., Peelen, L. M., et al. (2013). Effect of intensive care environment on family and patient satisfaction: A before–after study. *Intensive Care Med, 39*, 1626–1634. https://doi.org/10.1007/s00134-013-2966-0
8. Livecchi, T., & Morton, L. (2023). *Healing hearts and minds: A holistic approach to coping well with congenital heart disease.* Oxford University Press.
9. Hertenstein, M. J., Keltner, D., App, B., Bulleit, B. A., & Jaskolka, A. R. (2006). Touch communicates distinct emotions. *Emotion, 6*(3), 528–533. https://doi.org/10.1037/1528-3542.6.3.528. PMID: 16938094.
10. Field, T. M., Diego, M., & Hernandez-Reif, M. (2010). Preterm infant massage therapy research: A review. *Infant Behavioral Development, 33*(2), 115–124.
11. Bliss for babies born premature or sick (2023). *Locked out: The impact of COVID-19 on neonatal care.*
12. Wilson, E. O. (1984). *Biophilia.* Harvard University Press.
13. Weerasuriya, R., Henderson-Wilson, C., & Townsend, M. (2019). A systematic review of access to green spaces in healthcare facilities. *Urban Forestry and Urban Greening, 40*, 125–132. https://doi.org/10.1016/j.ufug.2018.06.019
14. iSupport Team. (2021). Getting it right first time and every time: Re-thinking children's rights when they have a clinical procedure. *Journal of Pediatric Nursing, 61*, A10–A12. https://doi.org/10.1016/j.pedn.2021.11.017
15. Morton, L., Cogan, N., Kornfält, S., Porter, Z., & Georgiadis, E. (2020). Baring all: The impact of the hospital gown on patient wellbeing. *British Journal of Health Psychology, 25*(3), 452–473.
16. Cogan, N., Morton, L., Georgiadis, E., Butler, S. H., Fleck, V. J., & Johnstone, J. (2024). Exploring the perspectives of healthcare professionals concerning the use and utility of the hospital gown to develop theoretically informed behaviour change interventions. *Public Health Open Access, 8*(1).
17. Kanejima, Y., Shimogai, T., Kitamura, M., Ishihara, K., Izawa, K. P. (2020). Effect of early mobilization on physical function in patients after cardiac surgery: A systematic review and meta-analysis. *International Journal of Environmental Research and Public Health, 17*(19):7091. https://doi.org/10.3390/ijerph17197091
18. Cogan, N., Morton, L., Georgiadis, E., Butler, S. H., Fleck, V. J., & Johnstone, J. (2024). Exploring the perspectives of healthcare professionals concerning the use and utility of the hospital gown to develop theoretically informed behaviour change interventions. *Public Health Open Access, 8*(1).
19. Doherty, M., McCowan, S., & Shaw, S. C. (2023). Autistic SPACE: A novel framework for meeting the needs of autistic people in healthcare settings. *Br J Hosp Med (Lond), 84*(4), 1–9. https://doi.org/10.12968/hmed.2023.0006. Epub 2023 Apr 17. PMID: 37127416.
20. Hirvikoski, T., Mittendorfer-Rutz, E., Boman, M., et al. (2016). Premature mortality in autism spectrum disorder. *Br J Psychiatry, 208*(3), 232–238. https://doi.org/10.1192/bjp.bp.114.160192
21. Doherty, M., McCowan, S., & Shaw, S. C. (2023). Autistic SPACE: A novel framework for meeting the needs of autistic people in healthcare settings. *Br J Hosp Med (Lond), 84*(4), 1–9. https://doi.org/10.12968/hmed.2023.0006. Epub 2023 Apr 17. PMID: 37127416.
22. Doherty, M., McCowan, S., & Shaw, S. C. (2023). Autistic SPACE: A novel framework for meeting the needs of autistic people in healthcare settings. *Br J Hosp Med (Lond), 84*(4), 1–9. https://doi.org/10.12968/hmed.2023.0006. Epub 2023 Apr 17. PMID: 37127416.
23. Doherty, M., McCowan, S., & Shaw, S. C. (2023). Autistic SPACE: A novel framework for meeting the needs of autistic people in healthcare settings. *Br J Hosp Med (Lond), 84*(4), 1–9. https://doi.org/10.12968/hmed.2023.0006. Epub 2023 Apr 17. PMID: 37127416.
24. Huddlestone, P. (2012). *Prepare for surgery, heal faster: A guide of mind–body techniques* (4th ed.). Angel River Press.

25. National Guideline Centre (UK). (2021). *Evidence review for pain management programmes for chronic pain (chronic primary pain and chronic secondary pain), chronic pain (primary and secondary) in over 16s: Assessment of all chronic pain and management of chronic primary pain: Evidence review C.* National Institute for Health and Care Excellence (NICE); Apr. (NICE Guideline, No. 193.). Available from https://www.ncbi.nlm.nih.gov/books/NBK569980/
26. Bray, L., Carter, B., & Snodin, J. (2016). Holding children for clinical procedures: Perseverance in spite of or persevering to be child-centered. *Res Nurs Health*, 39, 30–41. https://doi.org/10.1002/nur.21700
27. United Nations Convention on the Rights of the Child, November 20, 1989, https://www.unicef.org.au/united-nations-convention-on-the-rights-of-the-child
28. Bray, L., Carter, B., Kiernan, J., et al. (2023). Developing rights-based standards for children having tests, treatments, examinations and interventions: Using a collaborative, multi-phased, multi-method and multi-stakeholder approach to build consensus. *European Journal of Pediatrics*, 182(10), 4707–4721. https://doi.org/10.1007/s00431-023-05131-9
29. iSupport Team. (2021). Getting it right first time and every time: Re-thinking children's rights when they have a clinical procedure. *Journal of Pediatric Nursing*, 61, A10–A12. https://doi.org/10.1016/j.pedn.2021.11.017
30. Bray, L., Carter, B., & Snodin, J. (2016). Holding children for clinical procedures: Perseverance in spite of or persevering to be child-centered. *Res Nurs Health*, 39, 30–41. https://doi.org/10.1002/nur.21700
31. Brenner, M. (2013). A need to protect: Parents' experiences of the practice of restricting a child for a clinical procedure in hospital. *Issues in Comprehensive Pediatric Nursing*, 36, 1–2,5–16, https://doi.org/10.3109/01460862.2013.768312
32. UCSF. (2024). *The comfort promise: Preventing needle pain.* UCSF Benioff Children's Hospitals.
33. Campbell-Yeo, M., Eriksson, M., & Benoit, B. (2022). Assessment and management of pain in preterm infants: A practice update. *Children (Basel)*, 9(2), 244. https://doi.org/10.3390/children9020244. PMID: 35204964; PMCID: PMC8869922.
34. Campbell-Yeo, M., Eriksson, M., & Benoit, B. (2022). Assessment and management of pain in preterm infants: A practice update. *Children (Basel)*, 9(2), 244. https://doi.org/10.3390/children9020244. PMID: 35204964; PMCID: PMC8869922.
35. Leroy, P. L., Costa, L. R., Emmanouil, D., van Beukering, A., & Franck, L. S. (2016). Beyond the drugs: Nonpharmacologic strategies to optimize procedural care in children. *Curr Opin Anaesthesiol*, 29(Suppl 1), S1–13. https://doi.org/10.1097/ACO.0000000000000312. PMID: 26926330.
36. Jolly, J. (1981). *The other side of paediatrics: A guide to the everyday care of sick children.* Macmillan.
37. Carus, E. G., Albayrak, N., Bildirici, H. M., et al. (2022). Immersive virtual reality on childbirth experience for women: A randomized controlled trial. *BMC Pregnancy Childbirth*, 22, 354. https://doi.org/10.1186/s12884-022-04598-y
38. Marsac, L., Azale, M., & Dahmani, S. (2019). Evaluation of a virtual reality headset in the prevention of intraoperative anxiety in children. *61st Congress of the French Society of Anaesthesia and Intensive Care*, September 19–21.
39. Assaker, R., Azale, M., Nesa, C., Julien-Marsollier, F., & Dahmani, S. (2021). Effectiveness of virtual reality in reducing anxiety and pain during paediatric idiopathic scoliosis surgery. *63rd Congress of the French Society of Anaesthesia and Intensive Care*, September 23–25, 2021.

40. The Christie, NHS Foundation Trust. (2024). *The Christie is the first hospital in the UK to use VR distraction therapy for children having radiotherapy*. Press release posted June 17, 2024.
41. Czech, O., Wrzeciono, A., Rutkowska, A., Guzik, A., Kiper, P., & Rutkowski, S. (2021). Virtual reality interventions for needle-related procedural pain, fear and anxiety: A systematic review and meta-analysis. *J Clin Med, 10*(15), 3248. https://doi.org/10.3390/jcm10153248. PMID: 34362032; PMCID: PMC8347054.
42. Nightingale, F. (1858). *Notes on nursing: What it is, and what it is not*. Appleton and Company.
43. Filippa, M., Nardelli, M., Della Casa, E., et al. (2022). Maternal singing but not speech enhances vagal activity in preterm infants during hospitalization: Preliminary results. *Children (Basel), 9*(2), 140. https://doi.org/10.3390/children9020140. PMID: 35204861; PMCID: PMC8869818.
44. Loewy, J., Stewart, K., Dassler, A. M., Telsey, A., & Homel, P. (2013). The effects of music therapy on vital signs, feeding, and sleep in premature infants. *Pediatrics, 131*(5), 902–918. https://doi.org/10.1542/peds.2012-1367. Epub 2013 Apr 15. PMID: 23589814.
45. Hole, J., Hirsch, M., Ball, E., Meads, C. (2015) Music as an aid for postoperative recovery in adults: a systematic review and meta-analysis. *Lancet, 386*(10004):1659–1671. doi: 10.1016/S0140-6736(15)60169-6. Epub 2015 Aug 12. Erratum in: Lancet. 2015 Oct 24;386(10004):1630. doi: 10.1016/S0140-6736(15)61181-3. PMID: 26277246.
46. Harper, F. W. K., Heath, A. S., Moore, T. F., Kim, S., & Heath, E. I. (2023). Using music as a tool for distress reduction during cancer chemotherapy treatment. *JCO Oncol Pract, 19*(12), 1133–1142. https://doi.org/10.1200/OP.22.00814. Epub 2023 Jul 11. PMID: 37433094; PMCID: PMC10732503.
47. Porges, S. W., & Furman, S. A. (2011). The early development of the autonomic nervous system provides a neural platform for social behavior: A polyvagal perspective. *Infant and Child Development, 20*, 106–118. https://doi.org/10.1002/icd.688
48. Sanders, M. (2019). Stärkung des Sicherheitsschaltkreises: Anwendung der Polyvagal-Theorie auf die Arbeit in einer Intensivstation für Neugeborene (NICU). In S. W. Porges, D. Dana, & T. Kierdorf (Eds.), *Klinische Anwendungen der Polyvagal-Theorie: Ein neues Verständnis des Autonomen Nervensystems und seiner Anwendung in der therapeutischen Praxis* (pp. 389–406). Probst.
49. Stakemann, R., & Jordan, A.-K. (2021). Erkenntnisse aus der Polyvagal-Theorie und ihre Relevanz für die Musiktherapie mit Frühgeborenen. *Musiktherapeutische Umschau 42*(4), 376–386.
50. Loewy, J., Stewart, K., Dassler, A. M., Telsey, A., & Homel, P. (2013). The effects of music therapy on vital signs, feeding, and sleep in premature infants. *Pediatrics, 131*(5), 902–918. https://doi.org/10.1542/peds.2012-1367. Epub 2013 Apr 15. PMID: 23589814.
51. Haslbeck, F., et al. (2017). "Musik von Anfang an": Referenzrahmen zur Anwendung von Musiktherapie in der Neonatologie. http://www.musiktherapie.de/musiktherapie/arbeitsfelder/neonatologie.html
52. Stakemann, R., & Jordan, A.-K. (2021). Erkenntnisse aus der Polyvagal-Theorie und ihre Relevanz für die Musiktherapie mit Frühgeborenen. In: *Musiktherapeutische Umschau 42*(4), 376–386.
53. Haslbeck et al. (2020). Creative music therapy with premature infants and their parents: A mixed-method pilot study on parents' anxiety, stress and depressive symptoms and parent–infant attachment. *Environmental Research and Public Health, 18*(1), 1–18.
54. Nightingale, F. (1858). *Notes on nursing: What it is, and what it is not*. Appleton and Company.

55. Harper, C. M., Dong, Y., Thornhill, T. S., Wright, J., Ready, J., Brick, G. W., & Dyer, G. (2015). Can therapy dogs improve pain and satisfaction after total joint arthroplasty? A randomized controlled trial. *Clin Orthop Relat Res, 473*(1), 372–379. https://doi.org/10.1007/s11999-014-3931-0. Epub 2014 Sep 9. PMID: 25201095; PMCID: PMC4390934.
56. Hinic, K., Kowalski, M. O., Holtzman, K., & Mobus, K. (2019). The effect of a pet therapy and comparison intervention on anxiety in hospitalized children. *J Pediatr Nurs, 46*:55–61. https://doi.org/10.1016/j.pedn.2019.03.003. Epub 2019 Mar 7. PMID: 30852256.
57. Vaartio-Rajalin, H., Santamäki-Fischer, R., Jokisalo, P., & Fagerström, L. (2020). Art making and expressive art therapy in adult health and nursing care: A scoping review. *Int J Nurs Sci, 8*(1), 102–119. https://doi.org/10.1016/j.ijnss.2020.09.011. PMID: 33575451; PMCID: PMC7859537.

8. Chapter 5

1. Restauri, N., & Sheridan, A. D. (2020). Burnout and posttraumatic stress disorder in the coronavirus disease (COVID-19) pandemic: Intersection, impact, and interventions. *J Am Coll Radiol, 17*(7), 921–926. https://doi.org/10.1016/j.jacr.2020.05.021. Epub 2020 May 27. PMID: 32479798; PMCID: PMC7250786.
2. Cogan, N., Kennedy, C., Beck, et al. (2022). ENACT study: What has helped health and social care workers maintain their mental wellbeing during the COVID-19 pandemic? Adaptive coping, team resilience, help-seeking behaviour and work based supports. *Health and Social Care in the Community, 30*(6), e6656–e6673. https://doi.org/10.1111/hsc.13992.
3. Peterson, U., Demerouti, E., Bergström, G., Samuelsson, M., Asberg, M., & Nygren, A. (2008). Burnout and physical and mental health among Swedish healthcare workers. *J Adv Nurs, 62*(1), 84–95. https://doi.org/10.1111/j.1365-2648.2007.04580.x. PMID: 18352967.
4. Figley, C. R. (1995). Compassion fatigue: Toward a new understanding of the costs of caring. In B. H. Stamm (Ed.), *Secondary traumatic stress: Self-care issues for clinicians, researchers, and educators* (pp. 3–28). Sidran Press.
5. Rothschild, B. (2005). *Help for the helper: The psychophysiology of compassion fatigue and vicarious trauma.* WW Norton.
6. Pirelli, G., Formon, D. L., & Maloney, K. (2020). Preventing vicarious trauma (VT), compassion fatigue (CF), and burnout (BO) in forensic mental health: Forensic psychology as exemplar. *Professional Psychology: Research and Practice, 51*(5), 454–466. Advance online publication. http://dx.doi.org/10.1037/pro000029
7. Figley, C. R. (1995). Compassion fatigue: Toward a new understanding of the costs of caring. In B. H. Stamm (Ed.), Secondary traumatic stress: Self-care issues for clinicians, researchers, and educators (pp. 3–28). Sidran Press.
8. Pirelli, G., Formon, D. L., & Maloney, K. (2020). Preventing vicarious trauma (VT), compassion fatigue (CF), and burnout (BO) in forensic mental health: Forensic psychology as exemplar. *Professional Psychology: Research and Practice, 51*(5), 454–466. Advance online publication. http://dx.doi.org/10.1037/pro000029
9. Pirelli, G., Formon, D. L., & Maloney, K. (2020). Preventing vicarious trauma (VT), compassion fatigue (CF), and burnout (BO) in forensic mental health: Forensic psychology as exemplar. *Professional Psychology: Research and Practice, 51*(5), 454–466. Advance online publication. http://dx.doi.org/10.1037/pro000029
10. Cogan, N., Kennedy, C., Beck, et al. (2022). ENACT study: What has helped health and social care workers maintain their mental wellbeing during the COVID-19 pandemic? Adaptive coping, team resilience, help-seeking behaviour and work based supports.

Health and Social Care in the Community, 30(6), e6656–e6673. https://doi.org/10.1111/hsc.13992.
11. Riley, R., Kokab, F., Buszewicz, M., et al. (2021). Protective factors and sources of support in the workplace as experienced by UK foundation and junior doctors: A qualitative study. *BMJ Open, 11*(6), e045588. https://doi.org/10.1136/bmjopen-2020-045588. PMID: 34162643; PMCID: PMC8231035.Kimet al, 2020
12. Delgado, C., Roche, M., Fethney, J., & Foster, K. (2021), Mental health nurses' psychological well-being, mental distress, and workplace resilience: A cross-sectional survey. *Int J Mental Health Nurs, 30*, 1234–1247. https://doi.org/10.1111/inm.12874
13. Restauri, N., & Sheridan, A. D. (2020). Burnout and posttraumatic stress disorder in the coronavirus disease (COVID-19) pandemic: Intersection, impact, and interventions. *J Am Coll Radiol, 17*(7), 921–926. https://doi.org/10.1016/j.jacr.2020.05.021. Epub 2020 May 27. PMID: 32479798; PMCID: PMC7250786.
14. Polle, E., & Gair, J. (2021). Mindfulness-based stress reduction for medical students: A narrative review. *Canadian Medical Education Journal, 12*(2), 74–80. www.erudit.org/en/journals/cmej/1900-v1-n1-cmej06034/1077196ar/abstract/; https://doi.org/10.36834/cmej.68406. Accessed April 2, 2023.
15. Otto, M. C. B., Van Ruysseveldt, J., Hoefsmit, N., & Dam, K. V. (2020). The development of a proactive burnout prevention inventory: How employees can contribute to reduce burnout risks. *Int J Environ Res Public Health, 17*(5), 1711. https://doi.org/10.3390/ijerph17051711. PMID: 32151047; PMCID: PMC7084396.
16. Mohammadi, F., Naderi, Z., Nikrouz, L., Oshvandi, K., Masoumi, S. Z., Sabetsarvestani, P., & Bijani, M. (2024). Ethical challenges as perceived by nurses in pediatric oncology units. *Nursing Ethics, 31*(2–3), 268–280.
17. Dietl, J. E., Derksen, C., Keller, F. M., & Lippke, S. (2023). Interdisciplinary and interprofessional communication intervention: How psychological safety fosters communication and increases patient safety. *Frontiers in Psychology, 14*, 1164288.
18. Hoegh, J., Rice, G., Shetty, S., Ure, A., Cogan, N., & Peddie, N. (2024). Health and social care professionals' experience of psychological safety within their occupational setting: A thematic synthesis scoping review protocol. *COJ Nursing and Healthcare, 8*(5), 915–920.
19. Lackie, K., Hayward, K., Ayn, C., et al. (2023). Creating psychological safety in interprofessional simulation for health professional learners: A scoping review of the barriers and enablers. *Journal of Interprofessional Care, 37*(2), 187–202.
20. West, M. A. (2019). Compassionate leadership in health and care settings. In L. Galiana & N. Sansó (Eds.), *The power of compassion* (pp. 317–338). Nova Science Publishers.
21. West, M. A. (2019). Compassionate leadership in health and care settings. In L. Galiana & N. Sansó (Eds.), *The power of compassion* (pp. 317–338). Nova Science Publishers.
22. Atkins, P., & Parker, S. (2012). Understanding individual compassion in organizations: The role of appraisals and psychological flexibility. *Academy of Management Review, 37*, 524–546. 10.5465/amr.2010.0490.
23. West, M. A. (2021). *Compassionate Leadership: Sustaining Wisdom, Humanity and Presence in Health and Social Care*. The Swirling Leaf Press.

9. Chapter 6

1. Tucker, C. M., Marsiske, M., & Rice, K. G. (2011). Patient-centered culturally sensitive health care: Model testing and refinement. *Health Psychology, 30*, 342–350. https://doi.org/10.1037/a0022967.
2. Herman, K. C., Tucker, C. M., Ferdinand, L. A., Mirsu-Paun, A., Hasan, N. T., & Beato, C. (2007). Culturally sensitive health care and counseling psychology: An overview. *Counseling Psychologist, 3*, 633–649.

3. Herman, K. C., Tucker, C. M., Ferdinand, L. A., Mirsu-Paun, A., Hasan, N. T., & Beato, C. (2007). Culturally sensitive health care and counseling psychology: An overview. *Counseling Psychologist, 3*, 633–649.
4. Campinha-Bacote, J. (2002). The process of cultural competence in the delivery of healthcare services: A model of care. *Journal of Transcultural Nursing, 13*(3), 181–184.
5. Greenman, P. S., & Johnson, S. M. (2022). Emotionally focused therapy: Attachment, connection, and health. *Curr Opin Psychol, 43*, 146–150. https://doi.org/10.1016/j.copsyc.2021.06.015. Epub 2021 Jun 30. PMID: 34375935.
6. Steptoe, A., & Zaninotto, P. (2020). Lower socioeconomic status and the acceleration of aging: An outcome-wide analysis. *Proc Natl Acad Sci USA, 117*(26), 14911–14917, https://doi.org/10.1073/pnas.1915741117.
7. Dale, L. P., Cuffe, S. P., Kolacz, J., et al. (2022). Increased autonomic reactivity and mental health difficulties in COVID-19 survivors: Implications for medical providers. *Front Psychiatry, 13*, 830926. https://doi.org/10.3389/fpsyt.2022.830926. PMID: 35693957; PMCID: PMC9174530.
8. Bogart, K. R. (2020). *How Disability pride fights ableism: Reflections on the 30th anniversary of the Americans with Disabilities Act*. Accessed 10th August 2020, https://www.psychologytoday.com/gb/blog/disability-is-diversity/202008/how-disability-pride-fights-ableism?msockid=156833b14c57639026e926674d2d6282.
9. Rowe, M. (2015). *Citizenship and mental health*. Oxford University Press.
10. Crenshaw, K. W., Gotanda, N., Peller, G., & Thomas, K. (1995). *Critical race theory: The key writings that formed the movement* (p. 101). Faculty Books.
11. Baumeister, A., Chakraverty, D., Aldin, A., et al. (2021). "The system has to be health literate, too": Perspectives among healthcare professionals on health literacy in transcultural treatment settings. *BMC Health Serv Res, 21*, 716. https://doi.org/10.1186/s12913-021-06614-x
12. Gerhards, S. M., Schweda, M., & WeBel, M. (2023). Medical students' perspectives on racism in medicine and healthcare in Germany: Identified problems and learning needs for medical education, *GMS J Med Educ, 40*(2), Doc22.
13. National Institute for Health and Care Research. (n.d.). *Improving how we work with patients, carers and the public. NIHR strategic commitments for public partnerships 2025–2030*. Available from: https://www.nihr.ac.uk/about-us/what-we-do/Improving-how-we-work-with-patients-carers-and-the-public.htm. Accessed March 2024.
14. Holland, E., Matthews, K., Macdonald, S., et al. (2024). The impact of living with multiple long-term conditions (multimorbidity) on everyday life: A qualitative evidence synthesis. *BMC Public Health 24*, 3446. https://doi.org/10.1186/s12889-024-20763-8
15. Cleghorn, E. (2021). *Unwell women: A journey through medicine and myth in a man-made world*. Weidenfield & Nicolson.
16. Young, K., Fisher, J., & Kirkman, M. (2018). "Do mad people get endo or does endo make you mad?": Clinicians' discursive constructions of Medicine and women with endometriosis. *Feminism & Psychology, 29*(3), 337–356. https://doi.org/10.1177/0959353518815704 (Original work published 2019)
17. Schäfer, G., Prkachin, K. M., Kaseweter, K. A., & Williams, A. C. (2016). Health care providers' judgments in chronic pain: The influence of gender and trustworthiness. *PAIN, 157*(8), 1618–1625. https://doi.org/10.1097/j.pain.0000000000000536
18. Barth, C., Crestol, A., de Lange, A. M. G., & Galea, L. A. M. (2023). Sex steroids and the female brain across the lifespan: Insights into risk of depression and Alzheimer's disease. *The Lancet Diabetes and Endocrinology, 11*(12), 926–941.https://doi.org/10.1016/S2213-8587(23)00224-3

19. Nemiroff, L. (2022). We can do better: Addressing ageism against older adults in healthcare. *Healthcare Management Forum*, 35(2), 118–122. https://doi.org/10.1177/08404704221080882
20. de la Fuente-Núñez, V., Cohn-Schwartz, E., Roy, S., Ayalon, L. (2021). Scoping Review on Ageism against Younger Populations. *Int J Environ Res Public Health*, 18(8), 3988. doi: 10.3390/ijerph18083988. PMID: 33920114; PMCID: PMC8069403.
21. Morton, L. (2020). Using psychologically informed care to improve mental health and wellbeing for people living with a heart condition from birth: A statement paper. *Journal of Health Psychology*, 25(2), 197–206. https://doi.org/10.1177/1359105319826354
22. Howell, M., & Ford, P. (1992) [1980]. *The true history of the Elephant Man* (3rd ed.). Penguin Books.
23. Nair, A. (2020). *Public health campaigns and the "threat" of disability*. Welcome Collection.
24. Evans, S. E. (2004). *Forgotten crimes: The Holocaust and people with disabilities*. Ivan R. Dee.
25. Allport, G. W. (1954). *The nature of prejudice*. Addison-Wesley.
26. Earnshaw, V. A., & Quinn, D. M. (2012). The impact of stigma in healthcare on people living with chronic illnesses. *J Health Psychol*, 17(2), 157–168. https://doi.org/10.1177/1359105311414952. Epub 2011 Jul 28. PMID: 21799078; PMCID: PMC8919040
27. Mahajan, A. P., Sayles, J. N., Patel, V. A., et al. (2008). Stigma in the HIV/AIDS epidemic: A review of the literature and recommendations for the way forward. *AIDS*, 22(Suppl 2), S67–79. https://doi.org/10.1097/01.aids.0000327438.13291.62. PMID: 18641472; PMCID: PMC2835402.
28. Sayles, J. N., Ryan, G. W., Silver, J. S., Sarkisian, C. A., & Cunningham, W. E. (2007). Experiences of social stigma and implications for healthcare among a diverse population of HIV positive adults. *Journal of Urban Health*, 84(6), 814–828.
29. Quinn, D. M., & Chaudoir, S. R. (2009). Living with a concealable stigmatized identity: The impact of anticipated stigma, centrality, salience, and cultural stigma on psychological distress and health. *Journal of Personality and Social Psychology*, 97(4), 634–651.
30. Albrecht, G. L., & Devlieger, P. J. (1999). The disability paradox: High quality of life against all odds. *Soc Sci Med*, 48(8), 977–988. https://doi.org/10.1016/s0277-9536(98)00411-0. PMID: 10390038.
31. Office of National Statistics, United Kingdom. (2020). *Household income inequality, UK: Financial year ending 2021*.
32. Inclusive Futures. (2021). *A disability-inclusive response to COVID-19*. Inclusive-Futures-COVID-learnings.pdf (inclusivefutures.org).
33. Morton, L., Calderwood, C., Cogan, N., Murphy, C., Nix, E., & Kolacz, J. (2021). An exploration of psychological trauma and positive adaptation in adults with congenital heart disease during the COVID-19 pandemic. *Journal of Patient Experience*, 9(1), 82–94.
34. Morton, L., Calderwood, C., Cogan, N., Murphy, C., Nix, E., & Kolacz, J. (2021). An exploration of psychological trauma and positive adaptation in adults with congenital heart disease during the COVID-19 pandemic. *Journal of Patient Experience*, 9(1), 82–94.
35. Guggenbühl-Craig, A. (1998). *Power in the helping profession*. Spring.
36. Alzyoud, F. A., McCurry, M. K., & Hunter Revell, S. M. (2023). Patient abuse in healthcare: A theoretical synthesis. *Nursing Science Quarterly*, 36(1), 70–77. https://doi.org/10.1177/08943184221131969
37. Vedam S., Stoll K., Taiwo T. K., et al. (2019). The giving voice to mother's study: Inequity and mistreatment during pregnancy and childbirth in the United States. *Reproductive Health*, 16(1), 77. https://doi.org/10.1186/s12978-019-0729-2

38. Swahnberg K., Hearn J., & Wijma B. (2009). Prevalence of perceived experiences of emotional, physical, sexual, and health care abuse in a Swedish male patient sample. *Violence and Victims, 24*(2), 265–279. https://doi.org/10.1891/0886-6708.24.2.265
39. Alzyoud F., Khoshnood K., Alnatour A., & Oweis A. (2018). Exposure to verbal abuse and neglect during childbirth among Jordanian women. *Midwifery, 58*, 71–76. https://doi.org/10.1016/j.midw.2017.12.008
40. Johnstone, A., & Dent, C. (2015). *Investigation into the association of Jimmy Savile with Stoke Mandeville Hospital (The Stoke Mandeville Report)*. A Report for Buckinghamshire Healthcare NHS Trust.
41. British Medical Journal. (2023). Sexual safety incidents in the NHS: Results of a joint investigation by the BMJ and the Guardian. *British Medical Journal, 381*, 1105.
42. American Medical Association. (2021). *Organizational Strategic Plan to Embed Racial Justice and Advance Health Equity, 2021–2023* (pp. 5–6). American Medical Association. https://www.ama-assn.org/system/files/2021-05/ama-equity-strategic-plan.pdf
43. Zimmerman, M. S., et al. (2017). Global, regional, and national burden of congenital heart disease, 1990–2017: A systematic analysis for the Global Burden of Disease Study. *The Lancet Child and Adolescent Health*, Volume 4, Issue 3, 185–200.
44. "A Win for Patient Involvement: Congenital Heart Disease Standards in Scotland"—Health and Social Care Alliance Scotland (alliance-scotland.org.uk). https://www.alliance-scotland.org.uk/blog/opinion/a-win-for-patient-involvement-congenital-heart-disease-standards-in-scotland/
45. Royal College of Nursing, Scotland. (2024). *Once upon a time exhibition*.
46. Robertson, J. (1970). *Young children in hospital* (2nd ed.). Tavistock Publications.
47. Tucker, C. M., Roncoroni, J., Marsiske, M., Nghiem, K. N., & Wall, W. (2014). Validation of a patient-centered, culturally sensitive, clinic environment inventory using a national sample of adult patients. *J Transcult Nurs, 25*(1), 80–86. https://doi.org/10.1177/1043659613504111. Epub 2013 Oct 15. PMID: 24129544; PMCID: PMC4117241.
48. Rosen, L. T. (2021). Mapping out epistemic justice in the clinical space: Using narrative techniques to affirm patients as knowers. *Philosophy, Ethics, and Humanities in Medicine, 16*(1), 1–6.
49. Rosen, L. T. (2021). Mapping out epistemic justice in the clinical space: using narrative techniques to affirm patients as knowers. *Philosophy, Ethics, and Humanities in Medicine, 16*(1), 1–6.
50. Heggen, K. M., & Berg, H (2021). Epistemic injustice in the age of evidence-based practice: The case of fibromyalgia. *Humanit Soc Sci Commun 8*, 235. https://doi.org/10.1057/s41599-021-00918-3
51. National Institute for Health and Care Research. (n.d.). *Improving how we work with patients, carers and the public. NIHR strategic commitments for public partnerships 2025–2030*. Available from: https://www.nihr.ac.uk/about-us/what-we-do/Improving-how-we-work-with-patients-carers-and-the-public.htm. Accessed March 2024.
52. Holland, E., Matthews, K., Macdonald, S., et al. (2024). The impact of living with multiple long-term conditions (multimorbidity) on everyday life: a qualitative evidence synthesis. *BMC Public Health 24*, 3446. https://doi.org/10.1186/s12889-024-20763-8
53. Oliver, M. (1990). *The politics of disablement*. Macmillan Education.
54. Oliver, M. (2013). The social model of disability: Thirty years on. *Disability and Society, 28* (7), 1024–1026.
55. Burnham, J. (2012). Developments in social GRRRAAACCEEESSS: Visible-invisible and voiced-unvoiced. In I.-B. Krause (Ed.), *Culture and reflexivity in systemic psychotherapy: Mutual perspectives*. Karnac.

10. Chapter 7

1. BPS. (2017). *Position statement: Understanding and preventing suicide: A psychological perspective.* https://cms.bps.org.uk/sites/default/files/2022-06/Understanding%20and%20preventing%20suicide%20-%20a%20psychological%20perspective.pdf
2. Reeves, A. (2015). *Working with risk in counselling and psychotherapy.* SAGE.
3. Rogers, C. R. (1959). A theory of therapy, personality, and interpersonal relationships, as developed in the client-centered framework. *Psychology: A Study of a Science, 3,* 184–256.
4. Rogers, C. R. (1961). *On becoming a person.* Houghton Mifflin.
5. Hayes, S. C., Levin, M. E., Plumb-Vilardaga, J., Villatte, J. L., & Pistorello, J. (2013). Acceptance and commitment therapy and contextual behavioral science: Examining the progress of a distinctive model of behavioral and cognitive therapy. *Behav Ther, 44*(2), 180–198. https://doi.org/10.1016/j.beth.2009.08.002. Epub 2011 Jun 1. PMID: 23611068; PMCID: PMC3635495.
6. Hughes, L. S., Clark, J., Colclough, J. A., Dale, E., & McMillan, D (2017). Acceptance and commitment therapy (ACT) for chronic pain: A systematic review and meta-analyses. *The Clinical Journal of Pain, 33*(6), 552–568. https://doi.org/10.1097/AJP.0000000000000425
7. Palermo, T. M. (2009). Enhancing daily functioning with exposure and acceptance strategies: An important stride in the development of psychological therapies for pediatric chronic pain. *Pain, 141*(3), 189–190. https://doi.org/10.1016/j.pain.2008.12.012. Epub 2008 Dec 27. PMID: 19114294; PMCID: PMC2654190.
8. Fredrickson, B. L., Cohn, M. A., Coffey, K. A., Pek, J., & Finkel, S. M. (2008). Open hearts build lives: Positive emotions, induced through loving-kindness meditation, build consequential personal resources. *J Pers Soc Psychol, 95*(5), 1045–1062. https://doi.org/10.1037/a0013262. PMID: 18954193; PMCID: PMC3156028.
9. Segal, Z., Teasdale, J., & Williams, M. (2002). *Mindfulness-based cognitive therapy for depression.* Guilford Press.
10. Lucas, A. R., Klepin, H. D., Porges, S. W., & Rejeski, W. J. (2018). Mindfulness-based movement: A polyvagal perspective. *Integr Cancer Ther, 17*(1), 5–15. https://doi.org/10.1177/1534735416682087. Epub 2016 Dec 21. PMID: 28345362; PMCID: PMC5482784.
11. Ludwig, D. S., & Kabat-Zinn, J. (2008). Mindfulness in medicine. *JAMA, 300*(11), 1350–1352. https://doi.org/10.1001/jama.300.11.1350. PMID: 18799450.
12. Kabat-Zinn, J., Wheeler, E., Light, T., et al. (1998). Influence of a mindfulness meditation-based stress reduction intervention on rates of skin clearing in patients with moderate to severe psoriasis undergoing phototherapy (UVB) and photochemotherapy (PUVA). *Psychosom Med, 60*(5), 625–632. https://doi.org/10.1097/00006842-199809000-00020. PMID: 9773769.
13. Ehlers, A., & Wild, J. (2020). Cognitive therapy for PTSD. In L. F. Bufka, C. V. Wright, & R. W. Halfond (Eds.), *Casebook to the APA clinical practice guideline for the treatment of PTSD* (pp. 91–121). American Psychological Association. https://doi.org/10.1037/0000196-005
14. Foa, E. B., Hembree, E. A., & Rothbaum, B. O. (2019). *Prolonged exposure therapy for PTSD: Emotional processing of traumatic experiences, therapist guide* (2nd ed.). Oxford University Press.
15. Shapiro, F. (2014). The role of eye movement desensitization and reprocessing (EMDR) therapy in medicine: Addressing the psychological and physical symptoms stemming from adverse life experiences. *Perm J, 18*(1), 71–77. https://doi.org/10.7812/TPP/13-098. PMID: 24626074; PMCID: PMC3951033.

16. Corrigan, F., Fisher, J., & Nutt, D. (2011). Autonomic dysregulation and the window of tolerance model of the effects of complex emotional trauma. *Journal of Psychopharmacology, 25*(1), 17–25. https://doi.org/10.1177/0269881109354930
17. Ogden, P., Pain, C., & Fisher, J. (2006). A sensorimotor approach to the treatment of trauma and dissociation. *Psychiatric Clinics of North America, 29*(Issue 1), 263–279, https://doi.org/10.1016/j.psc.2005.10.012
18. Payne, P., Levine, P. A., & Crane-Godreau, M. A. (2015). Somatic experiencing: Using interoception and proprioception as core elements of trauma therapy. *Front Psychol, 6*, 93. https://doi.org/10.3389/fpsyg.2015.00093. Erratum in: *Front Psychol, 6*, 423. PMID: 25699005; PMCID: PMC4316402.
19. Dana, D., & Porges, S. W. (2018). *The polyvagal theory in therapy: Engaging the rhythm of regulation*. W. W. Norton & Company.
20. Sullivan, M. B., Erb, M., Schmalzl, L., Moonaz, S., Noggle, T J., & Porges, S. W. (2018). Yoga therapy and polyvagal theory: The convergence of traditional wisdom and contemporary neuroscience for self-regulation and resilience. *Front Hum Neurosci, 12*, 67. https://doi.org/10.3389/fnhum.2018.00067. PMID: 29535617; PMCID: PMC5835127.
21. Kaimal, G., Jones, J. P., Dieterich-Hartwell, R., & Wang, X. (2020). Long-term art therapy clinical interventions with military service members with traumatic brain injury and post-traumatic stress: Findings from a mixed methods program evaluation study. *Mil Psychol, 33*(1), 29–40. https://doi.org/10.1080/08995605.2020.1842639. PMCID: PMC10013461.
22. Hickman, B., Pourkazemi, F., Pebdani, R. N., Hiller, C. E., & Fong Yan, A. (2022). Dance for chronic pain conditions: A systematic review. *Pain Med, 23*(12), 2022–2041. https://doi.org/10.1093/pm/pnac092. PMID: 35736401; PMCID: PMC9714531.
23. Malpus, Z., Nazar, Z., Smith, C., & Armitage, L. (2023). Compassion focused therapy for pain management: "3 systems approach" to understanding why striving and self-criticism are key psychological barriers to regulating activity and improving self-care for people living with persistent pain. *British Journal of Pain, 17*(1), 87–102. https://doi.org/10.1177/20494637221133630
24. Au, T. M., Sauer-Zavala, S., King, M. W., Petrocchi, N., Barlow, .D. H., & Litz, B. T. (2017). Compassion-based therapy for trauma-related shame and posttraumatic stress: Initial evaluation using a multiple baseline design. *Behav Ther, 48*(2), 207–221. https://doi.org/10.1016/j.beth.2016.11.012. Epub 2016 Nov 29. PMID: 28270331.
25. Morton, L. (2011). Can interpersonal psychotherapy meet the psychological cost of life gifted by medical intervention? *Counselling Psychology Review, British Psychological Society, 26*, 3.
26. Greenman, P. S., & Johnson, S.M (2022). Emotionally focused therapy: Attachment, connection, and health. *Curr Opin Psychol, 43*, 146–150. https://doi.org/10.1016/j.copsyc.2021.06.015. Epub 2021 Jun 30. PMID: 34375935.
27. Yalom, I. D. (1980). *Existential psychotherapy*. Basic Books.
28. Conner, K. J., Acosta, V. M., Nouri, R., Tyler von Wrangel, M., Gramillo, E., & Conner, A. (2023). Psychotherapy experiences of U.S. adults with physical disabilities: Recommendations for affirmative practice. *The Counseling Psychologist, 51*(7), 970–1004. https://doi.org/10.1177/00110000231186824
29. Delgadillo, J. (2018). Worlds apart: Social inequalities and psychological care. *Couns. Psychother. Res., 18*, 111–113. https://doi.org/10.1002/capr.12168
30. Hall, G. C. N., Berkman, E. T., Zane, N. W., et al. (2021). Reducing mental health disparities by increasing the personal relevance of interventions. *Am Psychol, 76*, 91–103.
31. Khan, M. (2023). *Working within diversity: A reflective guide to anti-oppressive practice in counselling and psychotherapy*. Jessica Kingsley.

32. Khan, M. (2023). *Working within diversity: A reflective guide to anti-oppressive practice in counselling and psychotherapy*. Jessica Kingsley.
33. Huey, S. J., Jr., Park, A. L., Galán, C. A., & Wang, C. X. (2023). Culturally responsive cognitive behavioral therapy for ethnically diverse populations. *Annu Rev Clin Psychol, 19*, 51–78. https://doi.org/10.1146/annurev-clinpsy-080921-072750. Epub 2023 Feb 28. PMID: 36854287.
34. Hall, G. C. N., Berkman, E. T., Zane, N. W., et al. (2021). Reducing mental health disparities by increasing the personal relevance of interventions. *Am Psychol, 76*, 91–103.
35. McKenzie-Mavinga, I. (2016). *The challenge of racism in therapeutic practice: Engaging with oppression in practice and supervision*. Palgrave.
36. Hahm, H. C., Cook, B. L., Ault-Brutus, A., & Alegría, M. (2015). Intersection of race-ethnicity and gender in depression care: Screening, access, and minimally adequate treatment. *Psychiatric Services, 66*(3), 258–264. https://doi.org/10.1176/appi.ps.201400116
37. Steptoe, A., Zaninotto, P. (2020). Lower socioeconomic status and the acceleration of aging: An outcome-wide analysis, *Proc. Natl. Acad. Sci. U. S. A. 117* (26). 14911–14917, https://doi.org/10.1073/pnas.1915741117
38. Pickett, K., & Wilkinson, R. (2010). *The spirit level*. Penguin Books.
39. Meyer, I. H. (2003). Prejudice, social stress, and mental health in lesbian, gay, and bisexualpopulations: Conceptual issues and research evidence. *Psychological Bulletin, 129*(5), 674–697. https://doi.org/10.1037/0033-2909.129.5.674
40. Naeem, F., Phiri, P., Rathod, S., & Ayub, M. (2019). Cultural adaptation of cognitive-behavioural therapy. *BJPsych Advances, 25*(6), 387–395. https://doi.org/10.1192/bja.2019.15
41. Naeem, F., Phiri, P., Rathod, S., & Ayub, M. (2019). Cultural adaptation of cognitive-behavioural therapy. *BJPsych Advances, 25*(6), 387–395. https://doi.org/10.1192/bja.2019.15
42. Naeem, F., Phiri, P., Rathod, S., & Ayub, M. (2019). Cultural adaptation of cognitive-behavioural therapy. *BJPsych Advances, 25*(6), 387–395. https://doi.org/10.1192/bja.2019.15
43. Naeem, F., Phiri, P., Rathod, S., & Ayub, M. (2019). Cultural adaptation of cognitive-behavioural therapy. *BJPsych Advances, 25*(6), 387–395. https://doi.org/10.1192/bja.2019.15
44. Turner-Stokes, L., & Wade, D. T. (2020). Updated NICE guidance on chronic fatigue syndrome. *BMJ, 371*, m4774. https://doi.org/10.1136/bmj.m4774
45. Herman, J. L. (1998). Recovery from psychological trauma. *Psychiatry and Clinical Neurosciences, 52*, S98–S103. https://doi.org/10.1046/j.1440-1819.1998.0520s5S145.x
46. Herman, J. L. (1998). Recovery from psychological trauma. *Psychiatry and Clinical Neurosciences, 52*, S98–S103. https://doi.org/10.1046/j.1440-1819.1998.0520s5S145.x
47. Herman, J. L. (1998), Recovery from psychological trauma. *Psychiatry and Clinical Neurosciences, 52*, S98–S103. https://doi.org/10.1046/j.1440-1819.1998.0520s5S145.x
48. van der Kolk, B. A. (2014). *The body keeps the score: Brain, mind, and body in the healing of trauma*. Viking.
49. Lanius, R. A., Terpou, B. A., & McKinnon, M. C. (2020). The sense of self in the aftermath of trauma: Lessons from the default mode network in posttraumatic stress disorder. *European Journal of Psychotraumatology, 11*(1), Article 1807703. https://doi.org/10.1080/20008198.2020.1807703
50. Levine, P. A. (1997). *Waking the tiger: Healing trauma: The innate capacity to transform overwhelming experiences*. North Atlantic Books.

51. Ogden, P. (2015). *Trauma and the body: A sensorimotor approach to psychotherapy and sensorimotor psychotherapy: Interventions for trauma and attachment.* W. W. Norton.
52. Rothschild, B. (2000). *The body remembers: The psychophysiology of trauma and trauma treatment.* W. W. Norton & Company.
53. van der Kolk, B. A. (2014). *The body keeps the score: Brain, mind, and body in the healing of trauma.* Viking.
54. Motsan, S., Bar-Kalifa, E., Yirmiya, K., & Feldman, R. (2021). Physiological and social synchrony as markers of PTSD and resilience following chronic early trauma. *Depression and Anxiety, 38*(1), 89–99.
55. van der Kolk, B. A. (2014). *The body keeps the score: Brain, mind, and body in the healing of trauma.* Viking.
56. Porges, S. W. (2022). Polyvagal theory: A science of safety. *Front Integr Neurosci, 16*, 871227. https://doi.org/10.3389/fnint.2022.871227. PMID: 35645742; PMCID: PMC9131189.
57. Mair, H. (2020). Attachment safety in psychotherapy. *Counselling and Psychotherapy Research, 00*, 1–9.
58. van der Kolk, B. A. (2014). *The body keeps the score: Brain, mind, and body in the healing of trauma.* Viking.
59. Dana, D., & Porges, S. W. (2018). *The polyvagal theory in therapy: Engaging the rhythm of regulation.* W. W. Norton & Company.
60. Morton, L., Cogan, N., Kolacz, J., et al. (2022). A new measure of feeling safe: Developing psychometric properties of the Neuroception of Psychological Safety Scale (NPSS). *Psychological Trauma: Theory, Research, Practice, and Policy, 16*(4), 701–708. https://doi.org/10.1037/tra0001374
61. Cogan, N., Morton, L., Campbell, J., Irvine Fitzpatrick, L., Lamb, D., De Kock, J., Ali A., Young, D., Porges, S. (2025) Neuroception of psychological safety scale (NPSS): validation with a UK based adult community sample. *Eur J Psychotraumatol. 16*(1):2490329. https://doi.org/10.1080/20008066.2025.2490329
62. Poli, A., Cappellini, F., & Miccoli, M. (2023). The integrative process promoted by EMDR in dissociative disorders: Neurobiological mechanisms, psychometric tools, and intervention efficacy on the psychological impact of the COVID-19 pandemic. *Front Psychol, 14*, 1164527.
63. Goodman, M. L., Seidel, S. E., Springer, A., Elliott, A., Markham, C., & Serag, H. (2023). Enabling structural resilience of street-involved children and youth in Kenya: Reintegration outcomes and the flourishing community model. *Front Psychol, 14*, 1175593.
64. Bandeira, M., Graham, M. A., & Ebersöhn, L. (2023). The significance of feeling safe for resilience of adolescents in sub-Saharan Africa. *Front Psychol, 14*, 1183748.
65. Leconstant, C., & Spitz, E. (2022). Integrative model of human-animal interactions: A one health–one welfare systemic approach to studying HAI. *Front Vet Sci, 9*, 656833.50.
66. Poli, A., & Miccoli, M. (2024). Validation of the Italian version of the Neuroception of Psychological Safety Scale (NPSS). *Heliyon, 10*, e27625.
67. Cogan, N., Campbell, J., Morton, L., Young, D., & Porges, S. (2024). Validation of the Neuroception of Psychological Safety Scale (NPSS) among health and social care workers in the UK. *International Journal of Environmental Research and Public Health, 21*(12), 1551. https://doi.org/10.3390/ijerph21121551
68. Gendlin, E. T. (1996). *Focusing-oriented psychotherapy: A manual of the experiential method.* Guilford Press.
69. Maté, G. (2003). *When the body says no: The cost of hidden stress.* Vermilion.
70. Maté, G. (2003). *When the body says no: The cost of hidden stress.* Vermilion.

71. Gross J. J. (2002). Emotion regulation: Affective, cognitive, and social consequences. *Psychophysiology, 39*(3), 281–291. https://doi.org/10.1017/s0048577201393198. PMID: 12212647.
72. Hayes, S. C., Levin, M. E., Plumb-Vilardaga, J., Villatte, J. L., & Pistorello, J. (2013). Acceptance and commitment therapy and contextual behavioral science: Examining the progress of a distinctive model of behavioral and cognitive therapy. *Behav Ther, 44*(2), 180–198. https://doi.org/10.1016/j.beth.2009.08.002. Epub 2011 Jun 1. PMID: 23611068; PMCID: PMC3635495.
73. Dana, D. (2018). *The polyvagal theory in therapy: Engaging the rhythm of regulation*. W. W. Norton & Company.
74. Hayes, S. C., Levin, M. E., Plumb-Vilardaga, J., Villatte, J. L., & Pistorello, J. (2013). Acceptance and commitment therapy and contextual behavioral science: Examining the progress of a distinctive model of behavioral and cognitive therapy. *Behav Ther, 44*(2), 180–198. https://doi.org/10.1016/j.beth.2009.08.002. Epub 2011 Jun 1. PMID: 23611068; PMCID: PMC3635495.
75. Neff, K. D., & Germer, C. (2017). Self-compassion and psychological wellbeing. In J. Doty (Ed.), *Oxford handbook of compassion science*, 478–492. Oxford University Press.
76. Porges, S. W. (2022). Polyvagal theory: A science of safety. *Front Integr Neurosci, 16*, 871227. https://doi.org/10.3389/fnint.2022.871227. PMID: 35645742; PMCID: PMC9131189.
77. Beck, A. T., & Dozois D. J. (2011). Cognitive therapy: Current status and future directions. *Annu Rev Med, 62*, 397–409. https://doi.org/10.1146/annurev-med-052209-100032. PMID: 20690827.
78. Gilbert, P. (2014). The origins and nature of compassion focused therapy. *British Journal of Clinical Psychology, 53*(1), 6–41.
79. Bogart, K. R., Lund, E. M., & Rottenstein, A. (2018). Disability pride protects self-esteem through the rejection-identification model. *Rehabilitation Psychology, 63*(1), 155–159. https://doi.org/10.1037/rep0000166
80. Livecchi, T., & Morton, L. (2023). *Healing hearts and minds: A holistic approach to coping well with congenital heart disease*. Oxford University Press.
81. Livecchi, T., & Morton, L. (2023). *Healing hearts and minds: A holistic approach to coping well with congenital heart disease*. Oxford University Press.
82. Frank, A. (1995). *The Wounded Storyteller*. University of Chicago Press.
83. Stapleton, C. M., Zhang, H., & Berman, J. S. (2021). The event-specific benefits of writing about a difficult life experience. *Eur J Psychol, 17*(1), 53–69. https://doi.org/10.5964/ejop.2089. PMID: 33737974; PMCID: PMC7957853.
84. Morton, L. (2011). Can interpersonal psychotherapy meet the psychological cost of life gifted by medical intervention? *Counselling Psychology Review, British Psychological Society, 26*, 3.
85. Kovacs, A. H., Grace, S. L., Kentner, A. C., Nolan, R. P., Silversides, C. K., Irvine, M. J. (2018). Feasibility and Outcomes in a Pilot Randomized Controlled Trial of a Psychosocial Intervention for Adults With Congenital Heart Disease. *Can J Cardiol, 34*(6), 766–773. https://doi.org/10.1016/j.cjca.2018.02.023. Epub 2018 Mar 2. PMID: 29801741.
86. Livecchi, T., & Morton, L. (2023). *Healing hearts and minds: A holistic approach to coping well with congenital heart disease*. Oxford University Press.
87. Delaney, A. E., Qiu, J. M., Lee, C. S., Lyons, K. S., Vessey, J. A., & Fu, M. R. (2021). Parents' perceptions of emerging adults with congenital heart disease: An integrative review of qualitative studies. *J Pediatr Health Care, 35*(4), 362–376. https://doi.org/10.1016/j.pedhc.2020.11.009. Epub 2021 Feb 10. PMID: 33581995.

88. Morton, L., Cogan, N., Kornfält, S., Porter, Z., & Georgiadis, E. (2020). Baring all: The impact of the hospital gown on patient wellbeing. *British Journal of Health Psychology, 25*(3), 452–473.
89. Robertson, J. (1970). *Young children in hospital* (2nd ed.). Tavistock Publications.
90. Fortney, L., & Taylor, M. (2010). Meditation in medical practice: A review of the evidence and practice. *Prim Care, 37*(1), 81–90. https://doi.org/10.1016/j.pop.2009.09.004. PMID: 20188999.
91. Ai, A. L., Park, C. L., Bu Huang, Rodgers, W., & Tice, T. N. (2007). Psychosocial mediation of religious coping styles: A study of short-term psychological distress following cardiac surgery. *Personality and Social Psychology Bulletin, 33*(6), 867–882. https://doi.org/10.1177/0146167207301008
92. Vishkin, A., Ben-Nun Bloom, P., Schwartz, S. H., Solak, N., & Tamir, M. (2019). Religiosity and emotion regulation. *Journal of Cross-Cultural Psychology, 50*(9), 1050–1074. https://doi.org/10.1177/0022022119880341
93. Hebert, R., Zdaniuk, B., Schulz, R., & Scheier, M. (2009). Positive and negative religious coping and well-being in women with breast cancer. *J Palliat Med, 12*(6), 537–545. https://doi.org/10.1089/jpm.2008.0250. PMID: 19508140; PMCID: PMC2789454.
94. Hefferon, K., Grealy, M., & Mutrie, N. (2009). Posttraumatic growth and life-threatening physical illness: A systematic review of the qualitative literature. *British Journal of Health Psychology, 14*, 343–378.
95. Tedeschi, R. G., & Calhoun, L. G. (1996). The Posttraumatic Growth Inventory: Measuring the positive legacy of trauma. *J Trauma Stress, 9*(3), 455–471. https://doi.org/10.1007/BF02103658. PMID: 8827649.
96. Tedeschi, R. G., Shakespear-Finch, J., Taku, J., & Calhoun, L. G. (2018). *Posttraumatic growth: Theory, research, and applications*. Routledge.
97. Camus, Albert. (1952). *Return to Tipasa in Personal Writings*. Vintage.
98. Tedeschi, R. G., & Moore, B. A. (2021). Posttraumatic growth as an integrative therapeutic philosophy. *Journal of Psychotherapy Integration, 31*(2), 180–194. https://doi.org/10.1037/int0000250
99. Hayes, S. C., Levin, M. E., Plumb-Vilardaga, J., Villatte, J. L., & Pistorello, J. (2013). Acceptance and commitment therapy and contextual behavioral science: Examining the progress of a distinctive model of behavioral and cognitive therapy. *Behav Ther, 44*(2), 180–198. https://doi.org/10.1016/j.beth.2009.08.002. Epub 2011 Jun 1. PMID: 23611068; PMCID: PMC3635495.
100. Doran, G. T. (1981). There's a S.M.A.R.T. way to write management's goals and objectives. *Management Review, 70*(11), 35–36.

11. Appendix

1. Klagsbrun, J., Lennox, S.L., Summers, L. (2010). Effect of "Clearing a Space" on Quality of Life in Women with Breast Cancer. *United States Association for Body Psychotherapy Journal, 49*(2), 48–53.
2. Neff, K. D., & Germer, C. (2017). Self-Compassion and psychological wellbeing. In J. Doty (Ed.), *Oxford Handbook of Compassion Science*, 478–492. Oxford University Press.
3. Neff, K. D., & Germer, C. (2017). Self-Compassion and psychological wellbeing. In J. Doty (Ed.), *Oxford Handbook of Compassion Science*, 478–492. Oxford University Press.
4. Neff, K. D., & Germer, C. (2017). Self-Compassion and psychological wellbeing. In J. Doty (Ed.), *Oxford Handbook of Compassion Science*, 478–492. Oxford University Press.
5. Neff, K. D., & Germer, C. (2017). Self-Compassion and psychological wellbeing. In J. Doty (Ed.), *Oxford Handbook of Compassion Science*, 478–492. Oxford University Press.

6. Dreisoerner, A., Junker, N. M., Schlotz, W., Heimrich, J., Bloemeke, S., Ditzen, B., & van Dick, R. (2021). Self-soothing touch and being hugged reduce cortisol responses to stress: A randomized controlled trial on stress, physical touch, and social identity. *Comprehensive Psychoneuroendocrinology, 8*, 100091.
7. Bowen, S., Chawla, N., Grow, J., & Marlatt, G. A. (2021). *Mindfulness-based relapse prevention for addictive behaviors: A clinician's guide* (2nd ed.). The Guilford Press.
8. European Association for Children in Hospital (EACH) Charter. https://each-for-sick-children.org/each-charter/
9. iSupport. Rights-based standards for children having health care tests, treatments, examinations or interventions. https://www.isupportchildrensrights.com/english-version

Index

Figures are indicated by an italic *f* following the page number.

ableism, 31–36, 178
abuse, in hospitals, 169–171
acceptance and commitment therapy (ACT), 186, 219
ACHD. *See* adult congenital heart disease
ACT. *See* acceptance and commitment therapy
active listening, 89–94
   questions for patients to support mental health and well-being, 93
   skills exercises, 92
adult congenital heart disease (ACHD) support group, 213–215
adult healthcare, transition from childhood healthcare to, 98–100
affirmative action, 171
affirmative practice, 188
age-appropriate care, reflective exercise on, 101
ageism, 164–165
AHA. *See* American Hospital Association
Albrecht, G. L., 167
Album, Dag, 53
Alliance, The, 125–126
Allport, Gordon, 166
Allport's Scale, 166
allyship, 178
Alzyoud, F.A., 169
AMA. *See* American Medical Association
American Hospital Association (AHA), 172–173
American Medical Association (AMA) Organizational Strategic Plan to Advance Health Equity, 171
American Psychological Association (APA), 185
Anderson, Kirsty, 146
ANS. *See* autonomic nervous system
anticipated stigma, 34
anxiety, 13, 104, 110, 141–142, 205–206

APA. *See* American Psychological Association
arts-based therapies, 187
art therapy, 145–146
Ashdown, L., 57
ASKED. *See* Awareness, Skills, Knowledge, Encounter, and Desire
assertive communication, for people with LTCs, 212
asthma, 45
attachment theory, 26–27, 176, 188
autistic SPACE, 129–131
autonomic nervous system (ANS), 14–18, 73, 83, 85–86, 141, 144
avoidance behaviors, of patients with health anxiety, 104–105
Awareness, Skills, Knowledge, Encounter, and Desire (ASKED), 162

Baby Fae, 4
Bailey, Leonard, 4
Barnard, Christiaan, 3
Berg, H., 55, 178
beside manner, 60
Bevan, Aneurin, 172
biomedical model
   devaluation of individual patient experiences in, 55
   patient knowledge neglected in education, 57
biophilia hypothesis, 122
biopsychosocial model, 69
birth trauma, LTCs and, 18–24
body
   exercise and physical activity, 191
   helping clients work with, 206–207
   mind and, 43–46, 69, 193–194, 198–199
   in NPSS, 197
   under *le regard médical*, 43
   safety in mind and, 193–194

body (*Continued*)
  self-compassion for, 79–80, 204–205
  traumatic medical experiences for, 13–18
body image, 35, 37–39
body psychotherapy, 183, 192–193
Bogart, Kathleen, 35
Bowlby, John, 26–27, 176
BPS. *See* British Psychological Society
brain
  development, birth trauma and parenting in, 22
  responses to stress and trauma, 13, 14*f*, 105
Bray, Lucy, 135–136
Bristol Heart Institute, 97
British Medical Journal, 170
British Psychological Society (BPS), 185
Burnham, J., 179
burnout, 151–152, 155

Calgary-Cambridge Referenced Observation Guide (CCG), 82
Campbell-Yeo, M., 137
Campinha-Bacote Model, of culturally competent healthcare, 162
Camus, Albert, 218
CARE. *See* Consultation and Relational Empathy
Care Act of 2014 172
caregivers, support for, 100–101
Carter, Sue, 73
CBT. *See* cognitive-behavioral therapy
CCG. *See* Calgary-Cambridge Referenced Observation Guide
CFS. *See* chronic fatigue syndrome
CFT. *See* compassion-focused therapy
Chaney, S., 58
checking behaviors, 205–206
Cheng, M. Y., 60
childbirth-related post-traumatic stress disorder (CR-PTSD), 20
childhood illness, 73–75
  in education interruptions, 35
  epistemic injustice and, 56–57
  LTCs, psychological safety and, 83–85
  medical interruptions to secure attachment and, 25–31
  reflective exercise on children in hospital, 30–31
  soothing presence for patients with, 120–121
  traumatic experience with, 114–115, 134
childhood trauma, 17
child life specialists, 138–139
children
  child life specialists and health play specialists for, 138–140
  communicating with, recommendations for, 98–99
  establishing trust with, 95–96
  iSupport international rights based standards to support during medical procedures, 134–136
  Jolly on emotional well-being of, 138
  medical trauma of, 114–115, 134–136, 183–184
  music therapy for, 141–144
  pain management, 137
  teenagers, caring for, 96–98
  therapeutic play for, 138–140
  therapy animals for, 144–145
  transition from childhood to adult care, 98
Children's Charter, UK, 175
children's hospitals, 175–177
children's rights, 134–137, 175–177
child sexual abuse (CSA), 183–184
Christie, The, NHS Foundation Trust, 140–141
chronic diseases. *See* long-term conditions
chronic fatigue, 18, 52–53
chronic fatigue syndrome (CFS), 191–192
chronic pain, 8, 134, 186
cinemas, in hospitals, 146–147
clinical information, patient access to, 112–113, 125–126
cognitive-behavioral therapy (CBT), 108, 186, 205–206
cognitive defense strategies, 193–194
cognitive defusion, 186, 203–204
coming out as disabled, 206
committed action, 186, 219
communication training, 59
compassion
  building capacity for, 81
  defining, 77–78
  for health anxiety, 104
  in health outcomes, 79
  mindfulness practices, 82

in NPSS, 197
in psychologically informed healthcare, 73–82
self-compassion, 79–80, 186–187, 204–206
compassionate care, 78–81
active listening in, 89
in medical schools, 81–82
palliative, 80
compassionate communication, 79, 123
compassionate leadership, 156–158
compassion crisis in healthcare, 57–61
compassion fatigue, 152
compassion-focused therapy (CFT), 38–39, 39f, 187, 206
"Compassion in Practice" strategy, NHS, 58
complex PTSD, 105–106, 193
Concord Birth Trolley, 142
congenital heart conditions, 23–24, 35–36, 48, 168, 173–175, 213–215
connection, reintegration and, 209–211, 212f
Consultation and Relational Empathy (CARE) questionnaire, 82
co-regulation, psychological safety and, 82–87
COVID-19, 9, 27–28, 35, 153–154, 163–164, 167–169, 177
Crimean War, 50, 145
critical race theory (CRT), 164
CR-PTSD. See childbirth-related post-traumatic stress disorder
CRT. See critical race theory
CSA. See child sexual abuse
cultural humility, 177–178
culturally competent healthcare, Campinha-Bacote Model of, 162
culturally sensitive healthcare, 161, 164, 178
Cumper, Michael, 174

Dana, Deb, 196–197
death feigning mode, 15
dehumanization, 50
denial, 207–208
depression, 45, 103
red flag signs and symptoms, 110–111
sex differences in risk of, 164
Descartes, Rene, 43
Devlieger, P. J., 167
diabetes, 9, 18, 108

Dick, Alix, 145
difficult news, delivering, 94–95
dignity-focused care, 111
disability
coming out as disabled, 206
discrimination, stigma and, 165–167
human rights of people with, 173
LTC and, 4
social model of, 178
Disability-Inclusive Response to COVID-19, A, 167
disability paradox, 167
disability pride, 206
discrimination, 34–37, 162–167, 208
disease prestige, 52–53
disempowerment, in medical care, 46–47, 54, 123–125
distress, active listening and, 89–93
diversity, in therapeutic treatment, 188–191
Dixon, Katie, 135
DNA, 22
Doherty, Mary, 130
double gowning, 52

EACH. *See* European Association for Children in Hospital
ECHO. *See* European Children's Hospitals Organization
Edinburgh Hospital for Sick Children, 175
Ehlers-Danlos syndrome, 144
Elephant Man, The, 166
embodied experience, 45, 82, 194
EMDR. *See* eye movement desensitization and reprocessing
emotional focused therapy, 187
emotional preparation for surgery, 133
emotional regulation, 201–203
emotion wheel, 202
empathy, 78, 82
empowerment, 111–113, 123–125, 202, 215
ENACT Study, 153–154
Endometriosis UK report, 2023 44
Engel, George, 69
epilepsy, 9
epistemic injustice, 54–57, 178
Epstein, Ken, 101
Equality Act of 2010 173
establishing trust with children and teenagers, 95–99

European Association for Children in Hospital (EACH), 135, 176
European Children's Hospitals Organization (ECHO), 177
evidence-based therapeutic treatment modalities, 185–187
exercise, 191
existential psychotherapy, 187
experienced or enacted stigma, 34
experiential focusing, 198–199
exposure hierarchy, 206
eye movement desensitization and reprocessing (EMDR), 186–187, 193, 197

fawn response, 16
feeling ill, patient role and, 7–12
feelings, safe spaces for, 87–89
felt sense, 198–199
female health, 164
Fennell, Melanie, 37
fibromyalgia, 55
fight or flight mode, 14–15, 78, 109
finding meaning, 216–220
flashbacks, in PTSD, 106–107
Foucault, Michel, 43
Four I's of oppression, 163
Francis, Robert, 58
Frank, Arthur, 208
Frankl, Viktor, 217
Freud, Anna, 176
Fricker, Miranda, 55

GAD. *See* generalized anxiety disorder
Gajwani, R., 17
Gendlin, Eugene, 198–199
generalized anxiety disorder (GAD), 109
Germer, C., 204
germ theory, 50
Gilbert, Paul, 38–39
goal setting, 220
Going to Hospital with Mother, 176
Gong, C. L., 36
Gorry, Anthony, 144
Great Ormond Street Hospital for Children, 175
green spaces, in healthcare settings, 122–123
grief, loss, and anger, 207–208

Harper, F. W. K., 142
Hauser, D. J., 88
HCPC. *See* Health and Social Care Professions Council
healing healthcare spaces, 117–118
Health 2020, WHO, 65
Health and Social Care Professions Council (HCPC), 185
health anxiety, 104
Healthcare Improvement Scotland (HIS), 174
healthcare professionals, emotional and psychological health of
 burnout and, 151–152, 155
 case study, 159–160
 compassionate leadership in, 156–158
 compassion fatigue and, 152
 COVID-19 and, 152–154
 establishing healthy boundaries, 150
 organizational responsibilities and, 151
 psychologically safe working environments for, 155–156
 resilience at work, 154–155
 self-care, 150–151, 154–155
 stress and, 150
 vicarious trauma and, 152–153
healthcare settings, psychological impact of working in, 39–40
health inequalities, in pregnancy and childbirth, 21–22
health play specialists, 139–140
health privilege, 32, 36
Heggen, K. M., 55, 178
Herman, Judith, 192–193
hermeneutical injustice, 55, 178
hidden curriculum, 164
hierometer theory, 37
HIS. *See* Healthcare Improvement Scotland
Hitler, Adolf, 166
HIV/AIDs, 34, 167
holding and restraint, 123, 137
holistic care, embedding psychological support and, 127–129
holistic healthcare practice, 5
holistic support, 138
Holland, E., 10, 54
Holocaust, 166
Hôpital des Enfants Malades, 175
hospital attire, 49–52, 124–125

hospital environment, as healing spaces, 117–118
hospital environment, as inhospitable, 61–62
Huddleston, Peggy, 133
humanistic psychology, 77, 185
humiliation, in medical education, 60–61
Hupcey, J. E., 72
hyperarousal, 15, 78, 85–86
hypoarousal, 15–16, 78, 85–86, 89

ICD. *See* implantable cardioverter-defibrillator
ICU. *See* intensive care unit
immobilization response, 15–16
immune system, ANS and, 18
implantable cardioverter-defibrillator (ICD), 10
Inclusive Futures, 167
infant mortality, 176
inspiration porn, 34
institutional abuse, 169
institutionalized CSA, 183
intensive care unit (ICU), 63
internalized stigma, 34
interpersonal disputes, 187
interpersonal psychotherapy, 187
intersectionality, social inequalities and, 162–165
intimate partner violence (IPV), 22
IPV. *See* intimate partner violence
iSupport international rights based standards to support children during medical procedures, 134–136

Johnson, Magic, 167
Jolly, June, 138–139, 145
Jones, L., 57

Kalbacker, Meredith, 213–215
Kazak, A., 28
Khan, Miyira, 189
Kovacs, A. H., 213–214
Kumar, Jenny, 146

Lancet, the, 164
Leiden Charter, 176
Leroy, Piet, 95, 138
letter writing, therapeutic, 208–209
Li, W. W., 60
listening therapy, 144

Lister, Joseph, 50
Livecchi, Tracy, 213
long COVID, 9
long-term conditions (LTCs)
 in ableist world, 31–36
 administrative load of, 10
 assertive communication for people with, 212
 body image, self-esteem and, 35–39
 clinical information access for patients with, 112–113, 125–126
 cognitive defense strategies of people with, 193–194
 COVID-19, psychological trauma and, 168–169
 depression and, 45
 diagnosed during childhood, psychological safety and, 83–84
 disability and, 4
 discrimination against people with, 161–163, 165–167
 epistemic injustice and, 54
 facilitating coping for patients with, 131–134
 grief, loss, and anger and, 207–208
 health anxiety and, 104
 healthcare professionals with, 40
 invasive tests and procedures for, 9–10
 lived experience of, 178
 medical trauma and, 17–18, 80, 184, 186, 192–197, 201
 mental health and, 40–41, 45, 63, 103, 162–163
 MLTCs, 10–11
 oppression of people with, 163
 parenting, birth trauma and, 18–24
 physical activity for, 35, 37, 111, 191
 PPI and, 164
 psychologically informed healthcare for patients with, 5–6, 63–64, 69–71, 70*f*, 111
 PTSD and, 105
 quality of life for people with, 9
 reflective exercise on, 12
 reintegration and connection for people with, 210–211
 self-compassion for people with, 204–207
 self-management of, 111–112, 114, 125–126, 215
 sexual health and, 33–35

long-term conditions (LTCs) (*Continued*)
  spirituality, finding meaning and, 216–219
  stigma and, 34–34, 162–165, 167
  stress of, Maté on, 199–201
  symptoms of, 8–9
  therapeutic treatment modalities for, 185–187
  war and battle metaphors for, 88
  well-being of patients with, 63–65, 69–70, 70f
  workplace discrimination and, 35–36
loving kindness meditation, 186
LTCs. *See* long-term conditions
Lupus, 19
Lynch, David, 166

Maté, Gabor, 199–201
maternal mortality, 20
maternal stress, 22–24
Mazzarelli, A., 59
MCBT. *See* mindfulness-based cognitive-behavioral therapy
Meadsteam, Catherine, 141–142
meaning, finding, 216–220
medical alarms, 62–63
medical gaze, 43, 50–52
medical trauma
  body and, 13–18
  of children, 114–115, 134–136, 183–184
  CSA and, 183–184
  delivering difficult news and, 94–95
  developmental, 26–27
  LTCs and, 17–18, 80, 184, 188, 201
  polyvagal approaches to dealing with, 194–195
  recognizing, 106–107
  symptoms, 106–107
  therapeutic treatment for, 186–187, 192–197
  TIC and, 101
MediCinema, 146–147
meditation, 86–87
Mehta, K. K., 60, 81
mental health
  active listening questions to support, 93–94
  diagnosis, 188
  disparities, 189–191
  of healthcare workers during COVID-19, ENACT Study on, 153–154
  LTCs and, 40–41, 45, 63, 103, 162–163
  psychologically informed healthcare for, 63–65
  recognizing difficulties, 103
  social support in, 33, 210, 216
  stigma, 44, 189–190
Merrick, Joseph, 166
Meyer, I. H., 190
microaggressions, 34, 211
Mid-Staffordshire National Health Service Foundation Trust, 58
mind and body
  dualism, 43
  in focusing, 199
  link, 45, 69
  safety and, 193–194
mindfulness-based cognitive-behavioral therapy (MCBT), 186
mindfulness practices, 82, 86–87, 186
Minnis, H., 17
minority stress model, 190
MLTCs. *See* multiple long-term conditions
morbus mediterraneus, 164
Morton, Liza, 213–214
Mount Sinai Fuster Heart Hospital, 213–215
movement therapy, 187
multiple long-term conditions (MLTCs), 10–11
multiple sclerosis, 8, 18
music therapy, 141–144

Naeem, F., 190–191
narrative humility, 177–178
National Association of Health Play Staff, 139–140
National Healthcare Standards in Scotland for CHD, 173–175
National Health Service (NHS), 58, 140–141, 154, 170, 172, 174–175
National Institute for Health and Care Research (NIHR), 164, 178
Nazism, 166
Neaton, Karen, 21
needle phobia, 107–108
Neff, K. D., 204
neuroception, 14, 15f, 144

Neuroception of Psychological Safety Scale (NPSS), 6, 83–85, 197–198
neurodivergent traits and neurodivergent individuals, 17, 91
NHS. *See* National Health Service
Nietzsche, Friedrich, 217
Nightingale, Florence, 7, 50, 62, 117, 141, 144–145
Nightingale Wards, 117
NIHR. *See* National Institute for Health and Care Research
nonverbal safety signaling, 85–86
NPSS. *See* Neuroception of Psychological Safety Scale

obsessive compulsive disorder (OCD), 108–109
occupational therapists (OT), 71–72
OCD. *See* obsessive compulsive disorder
older adults, caring for, 100–101
oppression, 163, 189
Organizational Strategic Plan to Advance Health Equity, AMA, 171
OT. *See* occupational therapists

pain
  morbus mediterraneus stereotype about, 164
  music therapy for, 141–142
  of nonverbal infants, 29
  pediatric, 137–138
  therapy animals and, 144–145
pain management programs, 134
palliative care, compassionate, 80
panic disorder, 109
parenting
  childhood illness and, 23–30
  LTCs and, 18–24, 33
Pasteur, Louis, 50
patience and waiting, in healthcare journey, 47–49
patient and public involvement (PPI), 11, 54, 164
patient burden, 5, 8, 112
patient-centered care, 65
patient-centered culturally sensitive healthcare, 161
patient knowledge and expertise, 57
patient rights, 172–173
patient role, 7–12, 43, 49, 54, 215

patient testimony, 55
patient waiting, 123–124
Paul, Liz, 23–24
pediatric pain, 137–138
person-centered therapy, 77, 185–186
pet therapy, 145
phased intervention model of psychological treatment, 193
phobias, 107–108
Platt Report, 176
polyvagal music (PVM), 144
polyvagal theory (PVT), 14–16, 73, 86*f*, 144, 155–156
  in approaches to dealing with medical trauma, 194–195
  mindfulness-based movement practices informed by, 187
  NPSS and, 83, 197–198
  psychological safety and, 82–87, 155–156, 195–198
  in therapeutic treatments, 186–187, 194–197
  WAPs informed by, 158–159
Porges, Stephen, 14–15, 144, 195
post-Caesarean section shivering, 21
post-traumatic growth, 216–219
post-traumatic stress, 16–17, 28
post-traumatic stress disorder (PTSD)
  complex, 105, 193
  CR-PTSD, 20
  LTCs and, 103
  medical trauma and, 105, 107
  risk factors for, 105–106
  symptoms, 106–108
  treatment for, 193
postural orthostatic tachycardia syndrome (POTS), 18
POTS. *See* postural orthostatic tachycardia syndrome
PPI. *See* patient and public involvement
Primary Sjogren's syndrome, 19
prolonged exposure, 186
psychoeducation, 202, 211
psychologically informed healthcare
  affirmative action in, 171
  biopsychosocial model and, 69
  for childhood illness, 28–29
  compassion in, 73–82
  cultural humility in, 177

psychologically informed healthcare (*Continued*)
   on disempowering aspects of healthcare, 123
   emotional responses in, 88
   healing healthcare spaces in, 117
   for LTCs, 5–6, 63–64, 69–70, 70*f*, 111
   for mental health, 63–65
   on pain, 134
   on power of healthcare professionals over patients, 169
   reflective exercise for healthcare professionals on, 7, 223–224
   R.E.S.P.E.C.T. principles of, 71
   on support for healthcare professionals, 150
   as survival-focused healthcare, 44–46
   for well-being, 63–65, 69–70, 70*f*
psychological safety, 35
   co-regulation and, 83–87
   for doctors, 60
   LTCs diagnosed during childhood and, 83–85
   medical trauma and, 80
   nonverbal signaling, 85–86
   NPSS for measuring, 6, 83–85, 197–198
   PVT and, 83–87, 155–156, 195–198
   relational, 72–73
   of working environments for healthcare professionals, 155–156
psychological support
   holistic care and, 127–129
   in physical health teams, 184–185
PVM. *See* polyvagal music
PVT. *See* polyvagal theory

QPL. *See* Surgical Question Prompt List
quality of life, 8, 41

racial bias, clinician, 189
racism, 164
radical acceptance, 202
reassurance seeking, 205
regard médical, le, 43
reintegration, connection and, 209–211, 212*f*
relational safety, 71–73, 79
religiosity, 217
R.E.S.P.E.C.T. principles, of psychologically informed healthcare, 71

rheumatoid arthritis, 10
righteous anger, 208
Rimes, K. A., 37
Robertson, James, 176
Robertson, Joyce, 176
Rogers, Carl, 77, 185–186, 198
role transition, 187
Rosen, L. T., 55
Rowe, Michael, 163
Royal Children's Hospital in Melbourne, Australia, 117
Royal Hospital for Children in Glasgow, Scotland, 117–118

safeguarding, 172
Safe & Sound Protocol, 144, 195
safe spaces for feelings, 87–90
safety seeking behaviors, of patients with health anxiety, 104
San Francisco Department of Public Health (SFDPH), 101–102
Savile, Jimmy, 170
savoring, 220
Scarred FOR Life project, 146
SCCN. *See* Scottish Congenital Cardiac Network
Schwarz, N., 88
Scottish Congenital Cardiac Network (SCCN), 174
secure attachment, 25–31
self-actualization, 185–186
self-care
   for healthcare professionals, 150–151, 154–155
   in therapeutic treatment, promoting, 191–192
self-compassion, 79–80, 186, 204–206
self-esteem, 37–39, 103
self-management, of LTCs, 111–112, 114, 125–126, 215
sensory needs, predictability, acceptance, communication, and empathy (SPACE), for autistic patients, 129–131
sexual abuse, 169–171, 183
sexual health, 35
SFDPH. *See* San Francisco Department of Public Health
Shakur, Afeni, 172–173
shared decision-making, 112–114
shell shock, 105

Siegel, Dan, 26
sleep, in hospitals, 61–63, 119–120
smell, trauma and, 107–108
social connection, 71–73
social engagement system, 14, 78, 155
social exclusion, 162–163
social graces model, 179
social inequalities, intersectionality and, 162–165
social model of disability, 178
social networks, 210–211, 212f
social support, 33, 121, 187, 210–211, 216
sociometer theory, 37
sociostasis, 73
somatic therapeutic approaches, 187
Somerville Heart Foundation, 146
soothing presence, 120–121
soothing techniques, 203
sound and noise, in hospitals, 62–63
sound reduction bundles, 119
SPACE. *See* sensory needs, predictability, acceptance, communication, and empathy
speechless terror, 193
spirituality and finding meaning, 216–219
Stakemann, Ruth, 142–144
Steffens, N. M., 113
stigma, 34–35, 37, 44, 162–167, 187, 189–190
Stoke Mandeville Report, 170
story writing, in therapeutic treatment, 208
strengths-based therapeutic approach, 187
stress, 13–18
  of healthcare professionals, 150
  Maté on, 199–201
  maternal, 22
  minority stress model, 190
sudden cardiac arrest, 11
surgery, emotional preparation for, 133
Surgical Question Prompt List (QPL), 113
survival-focused healthcare, 44–46

Teenage Cancer Trust, 97
teenagers, caring for, 96–98
therapeutic life story work (TLSW), 55
therapeutic play, 139–140
therapeutic treatment
  affirmative practice, 188
  antioppressive, 189
  body psychotherapy, 183, 192
  case studies, 221–223
  CBT in, 186, 205–206
  diversity in, 188–189
  emotional regulation in, 201–203
  empowering self-management in, 215
  evidence-based modalities, 185–187
  finding meaning in, 216–220
  goal setting in, 220
  for grief, loss, and anger, 207–208
  letter writing in, 208–209
  for medical trauma, 186–187, 192–196
  mental health disparities and, 189–191
  NPSS in, 197–198
  polyvagal approaches to, 187, 194–197
  preparation for medical experiences in, 215–216
  reintegration and connection in, 209–211, 212f
  safety in mind and body of clients in, 193–194
  savoring in, 220
  self-care in, promoting, 191–192
  self-compassion in, 204–206
  social network mapping in, 212f
  story writing in, 208
therapy animals, 144–145
Thestrup, J., 95, 97
threat, drive, and soothing systems, 38–39, 38f, 206
TIC. *See* trauma informed care
TLSW. *See* therapeutic life story work
toolkit, therapeutic, 186
toxic positivity, 210–211
trauma. *See also* medical trauma; post-traumatic stress; post-traumatic stress disorder
  birth trauma, LTCs and, 18–24
  brain and, 13, 14f, 105
  childhood, 17
  of childhood illness, 114–115, 134
  compassion fatigue and, 152
  COVID-19 and, 168–169
  responses to, 14–16
  smell and, 107
  symptoms of, neurodivergent traits and, 17
  vicarious, 152–153
trauma informed care (TIC), 21, 101–103
trauma-informed CBT, 186

trauma-informed organizations, reflective exercise on, 103
Trauma-Informed Systems Initiative, of SFDPH, 102
Tronstad, O., 119
Trzeciak, S., 59
Tucker, C. M., 178
Tucker Culturally Sensitive Health Care Clinic Environment Inventory–Patient Form (T-CSHCCEI-PF), 178
Two-Year-Old Goes to Hospital, A, 176

UN-CDPR. *See* United Nations Declaration on Rights of Disabled People
unconscious bias, 177–178
United Nations Convention on the Rights of the Child (UNCRC), 135, 139, 176–177
United Nations Declaration on Rights of Disabled People (UN-CDPR), 173, 176–177

van der Kolk, Bessel, 193
Vedam, S., 169
vicarious trauma, 152–153
virtual reality (VR), in empathy training, 82
virtual reality distraction therapy (VRDT), 140–141
volunteers, in healthcare settings, 147
VR. *See* virtual reality
VRDT. *See* virtual reality distraction therapy

Walker, Alyson, 117–118
Wapling, Lorraine, 167
WAPs. *See* wellness action plans
ward rounds, 126–127
Washkansky, Louis, 3–4
WEIRD. *See* Western, Educated, Industrialized, Rich, and Democratic
well-being, 40–41
  active listening questions to support, 93
  emotional, of children, 138
  preparation for medical experiences for, 215–216
  psychologically informed healthcare for, 63–65, 69–70, 70f
wellness action plans (WAPs), 158–159
West, Michael, 156
Western, Educated, Industrialized, Rich, and Democratic (WEIRD), 54
white coat syndrome, 16
WHO. *See* World Health Organization
Wigg, L., 60
Wilson, Caroline, 146
Woolf, Virginia, 3
workplace discrimination, 36
World Health Organization (WHO), 8, 63–65, 177
World War II, 172

Young, Kate, 164

Zaidi, Ali N., 213

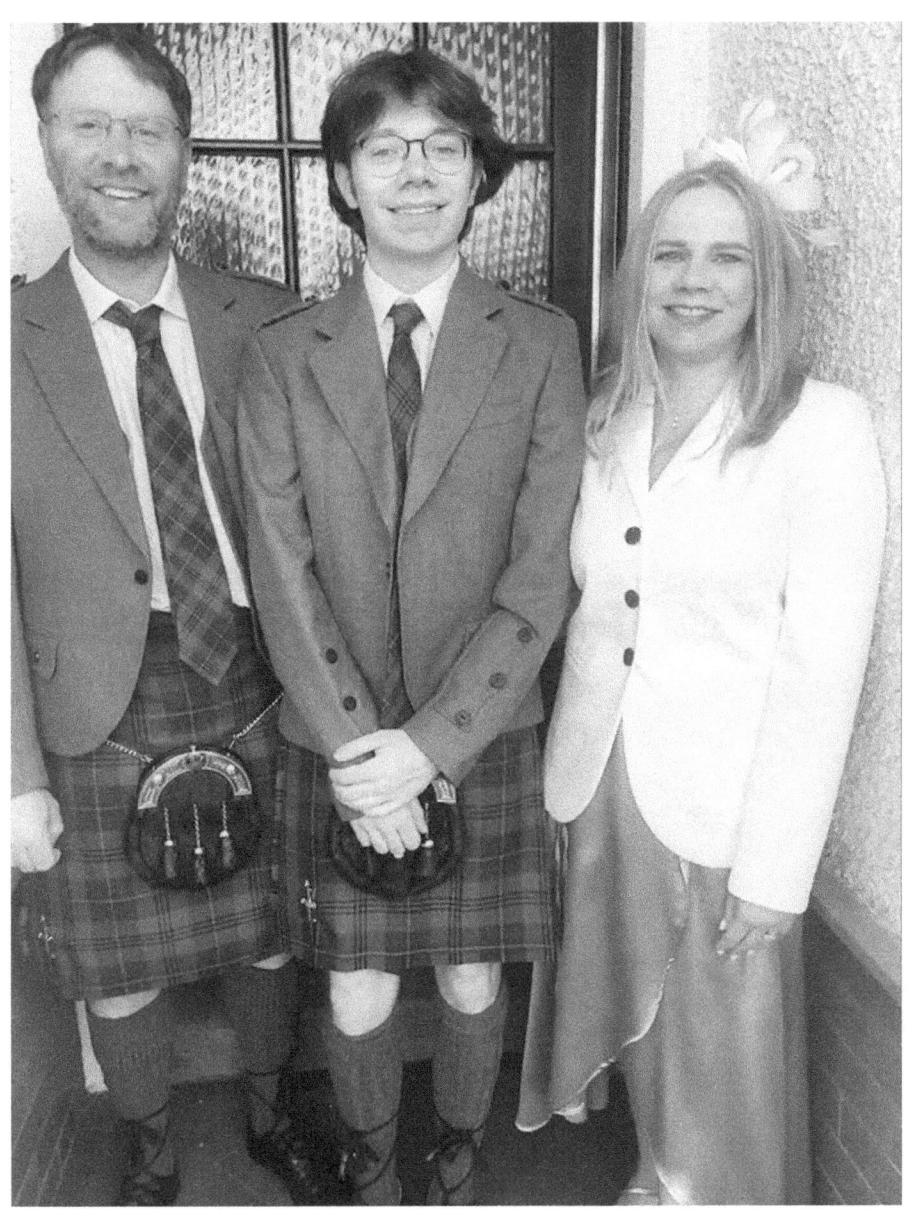

Liza with her husband Craig and son Dylan

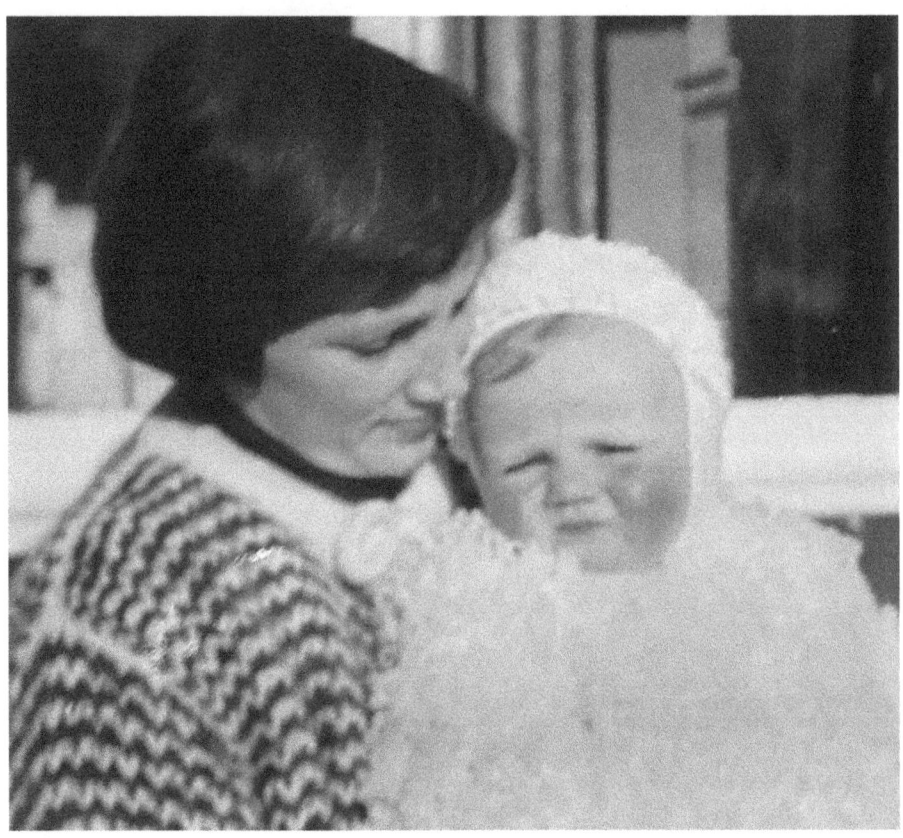

Liza as a baby with her mum, Liz (early 1980s)

www.ingramcontent.com/pod-product-compliance
Ingram Content Group UK Ltd.
Pitfield, Milton Keynes, MK11 3LW, UK
UKHW041850040126
466553UK00007B/56/J